Neuroreceptors

Neuroreceptors

Proceedings of the Symposium
Berlin (West), September 28–29, 1981

Editor
Ferdinand Hucho

Walter de Gruyter · Berlin · New York 1982

Editor
Ferdinand Hucho, Professor, Dr. rer. nat.
Free University Berlin
Department of Chemistry
Institute of Biochemistry
Fabeckstrasse 34
D-1000 Berlin 33
Germany

CIP-Kurztitelaufnahme der Deutschen Bibliothek

Neuroreceptors: proceedings of the symposium Berlin (West), September 26–29, 1981/ ed. Ferdinand Hucho. – Berlin; New York: de Gruyter, 1982.
ISBN 3-11-008855-X

NE: Hucho, Ferdinand [Hrsg.]

Library of Congress Cataloging in Publication Data

Neuroreceptors.

Bibliography: p.
Includes index.
1. Neurotransmitter receptors – Congresses. 2. Neural receptors – Congresses. 3. Acetylcholine – Receptors – Congresses.
I. Hucho, Ferdinand, 1939-
[DNLM: 1. Receptiors, Cholinergic – Congresses. 2. Receptors, Sensory – Congresses. WL 102.8 N49415 1981]
QP364.7.N46 599.01'88 82-1448
ISBN 3-11-008855-X AACR2

 Printing: Karl Gericke, Berlin. – Binding: Lüderitz & Bauer, Buchgewerbe GmbH, Berlin. – Cover Design: Taube Graphic, München. – **Printed in Germany.**

Preface

This volume contains reviews and original data on some of the neural receptors, which are at present the focus of interest. They were presented at a meeting held in Berlin on September 29 and 30, 1981. More than half of the volume deals with the nicotinic acetylcholine receptor, not merely because we consider this receptor the most interesting or the most important molecule of its kind, but also because we feel that its biochemical investigation is, for technical reasons, at present fairly advanced.

Whereas some of the other receptors presented here have not yet gone farther than the stage of hypothesis, others are already visible at least on autoradiograms, after radioactive labelling. The basic questions and the techniques for answering these appear to be very similar so that any exchange of ideas and experiences appears to be useful.

I would like to thank my co-workers for their help in organising this meeting; I thank the Publisher, de Gruyter, for the rapid publication of this volume, Frau Greiner for her help with the organization of this manuscript and the Deutsche Forschungsgemeinschaft for their financial support.

Ferdinand Hucho

Berlin, January 1982

List of participants:

Bakardjiev, Anastasia
Institut für Physiologische Chemie der Universität, Koelliker-str. 2, D-8700 Würzburg

Bandini, Giampiero
Institut für Biochemie der Freien Universität Berlin, Fabeck-str. 34-36, D-1000 Berlin 33

Barrantes, Francisco
Max-Planck-Institut für Biophysikalische Chemie, Postfach 968, D-3400 Göttingen

Bayer, Hermann
Institut für Biochemie der Freien Universität Berlin, Fabeck-str. 34-36, D-1000 Berlin 33

Bernhard, J.
Max-Planck-Institut für Biochemie, Am Klopferspitz 18a, D-8033 Martinsried

Betz, Heinrich
Max-Planck-Institut für Psychiatrie, Am Klopferspitz 18a, D-8033 Martinsried

Binder, Michael
Institut für Physiologische Chemie der Ruhr-Universität Bochum, D-4630 Bochum 1

Brühning, Gerold
Institut für Neuropsychopharmakologie der Freien Universität Berlin, Ulmenallee 30, D-1000 Berlin 33

Burgermeister, Wolfgang
Institut für Physiologische Chemie der Universität, Koelliker-str. 2, D-8700 Würzburg

Fels, Gregor
Max-Planck-Institut für Ernährungsphysiologie, Rheinlanddamm 201, D-4600 Dortmund

Graham, David
Max-Planck-Institut für Psychiatrie, Am Klopferspitz 18a,
D-8033 Martinsried

Gück, Stephan
Institut für Biochemie der Freien Universität Berlin, Fabeck-
str. 34-36, D-1000 Berlin 33

Hamill, Owen
Max-Planck-Institut für Biophysikalische Chemie, Postfach 968,
D-3400 Göttingen

Hucho, Ferdinand
Institut für Biochemie der Freien Universität Berlin, Fabeck-
str. 34-36, D-1000 Berlin 33

Kehr, W.
Schering AG, Müllerstr. 178, D-1000 Berlin 65

Kuhnen-Clausen, Dida
Fraunhofer-Institut für Aerobiologie, D-5948 Schmallenberg

Lauffer, Leander
Institut für Biochemie der Freien Universität Berlin, Fabeck-
str. 34-36, D-1000 Berlin 33

Layer, Paul
Max-Planck-Institut für Virusforschung, Spemannstr. 35, D-7400
Tübingen 1

Leicht, Wolfgang
Bayer AG, D-5600 Wuppertal-Elberfeld

Li, Ping-Lu
Kali-Chemie Pharma GmbH, D-3000 Hannover

Maelicke, Alfred
Max-Planck-Institut für Ernährungsphysiologie, Rheinlanddamm
201, D-4600 Dortmung

Müller, W.E.
Pharmakologisches Institut der Universität, Obere Zahlbacher-
str. 67, D-6500 Mainz

Neumann, Eberhard
Max-Planck-Institut für Biochemie, Am Klopferspitz 18a, D-8033 Martinsried

Pfeiffer, Friedhelm
Max-Planck-Institut für Psychiatrie, Am Klopferspitz 18a, D-8033 Martinsried

Prinz, Heino
Max-Planck-Institut für Ernährungsphysiologie, Rheinlanddamm 201, D-4600 Dortmund

Rohrer, Hermann
Max-Planck-Institut für Psychiatrie, Am Klopferspitz 18a, D-8033 Martinsried

Rommelspacher, Hans Josef
Institut für Neuropsychopharmakologie der Freien Universität, Ulmenallee 30, D-1000 Berlin 19

Spillecke, F.
Max-Planck-Institut für Biochemie, Am Klopferspitz 18a, D-8033 Martinsried

Stengelin, Siegfried
Institut für Biochemie der Freien Universität Berlin, Fabeckstr. 34-36, D-1000 Berlin 33

Sutter, Arne
Institut für Pharmakologie der Freien Universität Berlin, Thielallee 69, D-1000 Berlin 33

Verdenhalven, Jan
Institut für Biochemie der Freien Universität Berlin, Fabeckstr. 34-36, D-1000 Berlin 33

Watters, Diane
Max-Planck-Institut für Ernährungsphysiologie, Rheinlanddamm 201, D-4600 Dortmung 1

Whittaker, V.P.
Max-Planck-Institut für Biophysikalische Chemie, Postfach 968, D-3400 Göttingen

Witzemann, Veit
Max-Planck-Institut für Biophysikalische Chemie, Postfach 968,
D-3400 Göttingen

Wolff, Elmar
Max-Planck-Institut für Ernährungsphysiologie, Rheinlanddamm
201, D-4600 Dortmung 1

Zimmermann, Astrid
Institut für Pharmakologie der Freien Universität Berlin,
Thielallee 69, D-1000 Berlin 33

Contents

I. DIAZEPAM RECEPTOR

THE BENZODIAZEPINE RECEPTOR. A SUMMARY.

Walter E. Müller
Pharmakologisches Institut der Universität Mainz, Obere Zahlbacher Straße 67, D-6500 Mainz, Federal Republic of Germany

The Search for the Molecular Mechanism of Action of the Benzodiazepines.

Although the benzodiazepines are the most frequently prescribed group of drugs today the molecular mechanism, responsible for the pharmacological activity of the benzodiazepines, remained unclear for a long period of time. The concept which found increasing experimental support during the last years was the assumption of an enhanced or facilitated GABAergic transmission originated by the benzodiazepines. However, the mechanism by which benzodiazepines could enhance GABAergic transmission was not known.

Some properties of the benzodiazepines could suggest a receptor mediated mechanism of action, e.g. the pronounced structural specificity, the stereoselectivity, and the low dosages pharmacologically and clinically used. However, since the benzodiazepines do not interact with any of the already known neurotransmitters or neuromodulator receptors in the central nervous system the presence of a benzodiazepine-specific receptor with unknown physiological function had to be assumed. And indeed, Braestrup and Squires (1) and Möhler and Okada (2) reported first the presence of benzodiazepine specific, high-affinity binding sites for tritiated diazepam in the brain of rats and humans. These findings have been confirmed by many authors. Meanwhile, a few summaries about the properties of these "benzodiazepine receptors" have been published (1-6).

Neuroreceptors

General Properties of the Benzodiazepine Receptors.

Benzodiazepine receptors have been detected in the central nervous systems of nearly all vertebrate species investigated so far with fairly similar properties and with maximal densities usually found for neurotransmitter receptors in the CNS. Benzodiazepine receptors are absent in the brains of non-vertebrate species and in vertebrate tissues outside the CNS. Some major features of the benzodiazepine receptor in the human CNS are summarized in table 1, including maximal densities, regional distribution, and affinities of several benzodiazepine derivatives. As indicated in table 1, benzodiazepine receptors are widely but unevenly distributed in the human CNS. Similar but not identical regional distributions have been found for other mammalian species. Going from regional to cellular localization, several pieces of evidence suggest that benzodiazepine receptors are nearly exclusively located on neurons with only very small amounts on glia cells (1-6).

Benzodiazepine receptors are fairly specific for pharmacologically active benzodiazepine derivatives and are stereospecific in a way that the pharmacologically active isomer has the much higher affinity (table 1). Only few non-benzodiazepine drugs are known which bind to the benzodiazepine receptor at concentrations low enough to suggest the possibility of benzodiazepine-like effects or side-effects mediated through the benzodiazepine receptor (6). Some convulsants, e.g. pentetrazole, interact in convulsant concentrations with the benzodiazepine receptor suggesting that benzodiazepine opposite effects at the benzodiazepine receptor could be involved in their convulsive properties (7-9).

While all these findings strongly indicate the high specificity of this new receptor for benzodiazepine compounds high selectivity and even stereospecificity alone are not an absolute proof of the biological significance of these binding

Table 1: Properties of the benzodiazepine receptor in human brain.

Receptor densities:		
	Frontal cortex:	1.0 pmole per mg protein
	Nucleus caudatus:	0.4 pmole per mg protein
	Medulla:	0.2 pmole per mg protein
Receptor distribution:		
	High density areas:	Frontal cortex
		Cerebellar cortex
		Hippocampus
		Amygdala
	Medium density areas:	Hypothalamus
		Striatum
		Thalamus
		Retina
	Low density areas:	Pons
		Medulla oblongata
		Medulla spinalis
		Corpus callosum
Substrate specificity:		K_i (nmole/l)
	Triazolam	2
	Lorazepam	2
	Clonazepam	3
	Ro-II-6896 (3S)	4
	Diazepam	10
	Nitrazepam	20
	Flurazepam	20
	Oxazepam	30
	Bromazepam	40
	Prazepam	300
	Chlordiazepoxid	500
	Medazepam	1000
	Ro-II-6893 (3R)	2800

The data are taken from references (1-3).

K_i-values, the binding constants of the inhibitors, were calculated from the half-maximal inhibitory concentrations for specific ^{3}H-diazepam binding or specific ^{3}H-flunitrazepam binding.

sites. For example, specific high affinity binding of many drugs to membrane lipids and even glass fibre filters can be demonstrated and benzodiazepines bind with high affinity and pronounced stereospecificity to human serum albumin via a single binding site of receptor like specificity (10,11). Thus, the basic condition to accept these brain specific binding sites as the receptor which mediates the biological effects of the benzodiazepines must be a good correlation between affinity to these binding sites in vitro and pharmacological activity in vivo. And in fact, the correlations reported so far between receptor affinity and pharmacological or therapeutical activity for a large range of benzodiazepine derivatives are in general very good (1-4). Therefore, it is today generally accepted that the benzodiazepine receptor represents the physiological target which mediates the pharmacological and clinical effects of the benzodiazepines (1-6).

The Putative Endogenous Ligand(s)

Shortly after the discovery of specific benzodiazepine receptors the questions arose what is the physiological or biochemical function of these receptors and which compound(s) is (are) the native ligand(s) acting endogenously on this receptor? The parallelism to the opiate receptor is quite obvious. However, in large contrast to the opiate receptor where the search for an endogenous ligand led to the discovery of a new class of endogenously occurring compound, the endorphins, the question about the endogenous ligand of the benzodiazepine receptor is still open, since none of the candidates proposed (table 2) fulfils all criteria required. However, because of their sometimes extremely high affinity for the benzodiazepine receptor, ß-carbolines might give the most likely candidates, possibly in a way that the ß-carboline structure is the end-group of a small peptide. Since ß-carbolines have rather

Table 2: Putative endogenous ligands of the benzodiazepine receptor.

Compound	Status	Literature
Inosine and Hypoxanthine	Both compounds inhibit benzodiazepine receptor binding and have some pharmacological properties in common with the benzodiazepines. However, their affinities are very low (IC50 = ca. 1 mM). This, together with the low brain levels makes a significant occupation of receptors in vivo very unlikely.	(15,16)
Nicotinamide	Has benzodiazepine-like effects in vivo but a very low affinity (IC50 = ca. 3 mM). Brain levels are very low relative to its affinity.	(17)
Thromboxane A_2	Very unlikely.	(18)
Several proteins (mol.wt. 15000 - 70000)	Possibly too large to be neurotransmitters.	(19-21)
Ethyl ß-carboline-3-carboxylate	Very high affinity (IC50 = ca. 1 nM). Compound is not endogenous but an artefact of the isolation. The free acid (ß-carboline-3-carboxylic acid), the most likely precursor, has a three orders of magnitude lower affinity and also has not yet been identified in vivo.	(22)
Harmane (1-methyl-ß-carboline)	Has intermediate affinity (IC50 = ca. 10 µM). Antagonizes benzodiazepines competitively in vitro and in vivo. Present in mammalian brain, blood, and urine. However, the endogenous concentration in relation to the affinity might be too low to suggest a significant occupation of receptors in vivo. Binds also to other neurotransmitter receptors in a similar concentration range.	(14,23, 24)

IC50 = concentration which inhibits specific ^{3}H-diazepam or specific ^{3}H-flunitrazepam binding by 50 percent.

stimulating than depressing effects on the CNS it seems possible that the endogenous ligand is a CNS stimulating compound and the benzodiazepines are depressing antagonists (12-14).

Benzodiazepine Receptor Subclasses

All earlier studies using ^{3}H-diazepam or ^{3}H-flunitrazepam as ligands indicated the presence of only one population of benzodiazepine receptors with similar properties in all CNS regions. However, a variety of experimental observations suggests today the presence of multiple benzodiazepine receptors, e.g. polyphasic dissociation and polyphasic thermal inactivation curves, the presence of two soluble benzodiazepine receptor proteins, and Hill coefficients considerably different from unity in the case of the inhibition of benzodiazepine receptor binding by several triazolopyridazines, anxiolytic drugs with lower hypnotic potency compared to the benzodiazepines (25). While all these findings give rather indirect evidence for the presence of benzodiazepine receptor subclasses binding experiments with tritiated propyl ß-carboline-3-carboxylate for the first time directly indicate the presence of at least two subclasses or subpopulations of the benzodiazepine receptor (see the next chapter by Fehske and Müller in this volume).

Benzodiazepines and GABAergic Inhibition

As mentioned before, the most likely concept to explain the molecular mechanism of action of the benzodiazepines is the enhancement or facilitation of GABAergic inhibtion in many regions of the CNS by the benzodiazepines (26). This was first concluded from experiments indicating that benzodiazepines can enhance in a bicuculline sensitive manner presynaptic inhibition in the spinal cord which is mediated by GABA (26). In the meantime, it could be demonstrated that most of the biochemical, electrophysiological, pharmacological, and behavioral effects of the benzodiazepines can be blocked by GABA antagonists like bicuculline and/or depend on the presence of endogenous GABA (26). Since the benzodiazepines are not GABA receptor agonists, do not increase the neuronal release of GABA, and do not block the neuronal or glial reuptake of GABA, the mechanism how benzodiazepine enhance GABAergic transmission was not understood for a long period of time. Meanwhile, binding studies have provided some evidence that the enhancement of GABAergic inhibition takes place at the GABA receptor level although the final mechanism is still not yet known.

Many authors have reported that GABA and several other but not all GABAergic agonists stimulate the binding of benzodiazepines to the benzodiazepine receptor by increasing rather the affinity than by increasing the maximal number of binding sites (27,28). This effect can be specifically blocked by the GABA-receptor antagonist bicuculline. The next step, how the interaction of benzodiazepines with the receptor increases the response to GABA is much less clear but two interesting theories have been developed. 1. The interaction of benzodiazepines with the benzodiazepine receptor might interfere with the function of a protein, called GABA modulin, which shifts the GABA receptor from a high affinity to a low affinity state (28). Thus, in the presence of benzodiazepines more high affinity GABA receptors may be available and the GABA receptor occupation and therewith the response under a definite number of neuronally released GABA quanta is enhanced. 2. Benzodiazepine receptor occupation might modulate the effects of GABA on the chloride conductance by an allosteric mechanism without affecting itself the chloride conductance (3). If only one or both mechanisms together are present remains to be clarified.

The GABA Receptor - Benzodiazepine Receptor - Chloride Channel Unit as the Endogenous Target of Many Convulsants and Depressants

During the last few years, a variety of evidence has accumulated indicating that the GABA receptor, the benzodiazepine receptor, and the chloride channel form a functional unit in

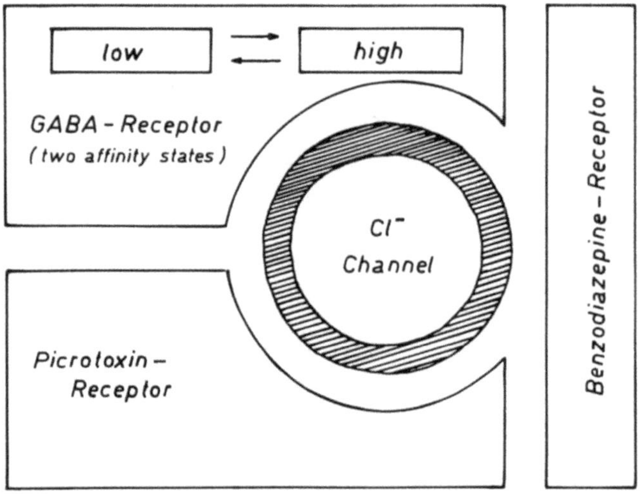

Fig. 1
Hypothetical model of the GABA receptor - benzodiazepine receptor - chloride channel unit. According to Olsen (29).

neuronal membranes of the CNS and that a broad range of CNS active drugs works via this system (9,29). It is quite clear for some time that GABA agonists increase the conductance of the chloride channel after binding to the GABA receptor, an effect which can be blocked competitively by direct GABA antagonists like bicuculline. Other GABA antagonists like picrotoxin do not interfere with the GABA receptor but block the conductance change of the chloride channel by binding to a specific site, presumably located very close to the chloride channel. More interestingly, some evidence exists that barbiturates in anesthetic concentrations directly increase chloride conductance by binding to the picrotoxin site (9,29, 30). In contrast to the barbiturates, the benzodiazepine do not directly alter the chloride conductance but only enhance the GABA initiated effect by one or both mechanisms mentioned in the last paragraph. On the other hand, in addition to the direct stimulation of the chloride conductance barbiturates seem to stimulate GABA and benzodiazepine receptor binding possibly also by interacting with the picrotoxin binding site. The biological significance of all these steps is not yet finally known. However, the data accumulated so far give some good evidence that mutual interactions within this functional unit could explain how many drugs act in the CNS (9,29,31).

Conclusions

As outlined above, our knowledge about the molecular mechanism of action of the benzodiazepine has increased considerably during the last few years. However, while some questions have been solved by the findings of a new benzodiazepine specific receptor many other questions are still open. Undoubtedly, it will take some more time until we understand completely how benzodiazepines work in the CNS.

References

1. Braestrup, C., Squires, R.F.: Brit. J. Psychiat. 133, 249-260 (1978).
2. Möhler,H., Okada,T.: Brit. J. Psychiat. 133,261-268 (1978)
3. Braestrup, C., Nielsen, M.: Arzneimittel-Forsch. 30, 852-857 (1980a)
4. Tallman, J.F., Paul, S.M., Skolnik, P., Gallager, D.W.: Science 207, 274-281 (1980)
5. Speth, R.C., Guidotti, A., Yamamura, H.I.: In "Neuropharmacology of central nervous system and behavioral disorders", ed. by G.C. Palmer, Academic Press,New York,1981.

6. Müller, W.E.: Pharmacology 22, 153-161 (1981).
7. Müller, W.E., Schläfer, U., Wollert, U.: Naunyn-Schmiedeberg's Arch. Pharmacol. 305, 23-26 (1978).
8. Antoniadis, A., Müller, W.E., Wollert, U.: Neuropharmacology 19, 121-124 (1980).
9. Paul, S.M., Marangos, P.J., Skolnick, P.: Biol. Psych. 16, 213-229 (1981).
10. Müller, W.E., Wollert, U.: Mol. Pharmacol. 11,52-60 (1975).
11. Müller, W.E., Wollert, U.: Pharmacology 19, 59-67 (1979).
12. Oakley,N.R., Jones,B.J.:Eur.J.Pharmacol. 68,381-382 (1980).
13. Cowen, P.J., Green, A.R., Nutt, D.J., Martin, I.L.: Nature 290, 54-55 (1981).
14. Rommelspacher, H., Nanz, Ch., Borbe, H.O., Fehske, K.J., Müller,W.E., Wollert,U.:Eur.J.Pharmacol. 70,409-416 (1981).
15. Marangos, P.J., Paul, S.M., Goodwin, F.K., Skolnick, P.: Life Sci. 25, 1093-1102 (1979).
16. Asano, T., Spector, S.: Acad. Sci. USA 76, 977-981 (1979).
17. Möhler, H., Polc, P., Cumin, R., Pieri, L., Kettler, R.: Nature 278, 563-565 (1979).
18. Ally, A.I., Manku, M.S., Horrobin, D.F., Karmali, R.A., Morgan, R.O., Karamazyn, M.: Neuroscience Letters 7, 31-34 (1978)
19. Davis, L.G., Cohen, R.K.: Biochem. Biophys. Res. Commun. 92, 141-148 (1980).
20. Coello, G.D., Hockenbery, D.M., Bosmann, H.B., Fuchs, S., Folkers, K.: Proc. Natl. Acad. Sci. 75, 6319-6323 (1978).
21. Woolf, J.H., Nixon, J.C.: Biochemistry 20,4263-4269 (1981).
22. Braestrup, C., Nielsen, M., Olsen, C.E.: Proc. Natl. Acad. Sci. 77, 2288-2292 (1980).
23. Rommelspacher, H., Nanz, C., Borbe, H.O., Fehske, K.J., Müller, W.E., Wollert, U.:Naunyn-Schmiedeberg's Arch. Pharmacol. 314, 97-100 (1980).
24. Müller, W.E., Fehske, K.J., Borbe, H.O., Wollert,U., Nanz, C.,Rommelspacher,H.:Pharmac.Biochem.Behav.14,693-699(1981).
25. Braestrup, C., Nielsen, M.: TINS 301-303 (1980b).
26. Haefely, W.E.: In "Psychopharmacology, a generation of progress", ed. by M.A. Lipton, A. DiMascio, K.F. Killam. Raven Press, New York, 1978.
27. Karobath, M., Sperk, G.: Proc. Nat. Acad. Sci. 76, 1004-1006 (1979).

28. Costa, E., Guidotti, A.: Ann. Rev. Pharmacol. Toxicol. 19, 531-545 (1979).

29. Olsen, R.W.: J. Neurochem. 37, 1-13 (1981).

30. Schulz, D.W., MacDonald, R.L.: Brain Res. 209, 177-188 (1981).

31. Sieghart, W., Placheta, P., Supravilai, P., Karobath, M.: In "GABA and benzodiazepine receptors", ed. by E. Costa, G. Di Chiara, G.L. Gessa. Raven Press, New York, 1981.

Acknowledgements

The author's studies cited in the present review have been supported by grants of the Deutsche Forschungsgemeinschaft.

CHARACTERIZATION OF THE INTERACTION OF ^{3}H-PROPYL-ß-CARBOLINE-3-CARBOXYLATE WITH THE BENZODIAZEPINE RECEPTOR IN THE BOVINE CENTRAL NERVOUS SYSTEM

Klaus. J. Fehske and Walter E. Müller
Pharmakologisches Institut der Universität Mainz, Obere Zahlbacher Straße 67, D-6500 Mainz, Federal Republic of Germany

Introduction

While the status of the ß-carbolines as endogenous ligands of the benzodiazepine receptor is still unclear (see the chapter by W.E. Müller in this volume) ß-carbolines have become important experimental tools in another respect related to the benzodiazepine receptor. In contrast to all the benzodiazepines investigated so far some ß-carbolines seem to have different affinities for at least two subclasses or subpopulations of the benzodiazepine receptor. This subclass specificity is mostly pronounced in the case of propyl ß-carboline-3-carboxylate (PrCC) (2,3,4). Using tritiated PrCC of high specific activity (^{3}H-PrCC) it is possible to demonstrate the presence of two subclasses of benzodiazepine binding sites in the bovine central nervous system including the retina (4) which also contains brain specific benzodiazepine receptors(5).

Saturation of Benzodiazepine Receptors with ^{3}H-PrCC

Saturable ^{3}H-PrCC binding can be demonstrated in different regions of the bovine central nervous system (CNS). Scatchard analysis of these binding data results in straight lines as revealed by regression analysis indicating a single population of PrCC sensitive binding sites (fig. 1). While the equili-

Neuroreceptors

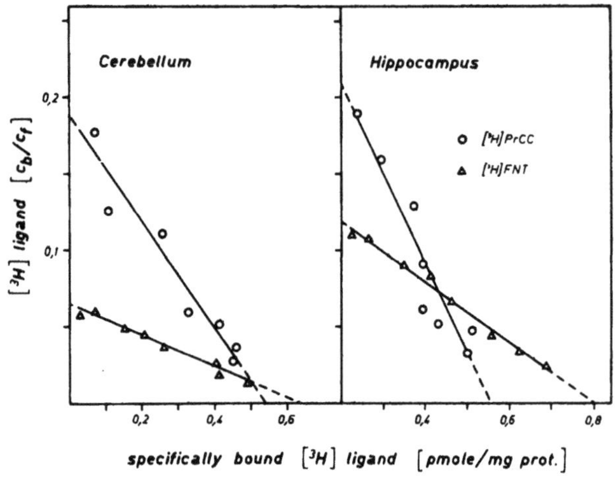

Fig. 1:
Scatchard plots of saturation experiments of specific ^{3}H-FNT and specific ^{3}H-PrCC binding in the bovine cerebellum and retina. The data are taken from reference (4).

brium dissociation constants of specific ^{3}H-PrCC binding are similar in the four regions investigated (tabel 1) pronounced differences of the maximal number of binding sites are evident for the four regions of the bovine CNS (table 1). A comparable distribution was found for the maximal number of binding sites of the benzodiazepine ligand ^{3}H-flunitrazepam (^{3}H-FNT) using Scatchard plots of saturation experiments (fig. 1, table 1). ^{3}H-FNT as ^{3}H-PrCC has similar dissociation constants in the four regions (table 1). However, in all regions more binding sites are available for ^{3}H-FNT than for ^{3}H-PrCC (table 1). Since diazepam (10 μM) was used as blank for both ligands one can assume the specific ^{3}H-FNT as well as specific ^{3}H-PrCC binding label exclusively benzodiazepine receptors (3). Thus, only about 60 % of the ^{3}H-FNT binding sites found in the cortex,hippocampus, and the retina are also available for ^{3}H-PrCC while this percentage is considerably higher in the cerebellum where about 80 % of the ^{3}H-FNT binding sites can also be labeled with ^{3}H-PrCC (table 1). Obviously, ^{3}H-PrCC interacts

Brain region	K_D [nM]		B_{max} [pmole/mg prot.]		n_H	
	$[^3H]$FNT	$[^3H]$PrCC	$[^3H]$FNT	$[^3H]$PrCC	$[^3H]$FNT	$[^3H]$PrCC
Calf						
Cerebellum	2.62	0.72	712	565 (79)	1.00	1.03
Cortex	2.66	0.67	1650	1018 (62)	0.96	0.94
Hippocampus	2.52	0.81	1322	787 (60)	0.99	0.98
Retina	2.24	0.69	692	437 (65)	0.98	1.04
Rat						
Cerebellum	1.4	0.9	63	57 (91)		
Cortex	1.5	0.8	121	86 (71)		
Hippocampus	1.3	1.2	94	53 (57)		

Table 1:

Characteristics of specific ^{3}H-FNT and specific ^{3}H-PrCC binding in the calf and rat CNS. The dissociation constants (K_D), and the maximal number of binding sites, and the Hill coeffients were calculated from saturation experiments by Scatchard or Hill analysis respectively. The data are taken from references (4) calf and (3) rat. Please note that the B_{max} values in the rat are calculated for mg wet tissue and not for mg protein (3).

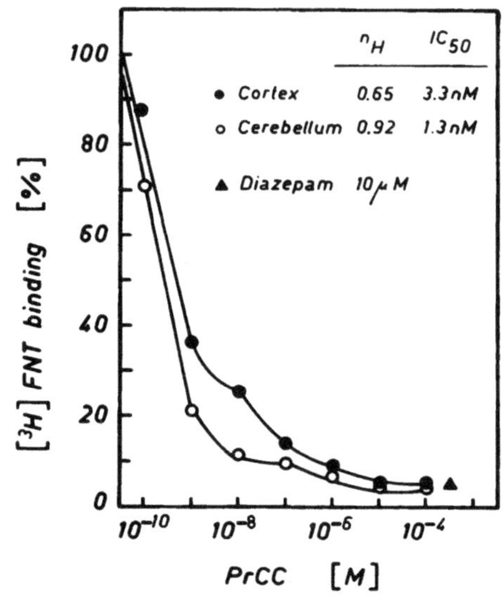

Fig. 2:
Inhibition of total ^{3}H-FNT binding in bovine cortex and cerebellum by increasing concentrations of PrCC and by diazepam (final concentration 10 μM). IC-50 = half maximal inhibitory concentration and n_H = Hill coefficient.Taken from reference(4).

in the concentration range investigated (0.1 - 5 nM) only with one subpopulation of the ^{3}H-FNT binding sites whose relative density is higher in the cerebellum than in the other three regions. This assumption is supported by the data given in fig. 2 where different displacement curves for total ^{3}H-FNT binding by unlabeled PrCC were found in the cortex and the cerebellum. While half-maximal inhibition occurs at only slightly different PrCC concentrations profound differences are obvious at PrCC concentrations higher than 1 nM. For example, at a concentration of 10 nM PrCC inhibits ^{3}H-FNT binding in the cerebellum by about 90 % but only by about 75 % in the cortex (fig. 2). However, at higher concentrations PrCC binds to all specific ^{3}H-FNT sites as indicated by the maximal displacement by PrCC which is similar to the inhibition observed in the presence of diazepam (10 μM), the blank usually employed to differentiate between specific and unspecific ^{3}H-FNT and ^{3}H-PrCC binding. In contrast to the Hill coefficients obtained from the saturation experiments (table 1) which are not different from one, the Hill coefficient for the inhibition of ^{3}H-FNT binding by PrCC is slightly smaller than one in the cerebellum and is considerably smaller than one in the cortex (fig. 2). These data are very well in agreement with the assumption of a different relative number of benzodiazepine receptors in both areas which are sensitive to PrCC. Furthermore, these data clearly indicate that PrCC also interacts with the second population of benzodiazepine receptors although at considerably higher concentrations.

Compared to some recent findings about the properties and distribution of PrCC sensitive benzodiazepine receptors in the RAT CNS (3) our data indicate some important differences between both species. While only 80 % of the total population of benzodiazepine receptors in the calf cerebellum belong to the PrCC sensitive type no differences where found in the rat cerebellum between total population and PrCC sensitive population (table 1). This species difference is less pronounced in the cortex with about 70 % of all sites sensitive to PrCC in the rat compared to 60 % in the calf and is absent in the hippocampus with 57 % sensitive to PrCC in the rat compared to 60 % in the calf (table 1). Interestingly, Young and Kuhar (6) reported substantial differences of the benzodiazepine receptor distributions between human and rat cerebellum which were more pronounced than the differences found for all other brain regions. Obviously, species differences of the properties of benzodiazepine receptors are more important in the cerebellum than in other areas of the CNS.

GABAergic Modulation

Many authors have reported that benzodiazepine receptor binding can be stimulated by GABA or other GABAergic agonists

	Cerebellum	Cortex	Hippocampus	Retina
	Specific $[^3H]$FNT Binding in Percent of Controls			
GABA 10 µM	155***	141**	132***	147***
GABA 1 µM	136**	121*	113*	134***
Bicuculline 50 µM	94	88	86	85
GABA 10 µM + Bicuculline 50 µM	98	92*	87	98
GABA 1 µM + Bicuculline 50 µM	87	87	84	86
	Specific $[^3H]$PrCC Binding in Percent of Controls			
GABA 10 µM	112**	108**	113**	114**
GABA 1 µM	110*	108**	112**	112**
Bicuculline 50 µM	91*	89	88**	86*
GABA 10 µM + Bicuculline 50 µM	95	84	94	91
GABA 1 µM + Bicuculline 50 µM	89	86	93	90

* $P < 0.05$, ** $P < 0.01$, *** $P < 0.001$

Table 2:
The effects of GABA and bicuculline on specific $[^3H]$FNT and on specific $[^3H]$PrCC binding in four regions of the bovine CNS. The data are taken from reference (4).

where these agents increase the affinity of the benzodiazepines rather than increase the maximal number of binding sites (7,8,9). Accordingly, GABA enhances specific ^{3}H-FNT binding to thoroughly washed menbranes of all four areas of the bovine CNS investigated (table 2). An about 50 % increase over controls at 10 µM GABA and an about 20 % increase over controls at 1 µM GABA were observed (table 3). All effects can be completely inhibited by the GABA receptor antagonist bicuculline at a final concentration of 50 µM (table 2). Similar to specific ^{3}H-FNT binding specific ^{3}H-PrCC binding can also be enhanced by GABA in all four regions. However, stimulation was only about 10 % over controls at 1 µM and could not be further increased by increasing the GABA concentration to 10 µM (table 2). Similar to specific ^{3}H-FNT binding the stimulation of specific ^{3}H-PrCC binding by GABA can be completely inhibited by bicuculline (table 2).

These observations could indicate that the PrCC sensitive subclass or subpopulation of the benzodiazepine receptor is less sensitive to GABAergic stimuli than the total receptor population. However, the alternative explanation that this observation is due to a much lesser sensitivity of a presumed ß-carboline conformation of the benzodiazepine receptor to GABAergic stimuli than a presumed benzodiazepine conformation can not be rouled out but is supported by very recent findings of the Braestrup group (10).

Substrate Specificity

Specific ^{3}H-FNT and specific ^{3}H-PrCC binding in the bovine cerebellum and retina, two regions with different relationships between PrCC sensitive and PrCC less sensitive benzodiazepine receptors, can be inhibited by a large variety of drugs and other compounds in a concentration dependent manner (table 3). These compounds include several benzodiazepine drugs, the

	IC_{50} [nM]			
	Cerebellum		Retina	
	[^{3}H]FNT	[^{3}H]PrCC	[^{3}H]FNT	[^{3}H]PrCC
Clonazepam	2.5	3.1	3.6	2.0
Ro 11-6896	11	16	9.3	14
Diazepam	19	20	10	9
Ro 11-6893	170	300	220	270
Chlordiazepoxid	920	1 310	1 200	960
R 15-1788	1.0	1.5	1.4	1.1
PK 9084	1 600	2 400	1 300	850
Fominobene	1 900	2 800	1 700	2 800
Glutethimide	26 000	30 000	29 000	39 000
Methaqualone	160 000	130 000	120 000	50 000
Cloxacilline	1 600 000	2 300 000	970 000	1 500 000
Pentetrazole	4 400 000	3 800 000	2 900 000	3 400 000
PrCC	1.8	1.5	3.2	1.8
ECC	0.8	1.3	0.8	0.5
MCC	1.4	1.8	2.0	0.9
Norharman	1 100	1 600	3 000	1 700
Harman	10 000	15 000	26 000	20 000
Tryptophanbenzylester	92 000	90 000	83 000	67 000
Inosine	500 000	620 000	520 000	720 000
Nicotinamide	2 800 000	3 900 000	4 500 000	2 100 000

Table 3:

Substrate specificity of specific [^{3}H]FNT and specific [^{3}H]PrCC binding in bovine cerebellum and retina. The concentrations which inhibit specific [^{3}H]FNT or specific [^{3}H]PrCC binding by 50% (IC_{50}) were determined by log probit analysis using 4-6 concentrations of the displacers.The data are taken from reference(4).MCC=Methyl ß-carboline-3-carboxylate.

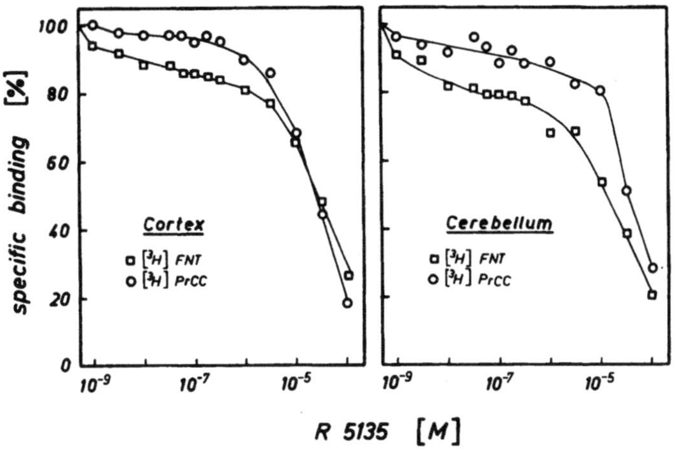

Fig. 3:
Inhibition of specific ^{3}H-FNT and specific ^{3}H-PrCC binding in bovine cortex and cerebellum by increasing concentrations of R 5135. The data are taken from reference (4).

the pharmacologically active and inactive enantiomers of a 3-methyl-benzodiazepine (Ro 11-6896 and Ro 11-6893) (11), the benzodiazepine antagonist Ro 15-1788 (12), several non-benzodiazepine drugs with putative benzodiazepine like (PK 9084, glutethimide, methaqualone) (13,14,15) or with putative benzodiazepine antagonistic (fominobene, cloxacillin, pentetrazole) (14,15,16) properties at the benzodiazepine receptor, several ß-carboline derivatives, tryptophanbenzylester, the most active compound out of a series of indole derivatives (17), and the two putative endogenous ligands inosine and nicotinamide (18,19). For all these quite heterogenous compounds very similar affinities for the binding sites labeled by specific ^{3}H-FNT binding or by specific ^{3}H-PrCC binding were observed, clearly indicating that both ligands label the same receptor.

Very recently, Hunt and Clements-Jewery (20) reported that the steroid derivative R 5135, besides its high affinity for the GABA as well as the glycine receptors, interacts with the benzodiazepine receptor in a biphasic manner. These findings are confirmed by the data of the present study (fig. 3) where R 5135 inhibits specific ^{3}H-FNT binding in bovine cortex and cerebellum in a biphasic fashion (fig. 3). But more important, the biphasic inhibition can not be demonstrated in the case of specific ^{3}H-PrCC binding in both regions (fig. 3) possibly indicating a higher affinity of R 5135 for the PrCC less sensitive than for the PrCC sensitive subpopulation of the benzodiazepine receptor.

Conclusion

The data reported in this communication (3,4) clearly indicate that specific ^{3}H-PrCC binding labels only one subclass or subpopulation of benzodiazepine receptors which is unevenly distributed in the bovine as well as the rat CNS.

Up to now, mainly indirect evidence has been presented for the presence of different benzodiazepine receptor subclasses (see the chapter by W.E. Müller in this volume). These subclasses might be of importance for the design of benzodiazepine like drugs with better specificities in respect to the pharmacological profile, e.g. anxiolytics without sedative side effects (21). Therefore, we think that the possibility to label only one of these subclasses, the BZ_1 or cerebellar type (1),fairly selectively by the specific binding of ^{3}H-PrCC is an important new experimental approach and a significant step forward. On the other hand, for the PrCC less sensitive subpopulation of benzodiazepine receptors, the BZ_2 or hippocampal type (1), specific ligands are not yet known. In this respect, our findings about the much higher affinity of the steroid derivative R 5135 for specific ^{3}H-FNT than for specific ^{3}H-PrCC binding could be the first experimental observation indicating a drug with higher affinity for the BZ_2 than for the BZ_1 subclass of the benzodiazepine receptor. However, the relevance of this observation in respect to the pharmacological profile of this new drug is not yet known (20).

These data clearly indicate that the characterization of subclasses of the benzodiazepine receptors is not only of theoretical interest to get further insight into the mechanisms how these drugs act on the CNS but is also of practical interest for the future development of better drugs.

Acknowledgements

These studies of the authors cited in this communication have been supported by a grant of the Deutsche Forschungsgemeinschaft.

References

1. Braestrup, C., Nielsen, M.: TINS, 301-303 (1980).
2. Nielsen, M., Braestrup, C.: J. Neurochem. 36,276-285(1981).
3. Braestrup, C., Nielsen, M.:J. Neurochem. 37,333-341(1981a).
4. Fehske, K.J., Zube, I., Borbe, H.O., Wollert, U., Müller, W.E.: submitted for publication.
5. Borbe, H.O., Müller, W.E., Wollert, U.: Brain Res. 182, 466-469 (1980).
6. Young, W.S., Kuhar, M.J.: J. Pharmacol. exp. Ther. 212, 337-346 (1980).
7. Costa, E., Guidotti, A.: Ann. Rev. Pharmacol. Toxicol. 19, 531-545 (1979).
8. Sieghart, W., Placheta, P., Supravilai, P., Karobath, M.: In "GABA and benzodiazepine receptors". Costa, E., Di Chiara, G., Gessa, G.L. (eds.).Raven Press, New York(1981).
9. Olsen, R.W.: J. Neurochem. 37, 1-13 (1981).
10. Braestrup, C., Nielsen, M.: Neurosc. Lett. suppl. 7, 57 (1981b).
11. Möhler, H., Okada, T.: Brit. J. Psychiat. 133, 261-268 (1978).

12. Hunkeler, W., Möhler, H., Pieri, L., Polc, P., Bonetti, E.P., Cumin, R., Schaffner, R., Haefely, W.: Nature 290, 514-516 (1981).

13. Le Fur, G., Mizoule, J., Burgevin, M.C., Ferris, O., Heaulme, M., Gauthier, A., Guérémy, C., Uzan, A.: Life Sci 28, 1439-1448 (1981).

14. Antoniadis, A., Müller, W.E., Wollert, U.: Neuropharmacology 19, 121-124 (1980a).

15. Müller, W.E., Schläfer, U., Wollert, U.: Naunyn-Schmiedeberg's Arch. Pharmacol. 305, 23-26 (1978).

16. Antoniadis, A., Müller, W.E., Wollert, U.: Ann. Neurol. 8, 71-73 (1980b).

17. Fehske, K.J., Müller, W.E., Platt, K.L., Stillbauer, A.E.: Biochem. Pharmacol., in press.

18. Marangos, P.J., Paul, S.M., Goodwin, F.K., Skolnick, P.: Life Sci 25, 1093-1102 (1979).

19. Möhler, H., Polc, P., Cumin, R., Pieri, L., Kettler, R.: Nature 278, 563-565 (1979).

20. Hunt, P., Clements-Jewers, S.: Neurpharmacol. 20, 357-363 (1981).

21. Albright, J.D., Moran, D.B., Wright, W.B., Collins, J.B., Beer, B., Lippa, A.S., Greenblatt, E.N.: J. med. Chem. 24, 592-600 (1981).

THE IN VIVO OCCURING ß-CARBOLINES INDUCE A CONFLICT-AUGMENTING EFFECT WHICH IS ANTAGONIZED BY DIAZEPAM: CORRELATION TO RECEPTOR BINDING STUDIES

H.Rommelspacher, G.Brüning, G.Schulze, and R.Hill
Department of Neuropsychopharmacology, Free University, Ulmenallee 30, D-1000 Berlin 19

Introduction

ß-carbolines are formed in vitro by a Picted-Spengler type of chemical reaction between indolealkylamines and aldehydes. They are widespread in the flora and in recent years their presence was demonstrated in several organs of mammals including the brain. The substances elicit a number of effects in humans, among them hallucinations, some symptoms of inebriation, autistic tendencies, euphoric mood changes, and aggressive behavior. In animals the compounds act as 5-hydroxytryptamine-agonists and dopamine-antagonists both in vitro and in vivo. In several behavioral tests the ß-carbolines elicit effects which cannot be accounted for 5-hydroxytryptamine/dopamine systems (for review see Rommelspacher 1981).

Recently, it was shown that ß-carbolines displace competitively (3H)-flunitrazepam from its specific binding sites on brain membranes (Braestrup et al. 1980, Rommelspacher et al. 1980). Since the ß-carbolines occur in vivo it was of interest to see, if they occupy the same receptor site as the benzodiazepines to elicit their pharmacodynamic effects. In pharmacological experiments it could be shown that the ß-carbolines induce convulsions. The convulsive potency of the various substances correlates well with their displacing potency in the binding experiments, with the exception of norharmane (Cowen et al. 1981, Müller et al. 1981, Rommelspacher et al. 1981). Thus, the ß-carbolines act opposite to the benzodiazepines under these conditions.

In the present contribution these studies are extended on a

conflict-punishment procedure presumably an animal model for the anxiolytic effect of the benzodiazepines in humans. The experiments revealed an antagonism between the ß-carbolines and benzodiazepines. The antagonistic potency of the ß-carbolines correlated with that in receptor binding experiments using whole brain membranes as performed previously. These studies are now refined in such a way that membranes from small brain regions are utilized.

Materials and Methods

1. Materials

Male Wistar rats (200 - 400 g) were used for the conflict-test and female Wistar rats (200 - 220 g) for receptor binding experiments. The male rats were housed individually and had tap water available ad libitum. The drugs were dissolved in 10% cremophor (Bayer, Leverkusen, FRG) in 0.9% NaCl (w/v). Controls were treated with vehicle only. The following substances were administered: harmane HCl, norharmane HCl (Sigma, Munich, FRG), diazepam (gift of Dr. Kapp, Hoffmann La Roche, Grenzach, FRG), ethyl-ß-carboline-3-carboxylate (gift of Dr. Schmiechen, Schering, Berlin, FRG and of Dr. Braestrup, Ferrosan, Kopenhagen, Denmark), (3H)-flunitrazepam (FNM, 84 Ci/mmol; Amersham Buchler, Braunschweig, FRG). Tetrahydronorharmane (THN) was synthesized as described by Vejdelek et al. (1961). Identity and purity of the compound were ascertained by the melting point at 281 - 288°C and the identity of the mass spectrum with that described in the literature.

2. Conflict-punishment procedure

The experiments were performed essentially as described by Cook and Davidson (1973). Male Wistar rats were fed by a food delivery meter in the experimental sessions and supplementary feeding at the end of each day. The experimental chamber measured 28x29x26 cm and contained a response lever and food-delivery apparatus, an electrifiable grid floor, a stimulus light which illuminated the chamber and a noise generator. The experimental chamber was enclosed by a sound-stable, ventilated box. Lever-press responses were reinforced by delivery of 45 mg Noyes food pellets. The experiment was automatically programmed and recorded by a Massey Dickinson steering apparatus and data recorder (Heinz Albrecht, Munich, FRG). The intensity of foot-shock punishment, delivered by a Getra shock generator and scrambler, was adjusted for each rat during training (range 0.5 - 1.3 mA; 1 sec duration) as well as every fourth to fifth weeks during the experimental period, to achieve an optimal degree of suppression.

The rats were trained to respond on a fixed ratio schedule of ten lever-press responses for each food reinforcement (FR 10) in the presence of flash light. The FR 10 lasted 2 minutes and was alternated with 5 minute periods of a variable interval schedule (VI, 30 sec) of reinforcement, in the presence of steady light. The possibility to get a pellet was signaled by a short tone. Daily experimental sessions consisted of 6 periods of the FR 10 (punishment) component and 7 periods of the VI 30 sec (non-punishment) component. They were conducted at the same time of the day and were preceeded by p.o. injection of diazepam and vehicle respectively and i.p. injection of the ß-carboline and vehicle respectively 30 min before placing the rat into the experimental chamber. At least one week elapsed between treatment. The experimental sessions were conducted at five days of the week.

For statistical analysis, each rat was used as its own control. The average number of responses on the day before the day of punishment in each of the two schedule components, was compared to the number of responses in these components at the day of punishment. The difference in percent of the respective pressing-rates was calculated. Statistical significance of differences between the mean values was determined using a two-tailed Students t-test.

3. Receptor-binding studies

Female rats were decapitated, their brains removed from the skull, and various brain regions dissected under a microscope for microsurgery (Zeiss, Oberkochen, FRG). The tissue was homogenized in 50 mmol/l Tris HCl buffer pH 7.4 and centrifuged at 48000 g for ten minutes. The membranes were stored at -20°C for at least 18 h and used for binding assay within one week. Specific (3H)-flunitrazepam binding was determined essentially as described by Braestrup and Squires (1977) and Rommelspacher et al. (1980). Tissue homogenates (0.5 - 2.0 mg protein/ml) were incubated in Tris HCl buffer with 0.3 mmol/l (3H)-flunitrazepam and various concentrations of the ß-carbolines in a total volume of 200 µl for 30 min on ice. The incubation period was terminated by adding 4 ml of ice-cold buffer and rapid filtration under vacuum on Whatman GF/B filters. The procedure was followed by two 4 ml washes with buffer. The radioactivity trapped by the filters was counted in a Packard liquid scintillation counter using Biofluor (New England Nuclear, Dreieich, FRG) as scintillation fluid. Unspecific binding was determined by incubation in the presence of 5 µmol/l diazepam. The counts were less than 10% of whole radioactivity. The amount of protein was measured by the method of Lowry et al. (1951) using bovine serum albumin as the standard.

Results

1. Interactions of diazepam and the ß-carbolines in the conflict-punishment procedure

Male Wistar rats were trained as described under methods to press a lever in a VI 30 sec, FR 10 schedule with food as reinforcer. This period lasted two to three months. No animal was eliminated from the group putting up with a longer lasting training period and a larger interindividual deviation as reported by others. At the end of the training period, the animals were exposed to a shock during FR 10 period at one day of the week (fig. 1 and tab. 1). In the figure an example is drawn for one animal. The vehicle-treated rat presses the lever seldom

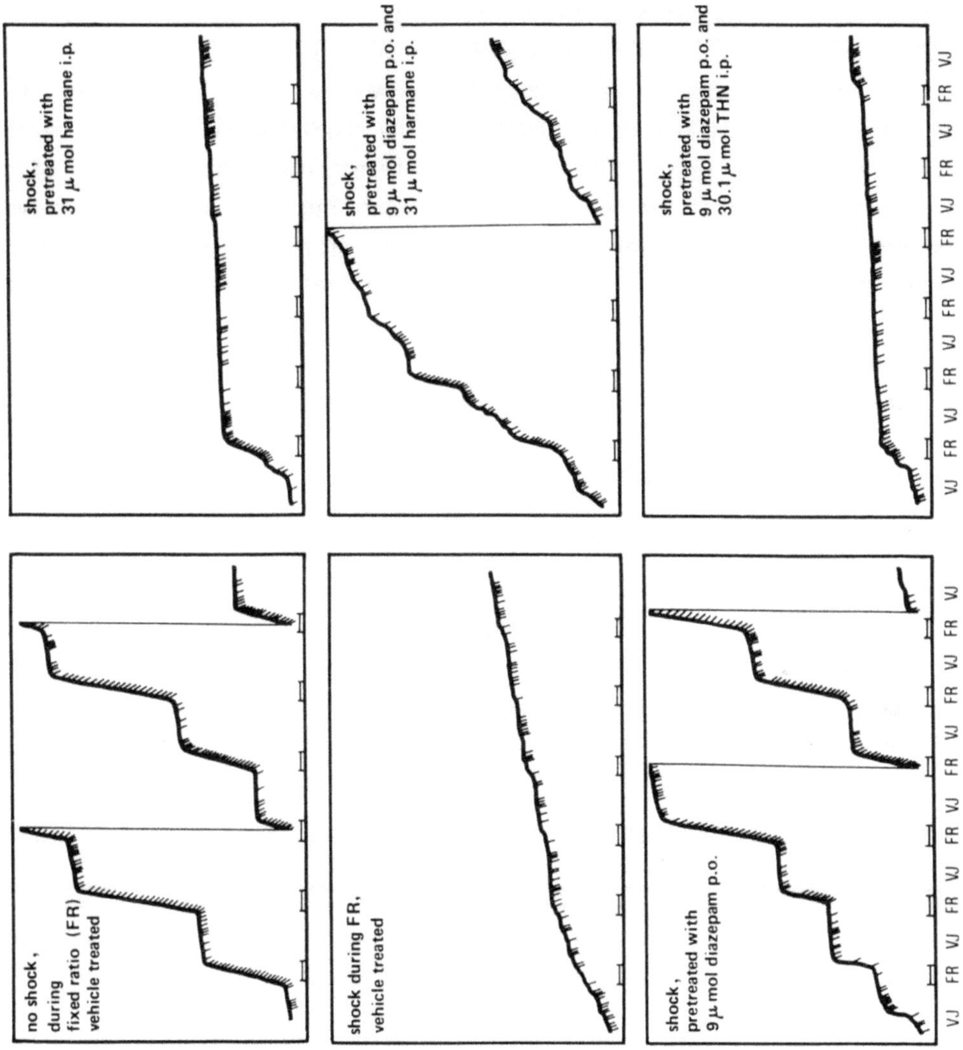

Fig. 1: Conflict punishment procedure following various treatments. The graph shows the registration from one rat.

during VI 30 sec as demonstrated by the flat course of the curve and more often during FR 10 as the curve becomes steeper (upper left drawing). The little marks indicate the reinforced lever pressings. On days, when the rat receives shock and food during FR 10, the characteristic FR 10 element disappears (middle left). The effect is attenuated by pretreatment with diazepam (lower left) but not by harmane (upper right) as well as diazepam and THN (lower right) reverses the effect of diazepam alone. Table 1 demonstrates that the VI 30 sec element does not change indicating that the motor activity of the rats is not essentially affected by the various treatments.

Tab. 1: Conflict punishment procedure

	VI 30 sec	FR 10
Controls	80.4 +/- 6.9	15.6 +/- 3.3
Diazepam	93.4 +/- 5.8	34.8 +/- 4.8*
Harmane	84.1 +/- 6.4	13.7 +/- 2.0
THN	97.1 +/- 7.4	12.9 +/- 2.1
Diazepam + Harmane	102.1 +/- 6.2	16.7 +/- 1.9
Diazepam + THN	73.9 +/- 8.2	11.6 +/- 1.9

Mean of the lever-pressing rate +/- SEM. 16 to 24 rats were pretreated 30 min before placing them into the experimental chamber with 8,8 µmol/kg diazempam p.o., 30.1 µmol/kg THN i.p., and 30.0 µmol/kg harmane i.p. respectively. Controls were treated with vehicle p.o. and i.p.
* $p<0.01$

These experiments do not allow to conclude that the ß-carbolines augment the conflict for the rat by themselves. The intensity of the shock is presumably too high to lower the pressing rate further as that of controls. Therefore, the experiments were continued in such a way that the vehicle-treated animals pressed the lever 77% during FR 10 at the "shock-day" compared to the day before. The results are presented in table 2. The values are given as the difference between the percentage of vehicle-treated controls and the percentage of drug-treated animals in

Tab. 2: Conflict-punishment procedure - mild shock conditions

	vehicle		Diazepam 8,8 µmol/kg	
	VI 30 sec	FR 10	VI 30 sec	FR 10
vehicle	reference values		3.4 ± 6.7	38.8 ± 6.4 (16)*
THN (7.5 µmol/kg)	1.0 ± 5.6	20.7 ± 11.1 (7)*	-12.0 ± 8.8	13.7 ± 10.9 (7)
THN (15.1 µmol/kg)	8.7 ± 4.4	40.5 ± 5.0 (10)*	11.2 ± 5.3	16.2 ± 6.9 (6)*
THN (30.1 µmol/kg)			13.3 ± 5.9*	65.6 ± 3.9 (9)*
Harmane (7.7 µmol/kg)	-4.8 ± 8.7	3.3 ± 7.2 (9)	-14.8 ± 12.5	-2.0 ± 7.6 (11)
Harmane (15.3 µmol/kg)	14.9 ± 3.9*	21.4 ± 13.0 (7)*	-2.3 ± 3.7	-0.7 ± 7.1 (7)
Norharmane (15.3 µmol)	-0.5 ± 2.6	23.6 ± 9.3 (7)*	-7.6 ± 11.1	-4.6 ± 7.7 (7)
Ethyl-norharmane-3-carboxylate (41.7 µmol/kg)	1.0 ± 4.1	41.9 ± 5.9 (10)*	11.8 ± 15.5	48.2 ± 10.0 (5)*

Differences (absolute values) between the pressing-rates of vehicle and drug treated rats. Each animal served as its own control. The rats were treated 30 min before placing them into the experimental box. The average pressing rate of controls was calculated 77.2 ± 3.9% (42) for the FR 10 component and 102.9 ± 2.1% for the VI 30 sec component at the "shock day" compared with the day before, when the rats had been treated with saline without shock during the FR 10 segment. Values presented are the means ± SEM of the number of rats given in parentheses.

*$p < 0.01$

each case referring to the pressing rate of the day before without shock.

Diazepam reduces the pressing-rate further as control rats under the "mild-shock" conditions. The effect is dose-dependent. Oral application of 10.6 µmol/kg diazepam lowers the pressing rate to 79.0% +/- 22.9 (VI 30 sec) and 56.0% +/- 11.7 (FR 10; 4 rats) and 12.3 µmol/kg diazepam to 85.6% +/- 21.5 (VI 30 sec) and 71.3% +/- 10.1 (FR 10; 3 rats). This action contrasts clearly to the results with a higher shock intensity. The four ß-carbolines act in the same direction (tab. 2). At least for THN and harmane the effect is dose-dependent. Even 7.5 µmol/kg THN i.p. causes a further reduction compared to control animals. Combined treatment with diazepam and various ß-carbolines leads to a pressing-rate in the control range, despite the observations that both classes of compounds reduce the pressing-rate in a conflict situation. The only exception is THN and diazepam. However, the same tendency was found under these treatments, too.

It is noteworthy that higher doses of THN overcome the conflict attenuating effect of the combined treatment (tab. 2).

To assess further the specificity of the drug effects the experiments were repeated with the only differences that the rats were placed 45 min after treatment into the experimental box. Under these conditions the ß-carbolines are partly metabolized (t 1/2, brain, for THN 115 min, unpublished). The effect of the ß-carbolines disappears, whereas that of diazepam is reduced compared with that seen after a 30 min interval.

2. Interaction of (3H)-flunitrazepam and the ß-carbolines on CNS-membranes

The observation that norharmane and harmane antagonizes the effect of diazepam completely at doses with which THN causes a clear cut but incomplete reduction of the pressing-rate back to control values, led to the question whether the effect correlates with receptor binding studies. To get a more detailed information, membranes from small brain regions and

Tab. 3 - Receptor-binding experiments

Brain region	IC 50 (µM) Norharmane	Harmane	T H N	n
Bulbus olfactorius	7.4 ± 2.0	50 ± 15	*2900 ± 260	4
Bulbus olfactorius accessorius	8.3 ± 3.2	58 ± 17	*3100 ± 300	3
Cortex	*10.4 ± 1.9	*61 ± 12	*3400 ± 110	5
Hippocampus	*10.6 ± 2.0	40 ± 10	*3300 ± 110	5
Gyrus dentatus	5.0 ± 2.0	23 ± 9	*2900 ± 270	4
Striatum	7.0 ± 2.2	24 ± 9	2400 ± 250	4
Septum	4.9 ± 2.8	24 ± 11	2100 ± 280	3
Cerebellum	2.7 ± 1.3	22 ± 3	2400 ± 120	5
Nucleus dentatus cerebelli	2.5 ± 3.9	18 ± 11	1600 ± 390	2
Nucleus arcuatus	10.2 ± 5.2	44 ± 15	2600 ± 480	2
Nucleus interpeduncularis	9.2 ± 4.9	60 ± 19	3600 ± 550	2
Colliculus superior	5.5 ± 2.4	32 ± 10	2200 ± 190	4
Colliculus inferior	6.5 ± 2.4	33 ± 10	2100 ± 1290	4
Tegmentum	5.1 ± 3.4	33 ± 12	2600 ± 300	3
Medulla spinalis	8.0 ± 3.8	35 ± 13	3000 ± 330	3

ß-carboline inhibition of (3H)-flunitrazepam receptor binding. The experiments were performed using published procedures as given under methods. IC 50 values, the concentrations which inhibit specific binding by 50% were determined by log-probit analysis, using five different concentrations of the displacers, each, performed in triplicate. The data are means ± SEM of individual determinations.

*$p<0.01$, referring to the data from the Nucleus dentatus cerebelli.

medulla spinalis were used for binding experiments. The binding of (3H)-flunitrazepam is antagonized by norharmane, harmane and THN as indicated by the IC 50 values given in table 3. Norharmane is most active on membranes from the N. dentatus of the cerebellum and the whole cerebellum. On membranes from midbrain regions (colliculus superior and inferior, tegmentum) and the septal area norharmane displays an intermediate potency, whereas in all other regions the ß-carboline shows a lower activity. Harmane is about one half order of magnitude less potent as norharmane in displacing (3H)-flunitrazepam. The differences in activity using the various regional membranes are similar as those of norharmane. THN displaced (3H)-flunitrazepam from its specific binding site in a millimolar concentration range. The differences among the various regions are comparable to those observed with norharmane and harmane respectively.

Discussion

The good correlation between the displacing potency of the ß-carbolines and their convulsive activity reported previously led to the assumption of a competitive antagonistic interaction of the ß-carbolines and the benzodiazepines at the receptor site of brain membranes in vivo and in vitro (Rommelspacher et al. 1980, 1981). In the present report the hypothesis was investigated further with respect to the anxiolytic effect using the conflict-punishment procedure according to Geller and Seifter (1960).

The experiments were performed under two different conditions: with a conventional intensity of the shock (as reported in the literature) and a mild intensity of the shock. The results differed in several respects.

Under "conventional conditions" harmane as well as THN antagonized the punishment-lessening effect of diazepam without clear differences in potency as it could have been expected from receptor-binding experiments. There is evidence that both GABA-ergic and 5-HT-ergic neurones are involved in the punishment-lessening activity of benzodiazepines.

GABA-mimetic drugs act similar as benzodiazepines in tests of "anti-anxiety" activity (Lal et al. 1980, Stein et al. 1975). The activity of 5-HT-ergic neurones can be reduced by benzodiazepines (Cook and Sepinwall 1975, Geller and Blum 1970, Geller et al. 1974, Graeff and Schoenfeld 1970, Robichand and Sidge 1969, Stein et al. 1973, Wise et al. 1973). A number of investigators have suggested that benzodiazepines may exert a primary action on the effectiveness of GABA transmission which in turn may regulate transmission at monoaminergic synapses; hence the benzodiazepines may affect 5-HT systems only indirectly (Costa et al. 1975, Haefely et al. 1975, Polc et al. 1974). The present finding under "conventional conditions" may be interpreted as actions on different neurones. Harmane with a relatively high affinity towards the (3H)-flunitrazepam binding site might act at the supramolecular GABA complex whereas THN exerts its action mainly by stimulating 5-HT transmission.

The results of the experiments under mild conditions seem to be contradictory. Both diazepam and ß-carbolines cause a reduction of the pressing rate. Combined treatment antagonizes both effects. Our explanation for these findings is based on two assumptions. Firstly, the mechanisms by which the rate is lowered differ for diazepam and the ß-carbolines and secondly, the neuronal activity in the brain (alertness) is lower under a mild conflict situation as under the conventional conflict situation. Under the later conditions activating as well as inhibiting neuronal mechanisms are stimulated by the strong conflict to which the rat is exposed (increased arousal state, Lader and Marks 1971, Groen 1975).

Under the mild conflict conditions the aversive stimulus namely the conflict has a minor impact on the animal and the conflict-lessening properties of diazepam are covered up. However, the sedative properties cause a reduction of the pressing rate in both components the VI and the FR in a dose-dependent manner. Tecce and coworkers (1978) point out that the predrug levels of distraction and arousal are important determinants of individual differences in response to diazepam. The ß-carbolines, on the other hand, act by increasing the conflict but not by increasing unspecifically the alertness since in this case the pressing-rate would increase above controls.

Following combined treatment the conflict - increasing effect of the ß-carbolines is antagonized by diazepam. This effect is dose-dependent and correlates possibly with findings in receptor-binding studies. The actions of harmane and norharmane are completely antagonized and those of the norharmane-ester to a lesser degree. The later compound shows a higher affinity to the benzodiazepine binding site. However, it is hydrolyzed fast in vivo (Braestrup et al. 1980). THN acts probably only in part via the benzodiazepine receptor as discussed above. Consequently the effect is not completely antagonized by diazepam.

In conclusion, the ß-carbolines are conflict-inducing endogenous compounds. Their action is attenuated by diazepam. It is conceivable that 5-HT-ergic mechanisms are involved in the effects of THN. The threshold dose for THN is lower as that for the other ß-carbolines investigated.

Summary

The effects of various ß-carbolines and diazepam as well as combined treatment were investigated in a conflict-punishment procedure. Two intensities of the shock were applied. In one situation vehicle-treated controls pressed the lever 13% compared to the non-shock day (conventional condition). In the other situation they pressed the lever 77% (mild condition). The results were compared to the displacing potency of the ß-carbolines in a (3H)-flunitrazepam binding assay using membranes from various brain regions.

The present results demonstrate that the conflict-lessening effect of diazepam depends probably on the arousal state of the brain. Under mild conflict conditions the sedative properties predominate, whereas under conventional conditions the conflict-lessening properties are more prominent. ß-carbolines augment the conflict for the animal. The effect is antagonized by diazepam. A correlation between these findings and those of receptor-binding studies possibly exists. However, THN acts not only via benzodiazepine receptors, but also via 5-HT-ergic mechanisms.

Acknowledgement

The study was supported by the Deutsche Forschungsgemeinschaft.

References

1. Braestrup, C., Nielsen, M., Olsen, C.E.: Proc. Natl. Acad. Sci. USA 77, 2288 (1980).

2. Braestrup, C., Squires, R.F.: Proc. Natl. Acad. Sci. USA 74, 3805 (1977).

3. Cook, L., Davidson, A.B.: In: The Benzodiazepines, eds. Garattini, S., Mussini E, Randall, L.O. (Raven Press, New York) pp 327-345 (1973).

4. Cook, L., Sepinwall, I.: In: Mechanism of Action of Benzodiazepines, eds. Costa, E., Greengard, P. (Raven Press, New York) pp 1-28 (1975).

5. Costa, E., Guidotti, A., Mao, C.C., Suria, A.: In: Mechanism of Action of Benzodiazepines, eds. Costa, E., Greengard, P. (Raven Press, New York) pp 113-130 (1975).

6. Cowen, P.J., Green, A.R., Nutt, D.J., Martin, I.L.: Nature 290, 54 (1981).

7. Geller, I., Blum, K.: Europ. J. Pharmacol. 9, 319 (1970).

8. Geller, I., Hartman, R.J., Croy, D.J.: Res. Comm. Chem. Pathol. Pharmacol. 7, 165 (1974).

9. Geller, I., Seifter, J.: Psychopharmacologia (Berlin) 1, 482 (1960).

10. Graeff, F.G., Schoenfeld, R.L.: J. Pharmacol. exp. Ther. 173, 277 (1970).

11. Groen, J.J.: In: Emotions, ed. Levi, L. (Raven Press, New York) pp 727-746 (1975).

12. Haefely, W., Kulcsar, A., Möhler, H., Pieri, L., Polc, P., Schaffner, R.: In: Mechanism of Action of Benzodiazepines, eds. Costa, E., Greengard, P. (Raven Press, New York) pp 131-151 (1975).

13. Lal, H., Shearman, G.T., Fielding, S., Dunn, R., Kruse, H., Theurer, K.: Neuropharmacology 19, 185 (1980).

14. Lader, M., Marks, J.: In: Clinical anxiety, Grune and Stratton, New York (1971).

15. Lowry, O.H., Rosebrough, N.J., Farr, A.C., Randall, R.J.: J. Biol. Chem 193, 265 (1951).

16. Müller, W.E., Fehske, K.J. Borbe, H.O., Wollert, K., Nanz, Ch., Rommelspacher, H.: Pharmacol. Biochem. Behav. 14, 693 (1981)

17. Polc, P., Möhler, H., Haefely, W.H.: Naunyn Schmiedebergs Arch. Pharmacol. 184, 319 (1974).

18. Robichaud, R.C., Sledge, K.L.: Life Sci. 8, 965 (1969).

19. Rommelspacher, H.: Pharmacopsychiat. 14, 117 (1981).

20. Rommelspacher, H., Nanz, Ch., Borbe, H.O., Fehske, K.J., Müller, W.E., Wollert, U.: Naunyn Schmiedebergs Arch. Pharmacol. 314, 97 (1980).

21. Rommelspacher, H., Nanz, Ch., Borbe, H.O., Fehske, K.J., Müller, W.E., Wollert, U.: Eur. J. Pharmacol. 70, 409 (1981),

22. Stein, L.: Arzneim. Forsch. Drug Res. 30, 868 (1980).

23. Stein, L., Wise, C.D., Belluzzi, J.D.: In: Mechanism of Action of Benzodiazepines, eds. Costa, E., Greengard, P. (Raven Press, New York) pp 29-44 (1975).

24. Stein, L., Wise, C.D., Berger, B.D.: In: The Benzodiazepines, ed. Garattini S. (Raven Press, New York) pp 299-326 (1973).

25. Tecce, J.J., Savignans-Bowman, J., Cole, J.O.: In: Psychopharmacology: A Generation of progress, eds. Lipton, M.A., Di Masció, A., Killam, K.F. (Raven Press, New York) pp 745-758 (1978).

26. Vejdelek, Z.J., Trcka, V., Protiva, M.: J. Med. Pharm. Chem. 3, 427 (1961).

27. Wise, C.D., Berger, G.C., Stein, L.: Biol. Psychiat. 6, 3 (1973).

II. NERVE GROWTH FACTOR RECEPTOR

SOME SECONDARY EVENTS AFTER NERVE GROWTH FACTOR (ßNGF)-BINDING TO PC12- AND DRG-CELLS

Paul G. Layer
Max-Planck-Institut für Virusforschung, Spemannstrasse 35, 7400 Tübingen, West Germany[x]

I. Introduction

Nerve growth factor (NGF) has become an important tool for probing the development and maintenance of the peripheral nervous system at the physiological and molecular level (for review see 1,2). To understand the different functions of NGF on a molecular level it is advisable to separate the whole action sequence into single steps and try to study them separately. This approach already led to many insights into the action-mechanism of NGF (3 - 8). I shall concentrate in this article on the description of secondary events which follow the binding to surface receptors within PC12- (pheochromocytoma cell (9)) and DRG-cells (dorsal root ganglia), including the internalization and lysosomal degradation of NGF by PC12- and DRG-cells, the down-regulation of ßNGF-receptors with PC12-cells, and crosslinking-experiments of ^{125}I-ßNGF to PC12-cells. The degradation data from PC12- and DRG-cells are compared. The significant differences between the two systems lead to some speculations about NGF's function as a "differentiation factor" and its possible role in tumor-genesis.

[x] The author wants to thank Dr. E. M. Shooter for his helpful and stimulating support throughout this whole project which was performed in his laboratory at the Dept. of Neurobiology, Stanford School of Medicine, Stanford CA. 94305, USA.

II. Interaction of ^{125}I-ßNGF with PC12-Cells

The first step in the interaction of Iß with PC12-cells is the binding of ßNGF to specific surface receptors (4,7). There appear to be two different kinds of binding sites for NGF on the PC12-cell which can be characterized by kinetic and steady-state-binding data, however the molecular nature of the different binding sites for NGF is not yet clear. (This has to be kept in mind when using the term "receptor" in this context.) In this first paragraph, I will first consider a few aspects of the secondary steps in the interaction of Iß with its target cells, which give us some insights into the ways by which the PC12-cell processes NGF after binding to the surface receptors.

An examination of the long-term binding curve of ^{125}I-ßNGF with PC12-cells (Fig.1A,B) shows the complexity of the system. Three distinct phases can be recognised: a steep rising phase during the first 60 - 90 minutes, after which the binding reaches a maximum, and then a declining phase which brings the binding value down to about 25 % of the 90-minute binding level (see Fig.1B). The binding stays at the low level for a long time (5 - 10th to 15 - 20th hours) and only after a full day it starts to increase very slowly again (recovery phase). This second increase can be blocked by cycloheximide indicating that it involves the synthesis of new receptors. It should be pointed out that the curve reflects the total cell associated radioactivity which includes intracellular material as well as material bound to specific receptors. How can we explain this complex binding curve? By a series of experiments and criteria it can be shown that this curve can be explained by a sequence of secondary steps which involve the internalization of NGF, it's degradation in lysosomes and the parallel down-regulation of surface receptors.

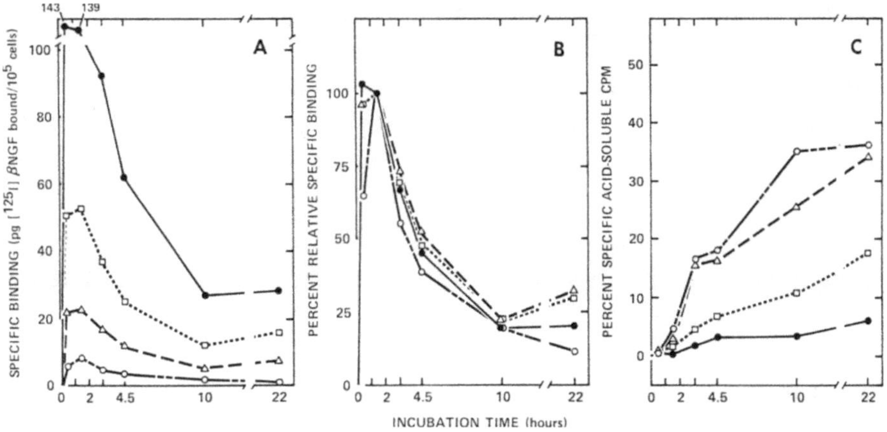

Fig.1: ^{125}I-ßNGF-concentration-dependence of binding and degradation of ^{125}I-ßNGF by PC12-cells (Longterm-binding-curve). 0.5 (O), 2.5 (Δ), 10 (□) and 50 (●) ng/ml ^{125}I-ßNGF are incubated with 3.5 ml cellsuspension in MEM/BSA (1.2 x 10^6 cells/ml, 35 mm dishes, 37 °C, 12 % CO_2). At the indicated time-points 400 µl-aliquots are taken out for determination of the specific binding and of the TCA-precipitability A: specific binding (= total-nonspecific binding, which is determined in parallel with an at least 1000-fold excess of cold NGF). B: relative binding. The data from A are plotted as percent of the according 90-minute value. C: specific TCA-solubility in the cellfree supernatants (further explanations of materials + methods see in 8, 15).

1. Internalization of NGF and degradation in lysosomes

Fig.1C shows that NGF is degraded during incubation with the PC12-cells. A number of findings suggest that this occurs mostly by lysosomal degradation (not all data shown, see 8). First of all, we could show that cell-external degradation is negligible (less than 10 %). No proteases in significant amounts are released from the cells before or during the incubation into the medium. Nor do increasing amounts of BSA in the medium influence the degradation. Secondly, the degradation is zero when the cells are incubated on ice, because the clustering-phenomenon is inhibited at this low temperature (10). Third, if we treat the cells with metabolic inhibitors like DNP, NaF or NaN_3 (-Glucose), which prevents the energy-dependent endocytosis process (11), we can effectively inhibit the degradation of NGF. Fourth, degradation can be effectively inhibited by a series of ammonium compounds like ammonium chloride or chloroquine which are well-known to inactivate lysosomal proteases (21).

2. Inhibition of secondary events influences the long-term binding characteristics

I have suggested that the complex nature of the longterm binding (Fig.1) is caused by secondary events such as internalization and lysosomal degradation. If this is true then it should be possible to change the binding curve significantly by blockage of these steps.

A. Effects of low temperature on the binding.

Fig.2 (●——●) shows the effect of low temperature on the binding curve and the degradation process over a time-period of 10 hours. The total specific binding on ice is only about 30 % of the maximal binding at 37 ^{o}C. There is no down-regulation but rather the binding reaches a saturation level. Degradation on ice is fully inhibited. This dramatic difference in the binding at low temperature and at 37° is quite remarkable and not fully understood. It is conceivable that the binding at 0° might reflect the real number of surface receptors for NGF and that the difference with the control curve is due to internalized NGF which accumulates inside the cell and therefore increases the level of "total" binding (more arguments for this "accumulation-hypothesis" are discussed below). The real number of surface receptors would then be only a fraction of that which is measured at 37 ^{o}C after about 60 minutes. Thus it may not be valid to determine the total number of binding sites on the cells at 37° from the total binding after about 60 minutes assuming that the binding reaches a certain steady-state-level, as has generally been the practice in this field.

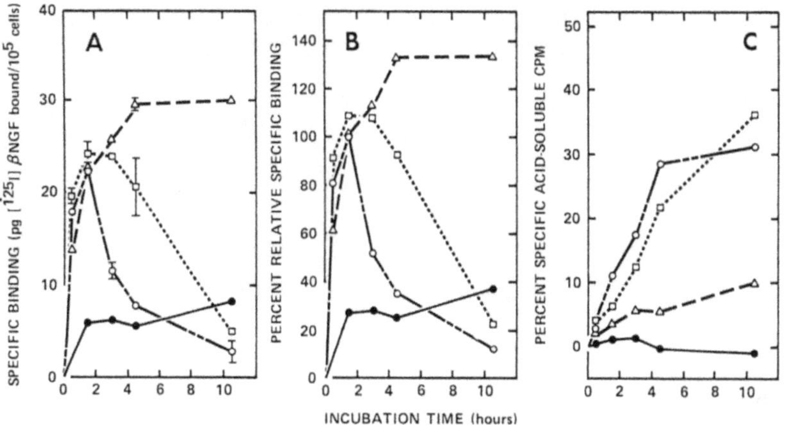

Fig.2: Effect of Chloroquine and low temperature on the binding-characteristics and the degradation of ^{125}I-ßNGF by PC12-cells. 3.5 ml cellsuspension (1.2 x 10^6/ml in MEM/BSA, 60 mm dishes) are incubated with 2.5 ng/ml ^{125}I-ßNGF. (O) is control at 37 °C, (□) 20 µM and (△) 100 µM Chloroquine is added 30 minutes before the addition of ^{125}I-ßNGF and is present throughout the experiment. (●) binding at 4 °C. Binding assays are done in triplicates.

B. <u>Effects of Chloroquine on the binding</u>.

In Fig.2 we see that Chloroquine, which inhibits the lysosomal proteases, increases the total binding at 37 °C (the effect being dose-dependent: at 100 µM the binding stays at more than 140 % of the control for several hours). This pronounced difference with the control curve indicates that NGF is being bound and accumulated inside the cell, but cannot be further processed through the cell because the final degrading step in the lysosomes is blocked. This Chloroquine-effect on the binding has been further investigated. The full lines in Fig.3A and B again show the effect of Chloroquine on the total binding at 37 °C and the difference between the two may reflect the difference in fully processed NGF within the two systems. If we examine the binding after a 20-minute cold-chase (see legend of Fig.3), in the absence of Chloroquine we find a fraction of about 1/3 which comes off the cells during the chase, whereas in the presence of Chloroquine this cold-chase

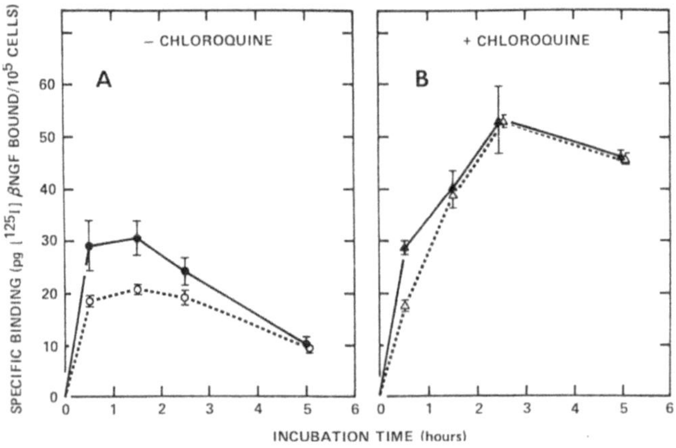

Fig.3: Time-course of specific "total" and "tight" binding of ^{125}I-ßNGF to PC12-cells in the presence and absence of 20 µM Chloroquine. 1 ml cellsuspension (0.75 x 10^6 cells/ml) in MEM/BSA are incubated with 2.8 ng/ml ^{125}I-ßNGF for the indicated time-intervals (single 30 mm-plates for each time-point, 37 °C/10 % CO_2), after which the cells are gently resuspended. Half the sample is used for determination of the "total" binding, the other half is incubated together with 2.75 µg/ml native ßNGF for 20 minutes on ice after which the restbinding (= "tight" binding) is determined. Data are corrected for nonspecific binding. A: control (- Chloroquine), (●) "total" binding (O) "tight" binding. B: 20 µM Chloroquine is added to the plates 20 minutes before the addition of ^{125}I-ßNGF. Chloroquine is present throughout the experiment (during the cold chase as well). (▲) total binding, (△) tight binding.

has no effect after 30 minutes. The "cold-chase-binding" is usually taken as a measure of how many "low-affinity"-sites are on the surface of the cell at a given moment. This interpretation certainly is not applicable in this experiment. Rather I think this result demonstrates that in the absence of Chloroquine part of the already degraded material dissociates from the cell during the chase on ice, an effect which is inhibited in the presence of Chloroquine. Only at the early time-point might we be dealing with "low-affinity"-sites on the surface.

3. Down-regulation of surface receptors

The experiment in Fig.4 demonstrates that the number of surface receptors is down-regulated after a first exposure of PC12-cells to ßNGF. The total specific binding after 90 minutes and 5 hours has been determined. After this first incubation period, we have washed the cells extensively to remove more than 90 % of the bound material. Then we add the same amount of ^{125}I-ßNGF as at the first incubation and again measure the binding after 90 minutes. The total specific binding after the second period is very much less than that after the first 90-minute-incubation. This demonstrates very clearly that the surface receptors for NGF have been down-regulated during the first 5 hours of incubation. The physiological significance of the down-regulation of receptors is so far poorly understood.

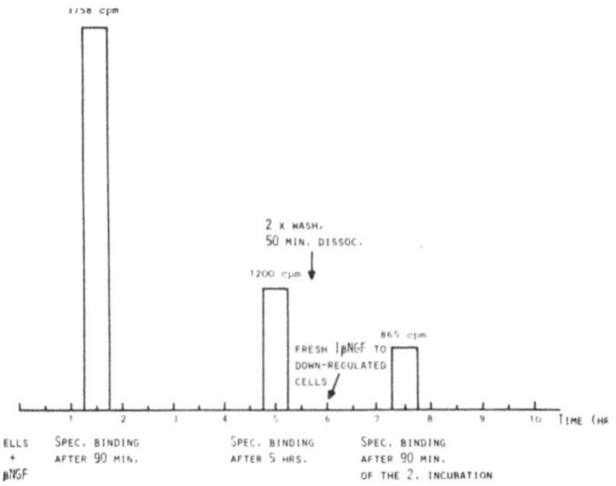

Fig.4: Rebinding of ^{125}I-ßNGF after down-regulation of PC12-cells. Naive PC12-cells (1.25 x 10^6 /ml, Vol. 1 ml) are incubated with ^{125}I-ßNGF (3.75 ng/ml) on 30 mm plates (37 $^{\circ}$C/12 % CO_2) and the specific binding is determined after 90 minutes and after 5 hours. On a parallel plate, naive cells at the same density are allowed to down-regulate by addition of 2.75 ng/ml of native ßNGF for the same time. Thereafter the supernatant is withdrawn, the cells are washed twice with fresh MEM/BSA and the medium is replaced again. Fresh ^{125}I-ßNGF (3.75 ng/ml) is now added again and the specific binding determined after another 90-minute-incubation.

4. Characterization of degradation products

We have further characterized the degradation products of NGF using immunoprecipitation, bioassay on DRG-single-neurons, SDS-PAA-electrophoresis and thin layer-chromatography of intact, partially and fully degraded NGF-samples. The results of these experiments showed that NGF is being degraded to single amino acids and that no intermediates can be found. The data from TCA, RIA and bioassay correlate quite well, so that the TCA-data can be taken as a real measure of the degradation. (Further discussion see 8).

5. The quantitation of the NGF-degradation process by PC12-cells

The amounts of NGF which can be processed by the PC12-cells are striking. In serum-free medium the degradation rate can reach up to 5 ng/10^6 cells x hour. The rate is slowed at high cell densities (e.g. at 6 x 10^6/ml the rate is about 30 - 40 % of that at 6 x 10^5/ml) and in the presence of serum (10 % FCS + 5 % HS decrease the rate to less than 50 %). The serum-sensitivity of the PC12-degradation can be explained by the assumption that in the presence of more serum the PC12-cell is shifted into a more proliferative state, in which protein-synthesis-rates are higher and the degradation-rates lower. This has been shown to be true for different other cell-types (e.g. WI38-fibroblasts, for review see 16). We have also observed a time-dependent increase of degradation after long exposure of the cells to ßNGF, which probably correlates with the increase in receptor-numbers on differentiated cells. In (12) we describe the quantitative aspects of the PC12-degradation and show that the PC12-cells always need a relatively high minimum concentration of ßNGF of about 2 ng/ml for biological response.

6. The NGF-receptor-molecule: an attempt at its characterization by crosslinking-experiments

Little is known about the molecular properties of the NGF-receptor (see 13, 14). To shed more light on this problem I have tried to crosslink the NGF-binding-site on PC12-cells with different chemical crosslinkers after incubation with ^{125}I-ßNGF. These crosslinkers included Suberimidate, Glutaraldehyde and a Nitro-azido-phenyl-derivatized ^{125}I-ßNGF. The latter was especially promising, since it retained some binding and biological activity and the molecule was photoactivatable after its derivatization. Yet the results with it were never very satisfying, because all photo-crosslinked radioactivity remained on top of the gels. A crosslinking-experiment with Glutaraldehyde is shown in Fig.5. All incubations were done on ice to inhibit secondary events after binding. After different times of incubation with ^{125}I-ßNGF the PC12-cells were washed and the Glutaraldehyde added. After

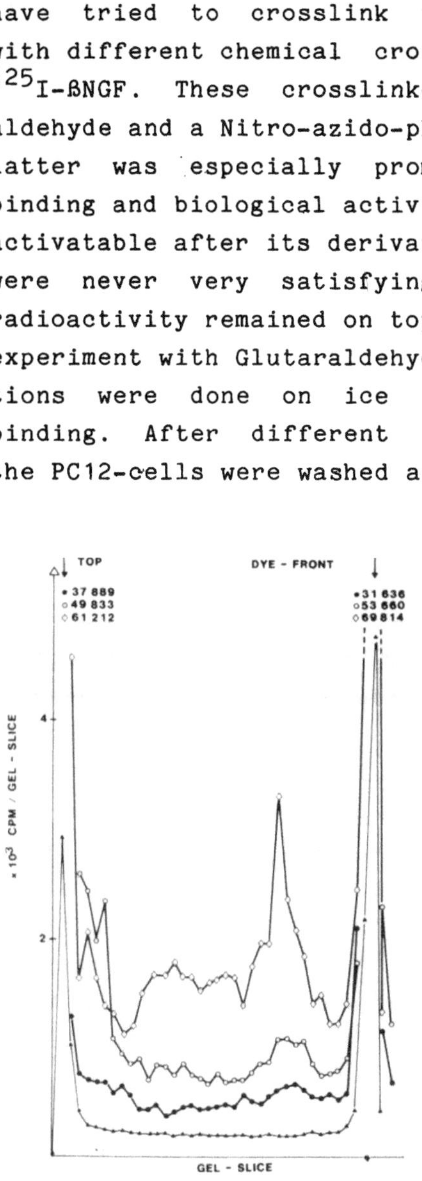

Fig.5: Crosslinking of specifically bound ^{125}I-ßNGF with PC12-cells. 2 x 10^6 cells/ml (1 ml vol.) in tubes are incubated on ice with 54 ng/ml ^{125}I-ßNGF (end cond.) for 10' (●), 30' (O) and 4 hours (◇). As a control (▲) one sample was preincubated with 1.69 µg/ml cold ßNGF for 10' on ice and then incubated for 4 hours with ^{125}I-ßNGF (4 x 10^6 cells/ml are used for the 4-hour-samples). The cells are washed now with PBS quickly and then 1 % Glutaraldehyde (end conc., Fisher) is added for 2 hours (on ice). After another wash the cell pellets are taken up in 50 µl Tris/SDS + 50 µl Lämmli-sample-buffer (+ mercapto-ethanol). The samples are boiled for 5 minutes and electrophoresed on a 5 % SDS-PAA-Lämmli-system (single tubes about 9 cm x 0.5 cm). The gels are cut into 2 mm-slices and counted for radioactivity.

SDS-extraction of the cells and a run of the material on 5 % PAA-gels, three main peaks were visible:

1. On top of the gel in the stacking gel and the first slice of the resolving gel one finds much radioactivity. This peak represents aggregates with huge molecular weights. We have found that a big fraction of this material is associated with the triton-insoluble pellet (e.g. it has nuclear or more likely cytoskeletal nature).

2. Another large fraction of the radioactivity runs with the dye-front and represents non-crosslinked, free ^{125}I-ßNGF-monomers (13 000 d).

3. A third peak shows up at a position of R_F = 0.71 - 0.73. Interestingly this peak increases with increasing incubation time. Calibration-curves show that this R_F-value corresponds to a molecular weight of 130 000. After subtracting 13 000 for one NGF-monomer we obtain 120 000 d as a tentative molecular weight of the NGF-binding-structure. Less pronounced peaks appear at positions of R_F = 0.53, 0.35 and 0.09 which possibly represent aggregates of the 120 000 d-structure. The controls in this experiment were: a) A 4-hour-incubation with ^{125}I-ßNGF in the presence of excess cold NGF (see Fig.5). Peak 3 is fully blocked under these conditions. b) No crosslinking after incubation with ^{125}I-ßNGF. Only the free NGF-monomer and a small peak on top of the gel is visible. This last peak might represent natural crosslinking of NGF. I have performed a similar experiment with Suberimidate in which I first solubilized the cell-material with 1 % Triton. Under these conditions the peak 1 on top of the gel is very much diminished, but the peak in the 130 000-position is still visible, although it should be mentioned that this peak was not easily resolvable in all experiments. We can therefore conclude that the 120 000 d-peak is likely to represent a specific NGF-binding-structure. More experiments are needed to further characterize the properties of this molecule.

III. Lysosomal Degradation of ßNGF by Dorsal Root Ganglion Cells (DRG)

Repeating the experiments described for the PC12-system we were able to show that single· cells from DRG (dorsal root ganglia) of 8-day chicken embryos would also degrade ßNGF in lysosomes. In Fig.6 the time-course of the degradation reaction of ^{125}I-ßNGF by dissociated DRG-cells is shown. The degradation is fully inhibited by the presence of a 100-fold excess of cold ßNGF, which shows that the degradation is a receptor-dependent process. Increasing concentrations of BSA do not affect the degree of degradation. The influence of different ammonium compounds (Chloroquine, Ammonium chloride and Methylamine) on the degrading system is demonstrated in Fig.7. All of these compounds as well as low temperature and metabolic inhibitors (data not shown, see 15) effectively inhibit the degrading capacity of the DRG-cells.

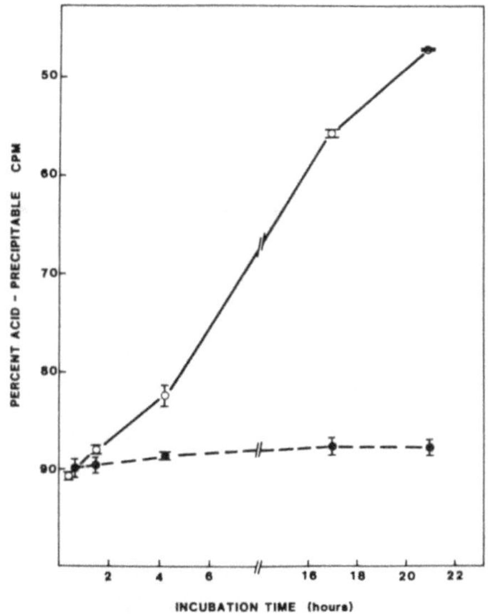

Fig.6: Time-course of ^{125}I-ßNGF-degradation by DRG-cells. 1 x 10^6/ml (1.5 ml total) dissociated single DRG-cells (non-separated) of 8-d chicken embryos are plated on 30 mm dishes in F12/FCS at 37 °C. After about 20 minutes the cells settle down and 2.5 ng/ml ^{125}I-ßNGF (final conc.) are added. On a parallel plate native ßNGF at a concentration of 275 ng/ml is added 10 minutes before for determination of the nonspecific degradation. Separate plates for each time-point are run. The TCA-precipitability in an aliquot of the cell-free supernatant is determined at the indicated points. (O) total degradation (●) nonspecific degradation.

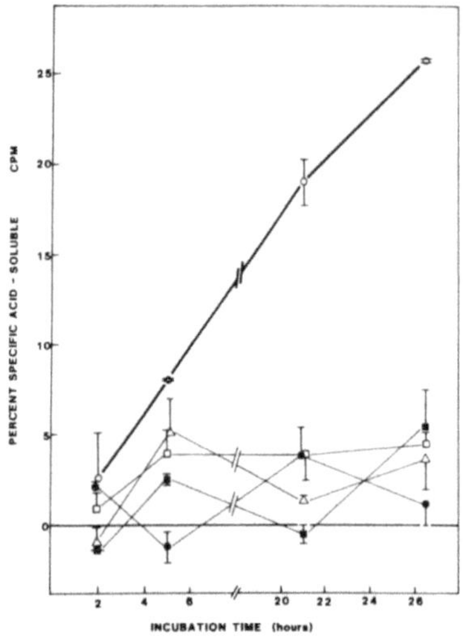

Fig.7: Effect of Ammonium compounds on the degradation of ^{125}I-ßNGF by DRG-cells. Separated (neuron-enriched) single DRG-cells at a concentration of 0.4 x 10^6 cells/ml in F12/FCS are used. After settling of the cells the indicated reagents and after another 20 minutes 1 ng/ml ^{125}I-ßNGF (final conc.) are added to start the incubation. Data are corrected for nonspecific degradation. (O) Control (□) + 20 µM Chloroquine, (△) + 50 µM Chloroquine, (●) + 10 mM Ammonium chloride, (■) + 20 mM Methylamine.

Does blockage of the lysosomal degradation also block the biological response to NGF?

This question has often been raised in terms of trying to understand the mechanism of action of NGF. In the experiments shown in Fig.8 we have found that there is still fiber-outgrowth from DRG-cells under conditions of almost fully blocked lysosomal degradation (presence of 20 uM Chloroquine). The

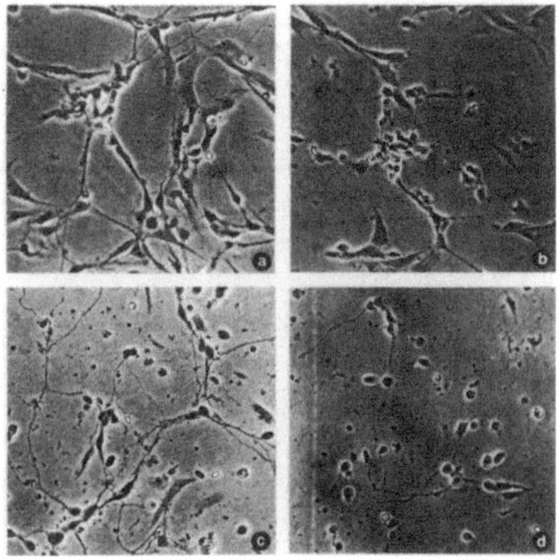

Fig.8: Biological response of single DRG-cells to ßNGF in the absence (6a,c) and presence (6b,d) of 20 µM Chloroquine. The photographs show representative sections of culture dishes with non-separated (6a,b) and separated (neuron-enriched) single DRG-cells (6c,d) after 20 hours incubation with ^{125}I-ßNGF.

response was better in a non-separated cell population (7a,b) than in a neuron-enriched population (7c,d). The toxic effects of Chloroquine raise problems in this culture system. However it is clear that the decrease of degradation caused by Chloroquine does not correlate with the decrease in the biological response. Experiments with less toxic lysosomal inhibitors which are now available should further clarify this important point.

IV. Comparison of the ßNGF-Degrading Capacities of PC12- and DRG-Cells

The PC12-cell is a tumor cell which is able to stop proliferation and differentiate into a sympathetic-like neuron after it is stimulated by a sufficient dosage of NGF. I have described the huge rates of internalization and lysosomal degradation which always appeared to me as being "abnormal" and possibly tumor-specific. For that reason I was interested to compare these rates with those from another NGF-responsive but non-tumorous cellsystem. I have chosen the DRG-system. In the following section the main qualitative and quantitative differences of the two systems will be worked out.

In Fig.9 the concentration-dependence of the degradation process of PC12 and DRG-single cells is compared. At low NGF-concentrations the PC12-curve reaches a degradation level of about 45 %, which corresponds to almost full degradation for this given ^{125}I-ßNGF-sample (full biological degradation in different ^{125}I-ßNGF-samples is reached between 25 % - 45 % TCA-precipitability). The steep and almost linear phases in the two curves correspond to different NGF-concentrations: for the DRG's significant amounts of NGF are degraded only at

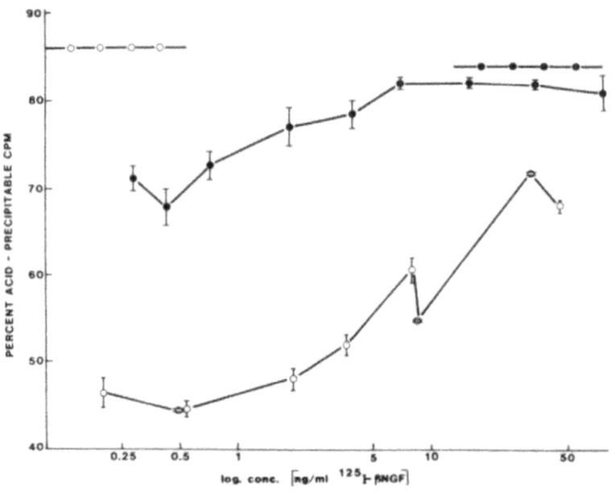

Fig.9: Concentration-dependence of ^{125}I-ßNGF-degradation by PC12- + DRG-cells. 3 x 10^5/ml (1.5 ml) dissociated, non-separated DRG-cells are plated on 30 mm culture dishes in F12/FCS. Increasing concentrations of ^{125}I-ßNGF are added and the plates are incubated for 16 hours at 37 °C. The TCA-precipitability is determined in aliquots of the total supernatant. Non-specific backgrounds (presence of excess cold ßNGF) were determined for the lowest and highest concentration and was 83 - 84 % (line on top; symbols for DRG: ●). The experiment with PC12-cells (O) was similar, but with the following modifications: 5 x 10^5cells/ml (1.5 ml vol.), incubation for 24 hours at 37 °C in MEM/BSA. Nonspecific backgrounds were 89 %.

relatively low concentrations (below 10 ng/ml), whereas in the case of the PC12-cells the linear phase is shifted to much higher values, e.g. 5 - 50 ng/ml. At high concentrations the DRG-curve reaches a plateau near the background level (the difference to this level is not Chloroquine-sensitive, indicating that some exterior proteolysis is involved). The PC12-curve in contrast shows even at 50 ng/ml quite significant amounts of specific degradation.

We have recalculated these data and plotted them as % NGF degraded/given NGF-concentration. This analysis of the efficiency of the degradation systems reveals that at high NGF-concentrations the PC12-cell degrades about 5 % of the given NGF/hour x 10^6 cells whereas the DRG-efficiency is close to zero (not measurable with our method). At lower concentrations both cell-types degrade relatively more than at higher concentrations but PC12-cells are still more efficient than DRG-cells (for methodological reasons the analysis becomes inaccurate in that concentration-range). In other words: at low-site-occupancy the PC12-cells degrade very effectively whereas the DRG-system is almost silent. Although we can only speculate about the underlying mechanism for the fast internalization and degradation of PC12-cells (e.g. direct and fast internalization of "low-affinity"-receptor-complexes, increased lysosomal activity serving as a "sink" for NGF, etc.), we can conclude that the low-affinity-sites of PC12cells somehow must be directly involved with this phenomenon.

In table I some differences between the two cellsystems are summarized:

Table I

	DRG	PC12
1. Max. spec. Degradation ng degrad./10^6 cells x hr.	30 - 80	> 5000
2. Degradation is Serum-	insensitive	sensitive
3. Full Chloroquine-inhibition at	20 µM	> 100 µM
4. Efficiency of degradation at low-site-occupancy	negligible	~ 5 %
5. Remarks:	Separated Neurons degrade only 1/4 of non-neuronal DRG-cells	

V. NGF-Degradation by PC12-Cells as a Model for Tumor-Genesis

How can we explain the huge degradation-rates of the PC12-cells? A simple answer would be that NGF is a foreign and abnormal protein for the PC12-cell, to which it is not supposed to respond biologically, because the normal fate of adrenal chromaffin cells (the origins of the PC12-line) is not to differentiate into regular sympathetic neurons. In fact it has been shown by Bradley, Hayflick and Schimke (17) that WI38 fibroblasts degrade "foreign, abnormal" proteins (protein analogues, erroneously synthesized proteins, etc.) much faster than "regular" proteins.

There are however other possible explanations. As I have mentioned above the PC12-cells need a lot of NGF to be biologically stimulated. We have determined a constant minimal value of about 2 ng/ml ßNGF being constantly required for the onset of differentiation by the PC12-cells (in terms of fiber-outgrowth)(12). This is already a physiologically quite high concentration and even if it were given in an in-vivo-situation, the fast degradation rate of PC12-cells would very quickly bring the NGF-level below the critical concentration.

At this point one might ask then if the PC12-cell as a tumor-cell would differentiate at all under normal conditions upon a given NGF-signal (e.g. the signal being a short NGF-wave)? Wouldn't it rather remain in the proliferative and non-differentiated state because it internalizes and degrades its own "differentiation-factor" NGF too efficiently? Therefore it is likely that the biological response of PC12- cells to ßNGF is a laboratory-artefact rather than being a real natural phenomenon.

What then is the physiological function of the NGF-receptors on the PC12-cell? Do they merely catch the NGF-molecules and transport them to the degrading system? At least part of them seem to serve this function. In this context the findings of Fabricant, de Larco and Todaro (18) are of interest: they have found that there are many NGF-receptors on certain melanoma and neuroblastoma-cells (all cells of neural crest origin) with especially high receptor-numbers present on metastatic melanomas. Some other tumors and non-tumerous cells showed no NGF-binding. Although again the real significance of these receptors is not known, one may ask by analogy if these increased numbers of receptors catch the "differentiation-factor" NGF and help to destroy it (as a "sink" for the differentiation-factor). This hypothesis could be formulated not only for NGF but in a more general way for other "differentiation-factors" (which are not known yet, but certainly will be found in the near future, (19))(see Fig.10):

"Any given stem cell needs a specific differentiation-factor (e.g. NGF) at a certain time and space in a minimal concentration and for a minimal time-period to undergo proper differentiation. If the cell has a defect in its internalization or degradation-mechanism (or both), it will degrade the factor too quickly and thus not respond biologically. It then remains in a proliferative state and thus it becomes a tumor-cell."

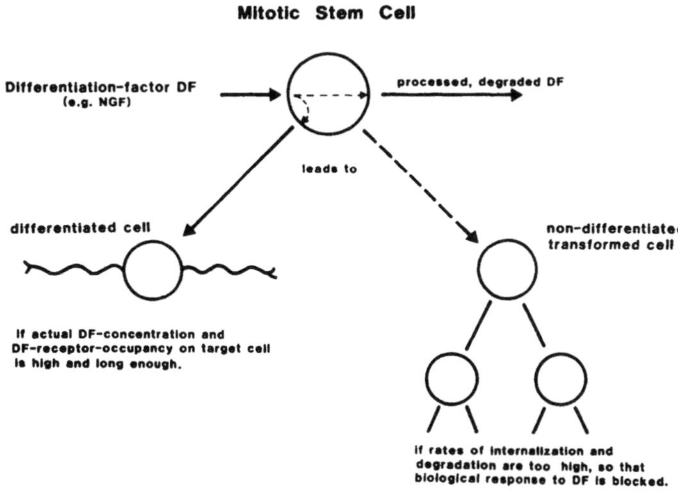

Fig.10:
A hypothesis of the involvement of "differentiation-factors" (e.g. NGF) in tumor-genesis. Explanation see text.

Arehart-Treichel asked in a review (20) "NGF may hold the key - but to what? Does the mysterious growth-triggering chemical figure in the cancer process?" I think that it might hold one key to it. The PC12-cell seems to be an attractive system in this respect, because it is a cell which is destined to remain in the proliferative state but with high amounts of NGF it can be brought to differentiation. The PC12/NGF-system could be a good starting model to prove or disprove my hypothesis and a further step for testing it could be the determination of degradation-rates for NGF in a series of tumor-cells and their non-transformed counterparts.

References

1. Mobley, W. C., Server, A. C., Ishii, D. N., Riopelle, R. J., Shooter, E. M.: New Eng. J. Med. 297, 1096-1104, 1149-1158, 1211-1218 (1977).
2. Thoenen, H., Barde, Y. A.: Physiol. Rev. 60, 1284-1335 (1980).
3. Sutter, A., Riopelle, R. J., Harris-Warrick, R. M., Shooter, E. M.: J. Biol. Chem. 254, 5972-82 (1979).
4. Landreth, G. E., Shooter, E. M.: Proc. Natl. Acad. Sci. USA 77, 4751-4755 (1980).
5. Yankner, B. A., Shooter, E. M.: Proc. Natl. Acad. Sci. USA 76, 1269-73 (1979).
6. Landreth G. E., Yankner, B. A., Layer P., Shooter E. M.: in "Deseases of the Motor Unit" ed. D. L. Schotland, Houghton Mufflin Prof. publishers.
7. Schechter, A. L., Bothwell, M. A.: Cell 24, 867-874 (1981).
8. Layer, P. G., Shooter, E. M.: submitted for publication to J. Biol. Chem. (1981).
9. Greene, L. A., Tischler, A. S.: Proc. Natl. Acad. Sci. USA 73, 2424-28 (1976).

10. Schlessinger, J., Shechter, Y., Willingham, M. C., Pastan, I.: Proc. Natl. Acad. Sci. USA 75, 2659-2663 (1978).

11. Goldstein, J. L., Anderson, G. W. A., Brown, M. S.: Nature 279, 679-685 (1979).

12. Gunning, P. W., Landreth, G. E., Layer, P., Ignatius, M., Shooter, E. M.: J. Neurosci. 1 (4), 368-379 (1981).

13. Costrini, N. V., Bradshaw, R. A.: Proc. Natl. Acad. Sci. USA 76, 3242-3245 (1979).

14. Costrini, N. V., Kogan, M. G.: Clin.Res. 28, 1738 (1980).

15. Layer, P. G., Rubenstein, J., Shooter, E. M.: manuscript in preparation

16. Rudland, P. S., Jimenez de Asua, L.: BBA 560, 91-133 (1979).

17. Bradley, M. O., Hayflick, L., Schimke, R. T.: J. Biol. Chem. 251, 3521-3529 (1976).

18. Fabricant, R. N., De Larco, J. E., Todaro, G. J.: Proc. Natl. Acad. Sci. USA, 565-569 (1977).

19. Edgar, D.: TINS Dec. 1979, 316-318.

20. Arehart-Treichel, J.: Science News 111, 330-335 (1977).

21. Sando, G. N., Titus-Dillon, P., Hall, C. W., Neufeld, E. F.: Exp. Cell Res. 119, 359-364 (1979).

Acknowledgements

I wish to thank Drs. Peter Frey, Peter Gunning, Gary Landreth, Arne Sutter, Paul Whitington, Bruce Yankner for helpful discussions and Mrs. Aiko Tanaka-Ingold for typing the manuscript. Financial support came from a DFG- (La 379/1+2) and a NATO-grant.

NERVE GROWTH FACTOR RECEPTOR ON SENSORY AND SYMPATHETIC NEURONS IN CULTURE

H. Rohrer, Y.A. Barde, D. Edgar and H. Thoenen
Max-Planck-Institut für Psychiatrie, Abteilung Neurochemie,
D-8033 Martinsried, FRG

Introduction

It is well established that during ontogenesis, the size of the field of innervation determines the extent of the development of the corresponding neurons (1,2,3). Demonstration of the specific uptake and retrograde axonal transport of nerve growth factor (NGF) by peripheral sympathetic and sensory neurons provided a paradigm for investigations into the mechanisms and messengers responsible for the trophic action of effector cells on innervating neurons (4).

The physiological importance of the retrograde axonal transport of NGF was inferred from the observation that interruption of this transport at a certain critical period of development leads to neuronal death, as does the neutralization of endogenous NGF by NGF antibodies at this stage (for reviews see 5,6). The injection of NGF antibodies into mammals in the prenatal period results in an extensive destruction of both sensory and sympathetic neurons whereas in the early postnatal phase this destructive effect is restricted to the sympathetic nervous system, and in adult animals to the impairment of specific neuronal functions such as a reduced synthesis of enzymes involved in adrenergic transmitter synthesis and by reduced levels of peptide transmitters in target neurons (5,6).

Neuroreceptors

The dependence of target neurons on NGF for survival can be demonstrated also <u>in cultures</u> of isolated neurons (7-12), and culture techniques have further shown that besides NGF other trophic factors - present in brain extracts or in media conditioned by C_6 glioma cells or chick heart muscle cells - are able to maintain the survival of chick sensory and sympathetic neurons (9,10,11), although the periods when neurons are maximally dependent differ according to the particular factor used (10,11).

It is the purpose in the present communication to describe the changing requirements of chick sensory and sympathetic neurons for different survival factors during development and to evaluate to what extent the dependence on NGF for survival of subpopulations of sensory and sympathetic neurons is reflected by the presence of specific NGF receptors.

<u>Age-dependent changes in the requirement of sensory and sympathetic neurons for different survival factors</u>.

The initial demonstration that survival factors present in media conditioned by glioma cells act on chick sensory neurons (9) and that medium conditioned by chick heart muscle cells acts on chick sensory, sympathetic and parasympathetic neurons (12) was followed by the quantitative analysis of the proportion of chick sensory (dorsal root ganglion) and sympathetic (paravertebral ganglion) neurons which depend on these factors and NGF during different developmental stages (10,11).

As summarized in Table I, the proportion of sensory and sympathetic neurons surviving with different factors added to the culture medium changes markedly during development.

Table I

A. Survival of cultured sensory neurons of different ages

Embryonic age, days	% neuronal survival in response to NGF	Brain extract	Brain extract + NGF
8	27 ± 2	17 ± 3	76 ± 6
10	42 ± 2	34 ± 1	69 ± 6
12	44 ± 0.5	51 ± 3	98 ± 6
14	25 + 0.2	47 ± 5	98 + 9
16	6 ± 0.4	73 ± 4	75 ± 0.7

B. Survival of cultured sympathetic neurons of different ages

Embryonic age, days	% neuronal survival in response to NGF	HCM	HCM + NGF
8	5 ± 2	16 ± 3	65 ± 7
10	25 ± 3	36 ± 6	84 ± 9
12	37 ± 6	45 ± 3	88 ± 11
14	30 ± 4	56 ± 9	92 ± 8
16	18 ± 3	55 ± 11	84 ± 9

Neurons were grown with NGF (5 ng/ml), rat brain extracts (25 mg wet weight/ml) or HCM plus 500 ng/ml NGF antibodies. Neurons were counted after 48 hr in culture. Results are expressed as percentages of surviving neurons ± SD.

The proportion of surviving sensory and sympathetic neurons in the presence of optimal concentrations of NGF is very low at embryonic day 8 (E8). It increases to a maximum of 44% in sensory and 37% in sympathetic neurons around E12 and afterwards declines.

In contrast, the percentage of plated sensory neurons surviving with rat brain extracts (RBE) increases steadily during development from about 10% at E8 to reach a final level of over 70% of plated neurons at E16. If RBE and NGF are combined a constant level of survival of about 80% from E8 to E16 is achieved.

The percentage of plated sympathetic neurons surviving with medium conditioned by chick heart muscle cells (HCM) also increases during development from about 16% at E8 to reach a maximal level at E14 of about 56%. Again a majority of the sympathetic neurons from 8-16 day old chick embryos can be kept alive in culture by the combination of NGF and HCM. The more than additive effect of the combination observed for instance at E8 leads to the conclusion that some neurons need two factors in order to survive in culture.

It is therefore possible to maintain the majority of all neurons present in a ganglion at a given developmental stage and also to select different neuronal subpopulations which represent either different stages of differentiation of the same neuronal type or different neuronal lineages. Besides the ability to survive with a given factor other properties seem to differ between these subpopulations: sympathetic neurons selected by HCM contain significantly higher levels of choline acetyltransferase than the population of sympathetic neurons kept alive in culture by NGF (11).

Presence of NGF receptors on sensory neurons in culture

The establishment of these culture systems made it possible to investigate the correlation between the ability of sensory neurons to survive with NGF and the presence of NGF receptors on these cells (13).

Specific receptors for NGF on cultured neurons were directly visualized (Fig.1) by an autoradiographic technique which consists of the incubation of cultured neurons with radio-iodinated NGF of high specific activity, fixation of the bound NGF after appropriate washing steps and processing the cultures for light microscopic autoradiography.

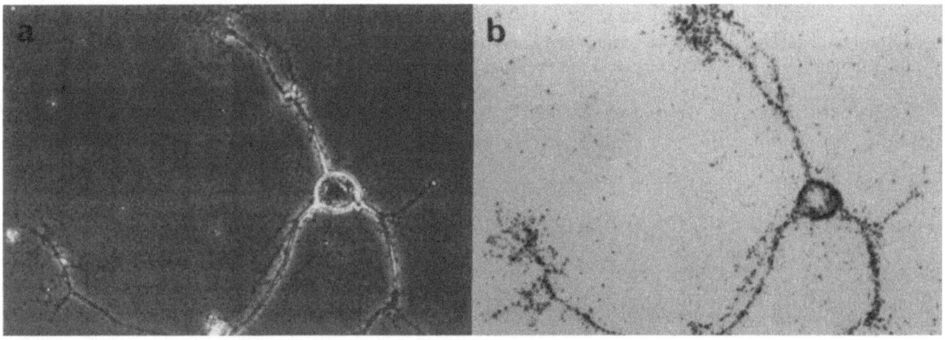

Fig. 1. Autoradiographic demonstration of NGF receptors in culture. E10 sensory neurons were cultivated with rat brain extract for 2 d. The cultures were incubated at 0°C with ^{125}I-NGF, washed, fixed and processed for autoradiography. a, phase contrast; b, bright field, Mag. x 800.

The silver grains are due to ^{125}I-NGF bound to the surface of neurites since the binding was carried out at 0°C to prevent internalization and degradation of NGF. NGF receptors are uniformly distributed over the neurites up to the fine filopodia of the growth cones.

Two types of NGF receptors on cell bodies of chick sensory neurons have been described (14), high affinity receptors (K_D (I) = 9.8×10^{-12} M at 2°C) and low affinity receptors (K_D (II) = 1.4×10^{-9} M at 2°C). Since NGF bound to any low affinity receptors with the binding characteristics of the site II receptors would virtually all dissociate during the washing procedure, we assume that the remaining grains represent NGF bound to high affinity receptors.

Two different populations of neurons could be distinguished; labeled neurons and unlabeled neurons (Fig.2). Cells were classified as unlabeled when the pattern of neurites could not be detected by the accumulation of grains above background (Fig.2b) under bright field illumination. The percentage of labeled cells was not influenced by increased exposure times.

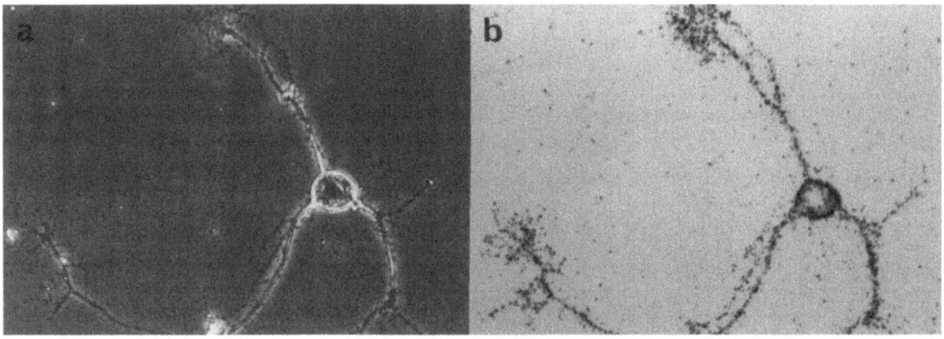

Fig. 2. E10 sensory neurons cultured in the presence of rat brain extract as in Fig. 1. In the vicinity of a strongly labeled neurite an unlabeled neuron can be seen. a, phase contrast; b, bright field. Mag. x 800.

The analysis of the percentage of sensory neurons which have NGF receptors at two embryonic ages, E10 and E16, clearly demonstrated (Table II) that at E10 not only the population of neurons which are surviving with NGF but also the population surviving with rat brain extract consists largely of cells with NGF receptors.

Table II

Percentage of sensory neurons labeled by ^{125}I-NGF

after 48h in the presence of	E 10	E 16
rat brain extract	82% $\pm$ 2	28% $\pm$ 8
NGF	95% $\pm$ 3	n.d.
NGF + rat brain extract	90% + 2	n.d.

If NGF and RBE are combined about 90% of the plated neurons survive and virtually all the sensory neurons are labeled. At this age only 40% of the neurons survive with NGF alone (Table I). The percentage of NGF receptor-bearing cells decreases drastically between E10 and E16 but at E16 still about 28% of the neurons surviving have NGF receptors whereas only about 6% of the plated neurons survive with NGF alone (Table I).

Sympathetic neurons from 8 to 16 day old chick embryos can be cultured with a high proportion of surviving cells in presence of the combination of heart conditioned medium and NGF (Table IB). When analyzed for the presence of NGF receptors by the autoradiography technique in contrast to the developmental decrease in the proportion of NGF receptor-bearing sensory neurons, 98-100% of the sympathetic neurons were labeled at all ages investigated.

For neurons from both sympathetic and sensory ganglia it was thus demonstrated that NGF receptors are present not only on the populations surviving with NGF but also on the populations which are not able to survive with NGF alone. Thus the survival effect of NGF cannot be strictly correlated with the presence of NGF receptors. The appearance of NGF receptors on young neurons might proceed the synthesis of the hormone binding to that receptor. On the other hand it must be pointed out, that the absence of a survival effect of NGF alone does not exclude the possibility that the receptors are involved in some other regulatory functions of NGF on these neurons, as well as mediating the survival ellicited by NGF acting together with another factor such as brain extracts or heart conditioned medium.

We investigated if the reduction in the proportion of receptor-bearing sensory neurons can also been observed with neurons brought into culture at E10 and cultivated until their age corresponded to that of E16 neurons. It was observed that the proportion of NGF receptor-bearing neurons decreased only by 20% - 30% when the neurons were cultivated in the presence of NGF. In contrast, E10 neurons cultured in the presence of rat brain extract kept their NGF receptors for about 4 days but then a drastic reduction in the percentage of labeled neurons occurred, resulting in a final percentage of labeled neurons of about 25% (13). Thus, neurons kept in culture with rat brain extract exhibit a similar time course for the disappearance of NGF receptors as *in vivo*.

The disappearance of NGF receptors in culture might be due to a factor present in rat brain extract or to an endogenous mechanism. Since the loss of receptors begins only after 4 days in culture the first assumption would mean that the neurons become susceptible to the repressive factor only after a time corresponding to E14. Alternatively, if the loss of receptors is due to an endogenous mechanism, the survival in the presence of rat brain extract would represent a permissive condition under which cells are able to reach a stage of maturation which is characterized by the loss of NGF receptors *i.e.* the rat brain extract functions only as a survival factor rather than an instructive factor.

Since NGF receptors disappear in culture to a similar extent in the presence of the combination of NGF and rat brain extract as with rat brain extract alone (unpublished observations) the possibility can be excluded that NGF has a positive regulatory function to maintain the production of its own receptor.

The decrease in the proportion of sensory neurons which have NGF receptors _in vivo_ and _in vitro_ described in this study is in agreement with the previous studies of Herrup and Shooter (16) who described a decrease in the number of NGF receptors on cells obtained from sensory ganglia of increasing age. They correlated this decrease with the loss of the ability of ganglia explants from embryos of increasing age to produce fiber outgrowth in response to NGF. Thus both studies show that sensory neurons from chick embryos (in contrast to sympathetic neurons) lose NGF receptors during development. We showed however that with respect to NGF receptors the population of sensory neurons is heterogenous and that a small but significant population of sensory neurons retains NGF receptors at E16. Since ganglia from embryos older than E16 cannot be dissociated without significant cell losses we were not able to determine if all sensory neurons eventually lose their receptors. The finding that sensory neurons selected and cultivated with rat brain extract show a similar time course of disappearance of NGF receptors between E10 and E16 as _in vivo_ provides the possibility to answer this question by cultivating these cells for longer time periods _in vitro_ and to analyse the mechanism of receptor elimination by brain extract.

After the short period of development where chick sensory neurons respond to NGF no biological effect of NGF has been demonstrated so far. The role of NGF receptors on E16 sensory neurons thus is not clear at present. In this context it is worth mentioning, that in _rat_ sensory neurons a function of NGF, after the period in which the survival effect is observed, has been described recently by the demonstration that the levels of substance P in sensory ganglia are affected by NGF and NGF antibodies (16-18). The presence of NGF receptors on rat sensory neurons during these later periods of development was inferred previously from the observation that sensory neurons in adult rats transport NGF retrogradely (19). Adult rat sympathetic neurons had previously been shown to respond to NGF by the induction of neurotransmitter synthesising enzymes (20).

Bovine adrenal medullary cells are another example for cells which show characteristic responses to NGF at early stages of development while those from adult animals lose their response although NGF receptors can be demonstrated on these non-responsive cells: NGF mediated fiber outgrowth was observed with cultured adrenal medullary cells from fetuses and NGF mediated induction of tyrosine hydroxylase was demonstrated in cells obtained from fetuses and calves (21). Both responses were absent in cells obtained from adult animals. NGF receptors with identical dissociation constant ($K_D = 1 \times 10^{-9}$M) were observed on cells at all stages of development from fetuses to adult cells (21). One can only speculate on the function of NGF receptors on adrenal medullary cells which retain their receptors in adult animals. For example it would certainly be worth investigating if the levels of enkephalins present in these cells are influenced by NGF.

The failure to see a biological effect in a tissue only means that the particular response tested for is lacking. In the case of sensory neurons from adult rats the discovery of the presence of NGF receptors (19) - indirectly demonstrated by the ability of the neurons to transport NGF retrogradely - preceded the discovery of a biological response (16-18). We would therefore suggest that all cells having NGF receptors be regarded as probable target cells.

References

1. Hamburger, V.: J. Comp. Neurol. 160, 535-546 (1975).
2. Hollyday, M. and Hamburger, V.: J. Comp. Neurol. 170, 311-320 (1976).
3. Landmesser, L. and Pilar, G.: J. Physiol. (London) 241, 715-736 (1974).
4. Hendry, I.A., Stoeckel, K., Thoenen, H. and Iversen, L.L.: Brain Res. 68, 103-121 (1974).
5. Greene, L.A. and Shooter, E.M.: Ann. Rev. Neurosci. 3, 353-402 (1980).
6. Thoenen, H. and Barde, Y.A.: Physiol. Rev. 60, 1284-1335 (1980).
7. Greene, L.A.: Devel. Biol. 58, 96-105 (1977).
8. Greene, L.A.: Devel. Biol. 58, 106-113 (1977).
9. Barde, Y.A., Lindsay, R.M., Monard, D. and Thoenen, H.: Nature 274, 818, (1978).
10. Barde, Y.A., Edgar, D. and Thoenen, H.: Proc. Natl. Acad. Sci. USA 77, 1199-1203 (1980).
11. Edgar, D., Barde, Y.A. and Thoenen, H.: Nature 289, 294-295 (1981).
12. Helfand, S.L., Riopelle, R.T. and Wessels, N.K.: Expl. Cell Res. 113, 39-45 (1978).
13. Rohrer, H. and Barde, Y.A.: Develop. Biol., (1982) in press.
14. Sutter, A., Riopelle, R.J., Harris-Warrik, R.M. and Shooter, E.M.: J. Biol. Chem. 254, 5972-5982 (1979).
15. Herrup, K. and Shooter, E.M.: J. Cell Biol. 67, 118-125 (1975).
16. Kessler, I.A. and Black, I.B.: Proc. Natl. Acad. Sci. USA 77, 649-652 (1980).
17. Otten, U., Goedert, M., Mayer, N. and Lembeck, F.: Nature 287, 158-159 (1980).
18. Goedert, M., Stoeckel, K. and Otten, U.: Proc. Natl. Acad. Sci. USA 78, 5895-5998 (1981).
19. Stoeckel, K., Schwab, M. and Thoenen, H.: Brain Res. 89, 1-14 (1975).
20. Thoenen, H., Angeletti, P.U., Levi-Montalcini, R. and Kettler, R.: Proc. Natl. Acad. Sci. USA 68, 1598-1602 (1971).
21. Naujoks, K.W., Korsching, S., Rohrer, H. and Thoenen, H.: Devel. Biol., submitted.

NERVE GROWTH FACTOR RECEPTORS ON NON NEURONAL CELLS OF DORSAL ROOT GANGLIA

Astrid Zimmermann and Arne Sutter

Department of Neurobiology, Stanford University Medical Center,
Stanford, Cal. 94305, USA, and
Pharmakologisches Institut der Freien Universität Berlin,
Thielallee 69/73, D-1000 Berlin 33, FRG

Abstract

The expression of receptors for nerve growth factor (NGF) was investigated autoradiographically using iodinated ßNGF on cultured chick sensory ganglia cells. Not only neurons but also a population of non neuronal cells of chick sensory ganglia carry NGF receptors on the cell surface. NGF appears to have no effect on the survival and the morphological differentiation of these NGF receptor positive non neuronal cells. The binding of ^{125}I-ßNGF to cell surface receptors on the non neuronal cells is specifically displaced by NGF but not by proteins either basic as NGF like cytochrome C or related to NGF as insulin and relaxin.

The NGF receptor positive flat cells interact with sensory neurons in a manner typical for Schwann cells. They contact, align themselves along, and finally ensheath the neurites. Concomitant with contact and alignment an increase in the proliferation of the NGF receptor positive flat cells is observed along the neurites.

Introduction

The formation of the myelin sheath, resulting from the interaction of neuron and oligodendrocyte in the central nervous system and of neuron and Schwann cell in the peripheral nervous system occurs in an ordered and defined manner in all parts of the nervous system during development, yet is little understood in molecular terms. In spite of very detailed ultrastructural information on the genesis of the myelin sheath and a lot of knowledge on its chemical composition (1) little is known about specific factors and cell surface components on neuronal or glial cells which mediate the initial cell-cell contact and the highly organized wrapping process during myelinization.

Culture systems of dissociated nervous system cells have the potential to permit studies on the dynamics of neuron-glia cell encounters and of contact behaviour between individual cells under well defined conditions. One problem of this approach lies in the identification of the cell types once the tissue has been dissociated into single cells. Cell morphology by itself has turned out to be a rather unreliable characteristic in vitro since it is easily influenced by the culture conditions (e. g. serum concentration, cAMP) (2). For these reasons it is important to obtain cell type specific markers, preferably of the cell surface, which allow the classification of individual cultured cells. In recent years antigens have been described which are characteristic for astrocyte or oligodendrocyte cell populations (3, 4, 5, 6). For Schwann cells the only known marker is the rat specific RAN-1 antigen (2). Traditionally in vitro studies on myelinization have not been done with single cells and did not include the use of cell type specific markers but rather utilized tissue explants, as for example the dorsal root ganglia (drg) (8). In such cultures the cellular organization of the ganglia is left intact and operational criteria (9) are employed to distinguish between fibroblasts and Schwann cells. Using explant cultures of rat drg and cytostatic agents to kill off the rapidly dividing non neuronal cells (classified as fibroblasts), Salzer and Bunge (10) were able to demonstrate that it is the membrane of the neurite which induces Schwann cell proliferation.

In order to learn about the action of ß nerve growth factor (ßNGF) which is an essential factor for survival and differentiation of sensory and sympathetic neurons in vivo and in vitro (11, 12) we have studied cultures of dissociated dorsal root ganglia in the past years. In such cultures it can be observed that the individual cells interact with each other in a very reproducible manner. Given sufficient density and time neuronal cell bodies will cluster and their neurites will form bundles. Some of the non neuronal flat cells interact with the neurites and ensheath them, while others - with the same morphology - do not interact but divide until a confluent flat cell layer is formed. In previous studies on the binding characteristics of ßNGF to cell surface receptors on chick sensory ganglia cells it was observed that not only neurons but also the non neuronal cell populations of the drg express specific binding sites for NGF (13). While on neurons NGF binding occurs to sites with two different affinities, only one binding affinity was observed on the non neuronal cells comprising Schwann cells and fibroblasts (14). To gain further insight into the cellular distribution of the NGF receptors we have employed autoradiographic techniques and analyzed cultured sensory ganglia cells of embryonic chick. In the following we will show that there is a differential distribution of NGF receptors within the flat cell population and further that the NGF receptor positive flat cells can be classified as Schwann cells on the basis of their characteristic interaction with the neurites of sensory neurons.

Materials and Methods

ßNGF was purified according to the procedure of Moore at al. (15) and iodinated as described by Sutter et al. (13). Neurons and non neuronal cells of the ganglia from eight day old chick embryos were separated by means of their differential adhesiveness to tissue culture plastic and cultured as described previously (14). Non neuronal cultures contained no neurons and neuronal cultures were $\geq$ 95% pure neuronal. For autoradiography the cultured cells were incubated with ^{125}I-ßNGF as described in the text, fixed, coated with NTB2 emulsion (Kodak) and developed 10 days later.

Results

Fig. 1 shows photomicrographs taken from neuronal and non neuronal cultures. As already described for sympathetic neurons, sensory neurons and PC12 cells (16, 17) NGF receptors were located on cell bodies, neurites and growth cones of the cultured neurons. In contrast to the results of Kim et al. (16) and Levi et al. (17) NGF receptors were also found in high density on flat cells of the sensory ganglia. Of the non neuronal cells shown in Fig. 1 two were labeled while the others were not. No obvious morphological difference between labeled and non labeled cells was observed. Spindle shape which has been widely used as a morphological marker for Schwann cells was more often associated with non labeled flat cells than with labeled ones. ßNGF binding to the flat cells was specific. All cell labeling was abolished when ^{125}I-ßNGF incubation was done in the presence of an excess of unlabeled NGF (Fig. 2). This is in agreement with receptor binding studies on cell suspensions in which specific cell labeling is abolished in the presence of excess unlabeled ßNGF (10^{-7} M) (14). High concentrations of proteins ($2\text{-}5 \times 10^{-7}$ M) with similar physicochemical properties like cytochrome C or proteins related to ßNGF like insulin or relaxin do not compete with ^{125}I-ßNGF binding to flat cells (data not shown). The percentage of non neuronal cells which bound ^{125}I-ßNGF in cultures without neurons was variable. It could be as high as 25% initially (12 h culture) - though generally it was much lower - and then decreased with time due to proliferation of receptor negative cells.

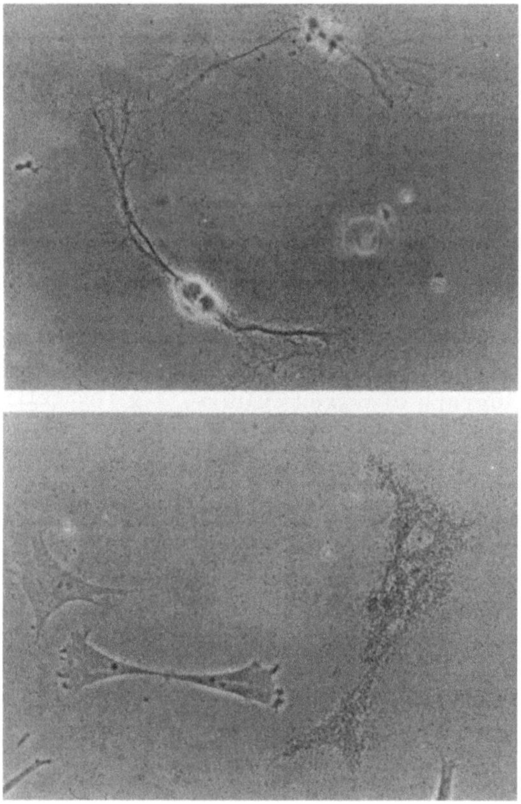

Fig. 1: Autoradiographs of separated neurons (upper photomicrograph) and non neuronal cells (lower photomicrograph) from sensory ganglia of eight day old chick embryos. The cells were cultured on polylysine coated 22 x 60 mm polystyrene cover slips (Lux) for 24 h. The slides were incubated with 10 ng/ml ^{125}I-ßNGF (55 cpm/pg) in PBS containing 1 mg/ml BSA for 20 min at 37°C, washed five times with incubation buffer, fixed with glutaralde-hyde/paraformaldehyde, washed extensively and dipped into NTB2 emulsion (Kodak), dil. 1 : 1. The slides were exposed for 10 days at 4°C, developed, mounted and analyzed under phase contrast. Photos were taken at 250 x with a Zeiss PM III.

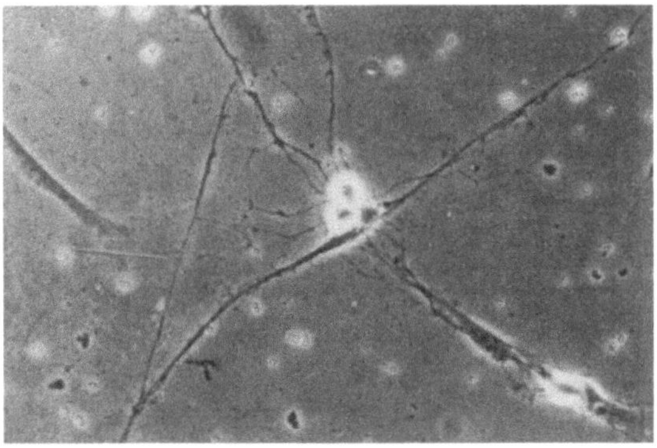

Fig. 2: Autoradiograph of mixed culture. 1×10^5 cells were plated per cover slip. The cells were incubated with 10 ng/ml ^{125}I-ßNGF and 10 µg/ml unlabeled ßNGF and processed as described in Fig. 1.

When mixed cultures (total dissociates of sensory ganglia) were observed over a period of several days it was apparent that the ^{125}I-ßNGF-labeled flat cells represented a class of cells which showed a very distinct behaviour towards the neurites of sensory neurons. This behaviour can be described in several stages. In stage I (Fig. 3, top) the cells grew in a random manner without special orientation with respect to each other. In stage II (Fig. 3, middle) NGF receptor positive flat cells showed increasing contact with the neurites and aligned themselves along the neurites while they grew in number. The receptor negative cells did not associate nor orient themselves in any specific way when in contact with neurites. The increase in NGF receptor positive flat cells along the neurites appeared to be due to increased proliferation (see also reference 10) rather than a change in phenotype from a receptor negative to a receptor positive cell (Zimmermann and Sutter, unpublished data). Following alignment the ensheathing process (stage III) (Fig. 3, bottom) started very rapidly. At this stage the Schwann cells along the neurites were no longer discernible as separate cells. Ultrastructural studies will be necessary to determine the degree of order of the wrapping process which is reached. Though the presence of the Schwann cell was no longer obvious in the "wrapped neurite"

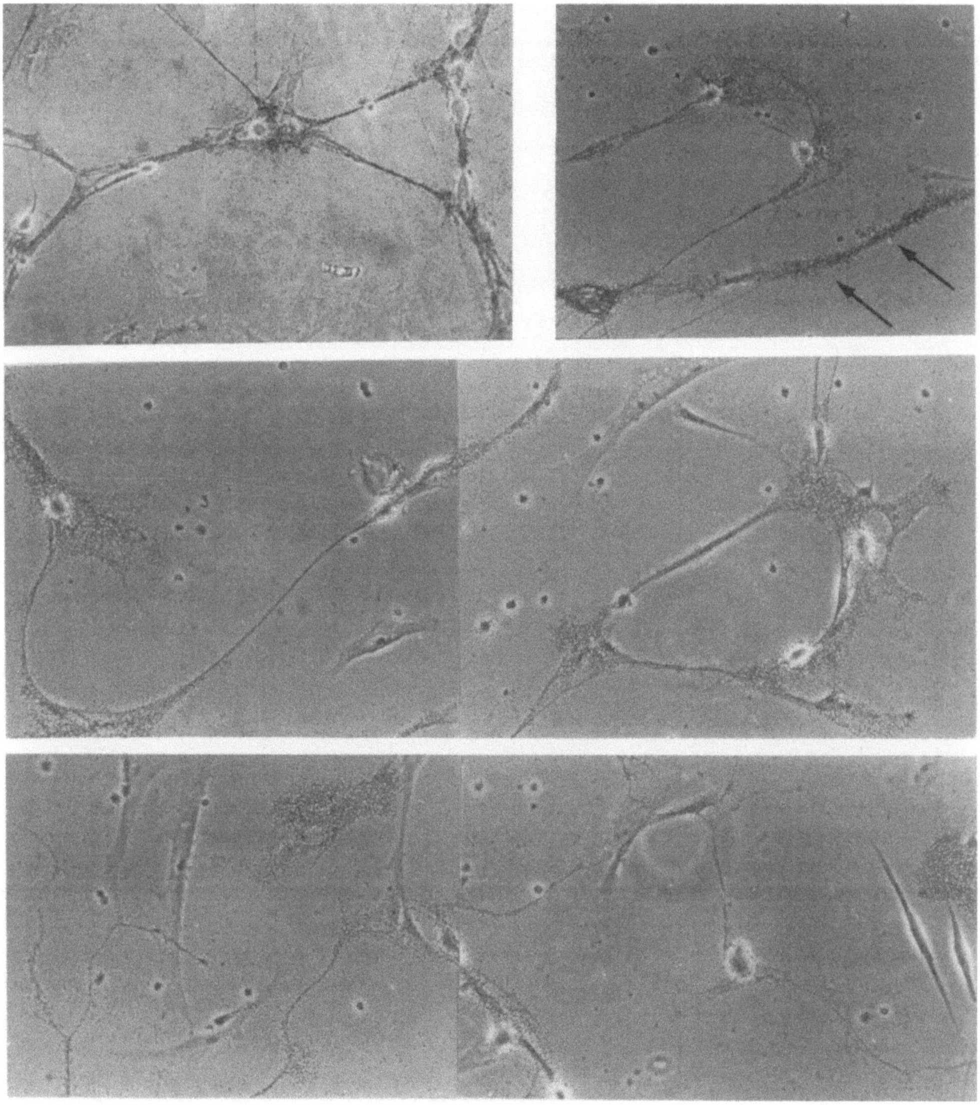

Fig. 3: Autoradiographs of mixed cultures. 1 x 10^5 cells were plated per cover slip. Labeling procedure as in Fig. 1. Stage I (top) is observed on the 1st day in culture. Stage II (middle) is typical for the 2nd day in culture. The photomicrograph bottom right reflects stage III (4 days in culture), the one bottom left shows an intermediate stage between II and III. Arrows indicate Schwann cell engaged with neurite.

stage represented all over the culture after four days, their presence can be detected by thymidine labeling prior to ensheathment in stage II (Fig. 4) and by immunofluorescence staining using anti-galactocerebroside anti-serum (data not shown). It has been suggested that not only oligodendrocytes but also Schwann cells when induced to myelinate become positive for galactocerebroside (18). If neurites degenerated, some Schwann cells regained their individual flat cell morphology. This generally occurred at a time when the culture was overgrown by receptor negative fibroblasts. NGF receptor positive cells then flattened out again and demarcated the original course of the neurites on top of the fibroblast layer (Fig. 5).

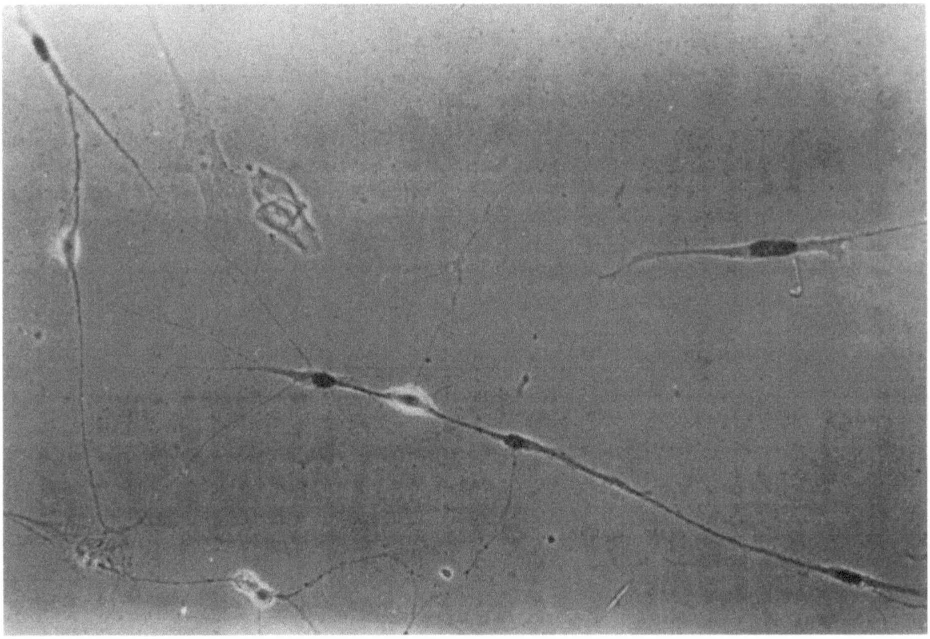

Fig. 4: Autoradiograph of ^{3}H-thymidine labeling (10 μCi/ml) for 24 h in stage II. Processing as in Fig. 1. Exposure time of dipped slides was 3 days.

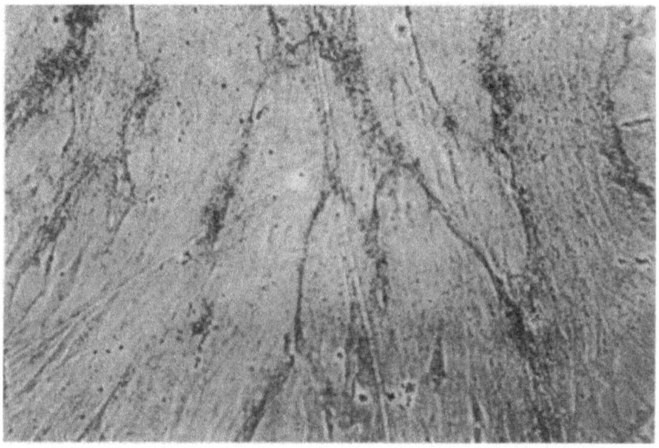

Fig. 5: Autoradiograph of a mixed culture after desintegration of neuronal network. Cell labeling was done as described in Fig. 1. Overgrowth of receptor negative flat cells and desintegration of the neuronal network starts to occur after a week in culture.

Discussion

What is the physiological role of NGF receptors on Schwann cells? At this point it is only possible to speculate. As far as we can say, ßNGF does not have any obvious effect on Schwann cell morphology or survival as it clearly has for the neurons. Whether NGF affects specific aspects of Schwann cell metabolism is an open field for future studies. It is of interest that cultures of non neuronal cells of sensory ganglia produce factor(s) with nerve growth factor activity. It is not known, though, whether these factors are produced by Schwann cells or fibroblasts. If in fact Schwann cells produce NGF (as e. g. C6 glioma cells apparently do (19)) one could envision NGF receptors on Schwann cells to serve as sensors of the extracellular NGF concentration and thereby as feedback regulators of NGF production. Alternatively if the fibroblasts produce NGF (as e. g. L929 cells apparently do (20)) Schwann cells could possibly regulate the actual quantities of NGF available to the neurons by their ability to bind and internalize NGF. The high grain density above the Schwann cells reflects a high NGF binding capacity. Looking at NGF receptors on Schwann cells in the context of NGF production it should be kept in mind that not only nervous system derived cells produce nerve growth factor like activities when put into culture (21). Monoclonal antibodies against ßNGF developed recently (22, 23) may allow to determine the degree of relatedness of nerve growth factor like activities with ßNGF. Aside from these thoughts on Schwann cell physiology it is very tempting to speculate that NGF receptors and ßNGF could be directly involved in the process of neuron-glia cell interaction. The dimeric ßNGF molecules could potentially be mediators of cell-cell contacts by binding to receptors on both cell types.

Acknowledgements

The authors are grateful to Dr. E. M. Shooter for his interest in this work and for his comments on the manuscript. The work was supported by grants from NINCDS (NS 04270) and the Deutsche Forschungsgemeinschaft

References

1. Morell, P.: Myelin, Plenum Press, New York and London (1977)
2. Brookes, J. P., Raff, M. C.: In Vitro 15, 772-778 (1979)
3. Dahl, D., Bignami, A.: Brain Res. 116, 150-157 (1976)
4. Eng, L. P., Vanderhaeghen, J. J., Bignami, A., Gerste, B.: Brain Res. 28, 351-354
5. Raff, M. C., Fields, K. L., Hakomori, S., Mirsky, R., Pruss, R. M., Winter, J.: Brain Res. 174, 283-308 (1979)
6. Lagenaur, C., Sommer, I., Schachner, M.: Dev. Biol. 79, 367-378 (1980)
7. Fields, K. L., Brookes, J. P., Mirsky, R., Wendon, L. M. B.: Cell 14, 43-51 (1978)

8. Peterson, E. R., Murray, M. R.: Dev. Biol. 2, 461-476 (1960)

9. Wood, P. M.: Brain Res. 115, 361-375 (1976)

10. Salzer, J. L., Bunge, R. P.: J. Cell Biol. 84, 739-752, 753-766, 767-778 (1980)

11. Levi-Montalcini, R., Angeletti, P. M.: Physiol. Rev. 48, 534-569 (1968)

12. Greene, L. A., Shooter, E. M.: Ann. Rev. Neurosci. 3, 353-402 (1980)

13. Sutter, A., Riopelle, R. J., Harris-Warrick, R. M., Shooter, E. M.: J. Biol. Chem. 254, 5972-5982 (1979)

14. Sutter, A., Riopelle, R. J., Harris-Warrick, R. M., Shooter, E. M.: Transmembrane Signaling, pp. 659-667, Alan R. Liss Inc., New York (1979)

15. Moore, J. B., Jr., Shooter, E. M.: Neurobiol. 5, 369-381 (1975)

16. Kim, S. U., Hogue-Angeletti, R., Gonatas, N. K.: Brain Res. 168, 602-608 (1979)

17. Levi, A., Shechter, Y., Neufeld, E. J., Schlessinger, J.: Proc. Natl. Acad. Sci. USA 77, 3469-3473 (1980)

18. Mirsky, R., Winter, J., Abney, E. R., Pruss, R. M., Gavrilovic, J., Raff, M. C.: J. Cell Biol. 84, 483-494 (1980)

19. Longo, A. M.: Dev. Biol. 65, 260-270 (1978)

20. Pantazis, N. I., Blanchard, M. H., Arnason, B. G. W., Young, M.: Proc. Natl. Acad. Sci. USA 74, 1492-1496 (1977)

21. Harper, G. P., Al-Saffar, A. M., Pearce, F. L., Vernon, C. A.: Dev. Biol. 77, 379-390 (1980)

22. Warren, S. L., Fanger, M., Neet, K. E.: Science 210, 910-912 (1980)

23. Zimmermann, A., Sutter, A., Shooter, E. M.: Proc. Natl. Acad. Sci. USA 78, 4611-4615 (1981)

III. DOPAMINE RECEPTOR

BIOCHEMICAL AND PHARMACOLOGICAL CHARACTERISTICS OF CENTRAL AND PERIPHERAL DOPAMINE RECEPTORS

W. Kehr

Research Laboratories of Schering, Berlin (West) and
Bergkamen, Federal Republic of Germany

Introduction

Since the discovery by Carlsson et al. (1) that dopamine (DA) - apart from being a precursor for noradrenaline and adrenaline - is a transmitter of its own, the receptor-mediated effects of this catecholamine have been studied extensively. The investigations were stimulated by two factors, namely the discovery that Parkinson's disease is associated with degeneration of the ascending dopaminergic fiber tract and the fact that blockade of dopaminergic transmission in the central nervous system is the common denominator of the mechanism of action of neuroleptics.

A. Central DA Receptors

Classically the appearance of certain behavioral symptoms is used as an indicator of the activity state of DA receptors in a particular brain area. In rodents, for example, the induction of stereotyped movements is considered as an indicator of striatal DA receptor stimulation whereas catalepsy is generally believed to indicate striatal DA-receptor blockade.

Some of these effects are the direct consequence of DA receptor stimulation or blockade at the effector cell, e.g. the inhibition of prolactin release is a direct consequence of DA receptor stimulation at mammotrophic cells of the pituitary gland. Other effects are only indirectly related to the state of DA receptors, e.g. activation of DA receptors in the nucleus accumbens of rodents induces transmission of information through a chain of complex neuronal circuits finally resulting in a stimulation of locomotor activity.

Apart from behavioral tests DA metabolites have been used to measure indirectly the activity of dopaminergic neurones and to evaluate DA receptor agonists and antagonists. This became possible by the observation of Carlsson and Lindqvist (2) that the neuroleptics haloperidol and chlorpromazine did not affect brain DA levels but markedly stimulated DA catabolism.

It was concluded from these observations that the activity of dopaminergic neurons is regulated in part by the activity of postsynaptic DA receptors via a neuronal feedback loop. Lateron, the determination of DA metabolites, DA synthesis rate or DA utilisation served as biochemical parameters to characterize DA receptor agonists and antagonists.

During recent years two factors have contributed decisively to our knowledge of postsynaptic dopaminergic transmission, firstly, the discovery that in some postsynaptic neurons the action of DA is mediated by cyclic adenosine monophosphate (c AMP) and secondly, the development of receptor binding assays which allow a more direct analysis of the interaction of agonists and antagonists with the membrane receptor.

1.DA-sensitive adenylate cyclase

Though DA-sensitive adenylate cyclase was discovered first outside the cns namely in the superior cervical ganglion of rabbits and calves (3) most subsequent experiments have been carried out on the cns of mammals. It should be noted, however, that DA-sensitive adenylate cyclase does not only exist in mammals but also e.g. in gastropodes and insects (for review see Ref. 4)

In mammalian brain DA-sensitive adenylate cyclase is found in brain areas which are innervated by dopaminergic neurons, i.e. striatum, olfactory tubercles, nucleus accumbens, median eminence, nucleus amygdaloideus centralis, frontal cortex and retina. From investigations of Bockaert et al. (5) it is known that the topography of DA-sensitive adenylate cyclase in the caudate nucleus is similar to the DA distribution and the high affinity DA uptake in this brain structure whereas the isoprenaline stimulated adenylate cyclase, i.e. the β-receptor linked cyclase is distributed evenly in the caudate nucleus. Similar studies have been carried out in the frontal cortex and the olfactory tubercles of the rat (for ref. s. 6). They show convincingly that the occurrence of DA-sensitive adenylate cyclase is correlated to dopaminergic innervation.

The existence of DA-sensitive adenylate cyclase in the substantia nigra, particularly in the zona reticulata (7, 8) may not fit into this correlation, since the substantia nigra does not contain classical dopaminergic synapses but rather dopaminergic cell bodies and dendrites. However, these dendrites are capable of synthesizing, storing and releasing dopamine (9,10) and thus it is not unexpected that DA-sensitive adenylate cyclase is found in the nigra on neurons passing through or terminating within this area.

Lesioning experiments utilizing 6-hydroxy-DA (6-OH-DA) clearly show that the activity of DA-sensitive adenylate cyclase is not associated with dopaminergic neurons - neither in the striatum nor in the substantia nigra (11, 12). However, utilizing the neurotoxin kainic acid, which is claimed to selectively destroy neuronal perikarya, a large decrease of DA-sensitive adenylate cyclase activity in the striatum was observed following intrastriatal injection, indicating the presence of adenylate cyclase in postsynaptic neuronal cell bodies (13).

Most studies on the characteristics of DA-sensitive adenylate cyclase have been carried out in cell-free preparation of the caudate nucleus. Since DA can stimulate the formation of cyclic AMP in vitro the postsynaptic receptor regulating the enzyme activity must be present in cell-free preparations and hence it was possible to study the structural requirements of receptor agonists and antagonists of the adenylate cyclase linked DA-receptor. Although many compounds, structurally related to DA were tested, none of the catecholamines was more active than DA itself. Epinine (N-methyl-dopamine) appears to be the only molecule with an intact catechol moiety which is equipotent to DA (6). Further substitution of the DA molecule is associated with a reduction of agonistic activity. Apart from DA derivatives some of the rigid or semirigid DA analogues possessing dopaminergic activity in vivo stimulate adenylate cyclase in vitro. Among these 2-amino-6,7-dihydroxy-tetrahydronaphtalene (6,7-ADTN) has the highest potency. The structure of 6,7-ADTN implies that the extended (trans) form and the β-rotamer is the preferred conformation of the flexible DA molecule stimulating adenylate cyclase (6).

Some DA analogues are not as active in vitro as expected from in vivo experiments. The intrinsic activity of apomorphine which is considered a classical DA-receptor agonist is not as marked as that of DA. As high concentrations of apomorphine are reached inhibitory effects are apparent (14) and in addition apomorphine can antagonize the stimulatory effect of DA on adenylate cyclase in cell-free preparations as well as in intact cells. Thus, apomorphine can be classified as partial agonist. Interestingly, apomorphine also shows partial agonistic activity in DA receptor binding studies (15).

Neuroleptic agents of the phenothiazine or butyrophenone type, which are known to block effects of DA-agonist, are potent competitive antagonists at DA-receptors linked to adenylate cyclase (16). The effect appears to be specific since α- and β-receptor blocking agents do not antagonize the effect of DA. The neuroleptics butaclamol and flupenthixol occur as optical isomers or stereoisomers. Only (+)-butaclamol and cis-flupenthixol which are active antipsychotics possess strong DA-antagonistic properties, whereas (-)-butaclamol and trans-flupenthixol which appear pharmacologically and clinically inactive are weak antagonists at the adenylate cyclase-linked DA-receptor (6). These observations strengthen the correlation between clinical efficacy of phenothiazines as antischizophrenics and their ability to inhibit DA-sensitive adenylate cyclase (6).

The hypothesis advocated some years ago that the adenylate cyclase itself were the DA receptor is not maintainable today. The characteristics of membrane binding sites for agonists and antagonists differ markedly from those of adenylate cyclase. It is not known in detail how the membrane receptor is coupled to adenylate cyclase. In any case guanyl nucleotides, specially guanosin triphosphate appear necessary for the coupling (17) - a general phenomenon proposed for the coupling between membrane receptors and adenylate cyclase (18).

2. Membrane binding sites

Investigations on the specific binding of radiolabelled DA-agonists and -antagonists to membranes have contributed a great deal to our knowledge of the characteristics of these receptor binding sites. These methods are mainly used to a) study the interaction of DA-agonists and -antagonists, b) analyse the location of binding sites, e.g. whether they are located pre- or postsynaptically and c) to compare receptor sites in various DA systems in the cns and the periphery.

Due to easy handling most binding experiments have been carried out on bovine striatal membrane. As far as this tissue is concerned there is good agreement that DA-agonists are much more potent than DA-antagonists to displace a DA-agonistic ligand from its receptor site, while DA-antagonists are more potent than DA-agonists to displace a DA-antagonistic ligand (19). These results have been interpreted in two ways. 1.) It was proposed that the DA-receptor was occurring in two conformational states, an agonistic and an antagonistic conformation (20). 2.) It was suggested by Titeler and Seeman (19) that two separate and independent binding sites exist, one for agonists and one for antagonists.

In favour of the latter hypothesis there is evidence that the specific binding of the DA-agonist ^{3}H-apomorphine is reduced in the presence of guanyl nucleotides whereas the specific binding of the DA-antagonists ^{3}H-haloperidol or ^{3}H-spiroperidol is not altered (21). Further, the existence of two independent receptor sites is supported by the fact that the receptor alkylating substance phenoxybenzamine is blocking the specific binding of ^{3}H-spiroperidol at low concentration, at which binding of ^{3}H-DA is left unchanged. Saturation experiments show that phenoxybenzamine reduces the number of binding sites while the affinity of e.g. ^{3}H-spiroperidol is unchanged (22).

Whichever of these hypotheses is correct some of the DA-agonists, such as apomorphine, N-n-propylnorapomorphine, 2-(N,N-dipropyl)-amino-5,6-dihydroxytetralin and bromocriptine have high affinity for both the agonist and antagonist receptor.

In contrast to bovine striatum results of DA-agonist binding experiments in rat striatum have to be interpreted with caution. While DA-antagonist show acceptable binding to rat striatal tissue, DA-agonists have consistently shown a binding which lacks stereospecificity and which is displaceable by the unlabelled compound only in high concentrations possibly reflecting binding to "non-specific" sites (23).

However, it has been shown recently that this "non-specific" binding site is occluded by the presence of a chelating agent (24). Under these conditions a binding site becomes demonstrable which shows stereospecificity and displacement by very low concentration of non-labelled agonist (24).

3.Location

Despite the above mentioned difficulties in relation to DA-agonist binding, such ligands (apart from antagonists) have been used in studies which have employed 6-OH-DA or kainic acid lesions in attempts to locate DA agonist/antagonist binding sites. The interpretation of lesion experiments is often hampered by the impossibility of obtaining a complete lesion, the possibility of denervation supersensitivity of postsynaptic receptors (masking presynaptic changes) and the possibility of transsynaptic changes. Thus, it is not surprising that divergent results have been reported from different laboratories. While Nagy et al. (25) observed a reduction of ^{3}H-apomorphine binding in striatum following 6-OH-DA-lesion of the nigrostriatal pathway and concluded that apomorphine labelled presynaptic sites on DA neuron, Creese and Snyder (26) reported an increase in ^{3}H-apomorphine binding after 6-OH-DA-lesion and suggested a postsynaptic location of the apomorphine binding site.

4.DA-autoreceptors

Despite the divergent results of radioreceptor ligand studies there is little doubt that DA-receptors located on the membrane of nigrostriatal DA neurons exist. The evidence for these so called DA-autoreceptors (27) is as follows. When the ascending nigrostriatal and mesolimbic fibers of rats are cut, the synthesis of DA is increased markedly and transiently in the terminal reticulum distal to the lesion. Under these conditions low doses of apomorphine inhibit DA synthesis and haloperidol antagonizes the effect of apomorphine indicating that the receptor-mediated feedback regulating DA synthesis is operative locally in striatum and mesolimbic structures and suggesting the involvement of presynaptic DA-autoreceptors (28). It is interesting that the receptor mediated feedback control of DA synthesis can also be shown in synaptosomal preparations in which neuronal or recurrent axonal loops can be excluded (29).

Further, DA-autoreceptors appear to play a role in regulating the amount of DA being released by nerve impulse. The field stimulation induced release of ^{3}H-labelled DA from striatal slices of rats or rabbits is reduced by DA-agonists like apomorphine or bromocriptine and enhanced by DA-receptor blocking agents (30, 31).

The third piece of evidence for the existence of DA-autoreceptors comes from electrophysiological experiments. When DA or apomorphine is applied microiontophoretically onto the surface of nigral DA neurons the firing rate in these neurons is depressed (32). Systemic administration of chlorpromazine or haloperidol abolish this local effect of DA suggesting that somato-dendritic DA-autoreceptor mediate the effect of DA (33). Taken together these receptors appear to be part of a homeostatic mechanism that regulates nerve impulse flow, transmitter synthesis and the amount of DA released from nerve endings.

The development of 3(3-hydroxyphenyl)N-n-propylpiperidine which has been reported to be a selective agonist for DA-autoreceptors (34) favours the view that pre- and postsynaptic DA-receptors have different properties. However, this hypothesis awaits further confirmation.

5. Heterogeneity of postsynaptic receptors

During recent years pharmacological and biochemical evidence has accumulated that at least two entities of postsynaptic DA-receptors exist which may also differ as regards their postsynaptic location.

One class of receptors is linked to adenylate cyclase whereas the other class is apparently not linked to an adenylate cyclase.According to Kababian (35) the adenylate cyclase linked receptor has been designated D_1receptor and the latter type D_2receptor. Though this subdivision is partly based on a negative and thus weak criterion namely the fact that a receptor is not linked to adenylate cyclase, the evidence for more than one type of postsynaptic DA receptor is convincing.

As mentioned above the synthesis and release of prolactin is under tonic inhibitory dopaminergic control. Dopaminergic agonists inhibit prolactin secretion by directly stimulating DA receptors on mammotrophic cells of the pituitary gland (36). However, there is no evidence that DA agonists stimulate the formation of cAMP in these cells. On the contrary,it is known that DA has an inhibitory effect on adenylate cyclase in human pituitary adenoma cells secreting prolactin (37).

The dopaminergic ergoline derivatives lisuride, lergotrile and bro-bromocriptine are potent inhibitors of prolactin secretion and these effects at the pituitary level can be completely abolished by pretreatment with DA-antagonists. At the DA-stimulated striatal adenylate cyclase, however, these ergolines themselves act as DA-antagonists. Since the action of DA at the mammotrophs of the pituitary does not appear to be linked to adenylate cyclase the respective DA receptors belong to the D_2type.

In the pituitary gland D_2receptors seem to occur also in the intermediate lobe where they play a role in the regulation of synthesis and release of a α-melanocyte stimulating hormone (α-MSH). It is known that β-adrenergic compounds stimulate the formation of cAMP and the consecutive release of α-MSH is thought to be linked to the increased formation of cAMP. Stimulation of DA-receptors which occur on these particular cells not only inhibits the spontaneous release of α-MSH but also attenuates the stimulatory effect of β-mimetics on α-MSH release as well as cAMP formation (35). These effects of DA can be considered specific since they are fully antagonised by butyrophenones and benzamides of which a prototype compound is sulpiride.

The classification of DA receptors in different brain areas is still at the very beginning. The blockade by sulpiride of apomorphine or 6,7-ADTN induced circling as well as stimulation of locomotor activity in rats and the lack of effect of sulpiride to block the DA-sensitive adenylate cyclase is considered as evidence for the occurrence of D_2-receptors in striatum (35). Since sulpiride is a potent DA antagonist also at pituitary DA receptors this compound appears to be a selective D_2-antagonist (Table 1).

Although haloperidol is a potent antagonist of DA-sensitive striatal adenylate cyclase, ^{3}H-haloperidol binding sites may not be indentical to those DA-receptors which are linked to adenylate cyclase. Lesion studies rather indicate that ^{3}H-haloperidol binding sites are not coupled to adenylate cyclase. As mentioned above kainic acid administered into the striatum drastically reduces the activity of DA-sensitive adenylate cyclase but does not or only marginally affect the number of striatal haloperidol binding sites. Elimination of cortico-striate afferents by cortical ablation, however, reduces the number of striatal ^{3}H-haloperidol binding sites while leaving DA-sensitive adenylate cyclase intact (46). This clear dissociation between ^{3}H-haloperidol binding site and DA-sensitive adenylate cyclase indicates that a substantial portion of striatal ^{3}H-haloperidol binding sites are located on axons of cerebral cortical afferents not linked to adenylate cyclase (and thus may be categorized as D_2receptor) whereas DA-sensitive adenylate cyclase is

Table 1: Comparison of dopamine receptor blocking properties of haloperidol and sulpiride

	Haloperidol	Sulpiride	Ref.
Antiemetic effect in dogs	+ +	+ +	38
Increase in serum prolactin in man	+ +	+ +	39
Blockade of apomorphine-induced circling in rats	+ +	+	40
Inhibition of 6,7-ADTN or apomorphine-induced locomotion in rats	+ +	+ +	41
Catalepsy in rats	+ +	-	42
Inhibition of DA-stimulated striatal adenylate cyclase	+ +	-	43
Displacement of ^{3}H-haloperidol	+ +	(+)	44
Displacement of ^{3}H-sulpiride	+ +	+ +	45

++ = strong, + = moderate, (+) = weak effect; - = no effect

confined to neurons intrinsic to the striatum.

Despite a great number of publications on receptor binding experiments the important question on the functional significance of the various binding sites for DA-agonists and antagonists in different brain areas remains to be answered.

B. Peripheral DA Receptors

DA-containing neuronal elements have been described in peripheral organs especially the kidney (47, 49). There is evidence that in these organs DA is synthesized and stored outside the sympathetic nerves and is functioning as a transmitter of its own. It is thus conceivable that also DA receptors exist in various peripheral organs. These receptors have not been investigated as extensive as the central

Table 2: Location and function of peripheral dopamine receptors

postsynaptic receptors	function of dopamine	Ref.
parathyroid gland	facilitation of hormone release	50
oesophagus, stomach, small intestine	relaxation, decrease of intestinal motility	51
pancreas, exocrine gland (?)	facilitation of secretion	51
cardiovascular system		
a) renal arteries b) coronary arteries c) cerebral arteries d) mesenteric arteries	vasodilation	52
presynaptic receptors		
sympathetic ganglia	induction of slow inhibitory postsynaptic potentials	51
terminal reticulum of noradrenergic sympathetic neurons	inhibition of noradrenaline release	53

DA-receptors.

As shown in Table 2, DA receptors occur postsynaptically on smooth muscle cells of the cardiovascular system, on smooth muscle cells of the gastrointestinal tract, on endocrine glands (parathyroid gland) and possibly on exocrine glands (pancreas, submandibular gland) and presynaptically on sympathetic noradrenergic neurons. In all organs investigated so far the vascular postsynaptic action of DA consists of a vasodilation. As long as the arterial systemic blood pressure is kept constant, DA-agonists increase the perfusion of these organs.This has been clearly shown for the kidney and in experiments of Goldberg et al. (51) the increase of renal blood flow has been used as a parameter to evaluate DA agonistic effects at postsynaptic receptors.

Dopamine, epinine and 6,7-ADTN are equipotent at the kidney DA-receptor, apomorphine is a very weak agonist ant the ergoline derivatives are inactive. Since 2-amino-5,6-dihydroxytetrahydronaphtalene (5,6-ADTN) is inactive and 6,7-ADTN one of the most potent agonists at the renal DA-receptor the flexible DA molecule appears to be active at the receptor only as β-rotamer and in its trans conformation. Among the neuroleptics sulpiride and bulbocapnine appear to be the most potent DA-antagonists followed by the butyrophenones and metoclopromide.

With regard to DA-sensitive adenylate cyclase activity investigations of the structure-activity relationship have not been carried out yet, though there is no doubt that a DA-sensitive adenylate cyclase does exist in kidney of various species. Whether postsynaptic DA-receptors in peripheral tissue can be subdiveded into D_1 and D_2 receptors remains to be clarified.

As shown in Table 2, presynaptic DA-receptors are known to occur in species including rat, guinea pig, rabbit, dog and possibly man. Activation of these receptors results in a down-regulation of noradrenergic transmission by an inhibition of impulse-induced release of noradrenaline (53). However, it has to be born in mind that some DA-agonists which have an affinity also to α-receptors may inhibit noradrenaline release by an activation of presynaptic α-receptors.

The rank order of potency of DA agonists at presynaptic DA receptors differs from that of postsynaptic DA receptors, e.g. 5,6-ADTN appears to be active at pre- but not at postsynaptic receptors whereas 6,7-ADTN is more active at post- than at presynaptic receptors (51, 54).

In addition, the observation that fluphenazine and sulpiride are far more potent as antagonists at presynaptic than at postsynaptic sites may indicate that pre- and postsynaptic peripheral DA-receptors are different entities.

Perspectives

Differentiation of various DA-receptors in the cns and peripheral organs is not only of theoretical interest but may create the basis for more selective intervention in pathophysiological processes and more selective therapie of schizophrenia, Parkinson's disease, diseases associated with hyperprolactinemia and cardiovascular diseases (55). By following the existing leads, it may be possible to use them as therapeutic principles in the near future.

References

1. Carlsson, A., Lindqvist, M., Magnusson, T., Waldeck, B., Science 127, 471 (1958).

2. Carlsson, A., Lindqvist, M., Acta Pharmacol.Toxicol. 20, 140, (1963).

3. Kebabian, J.W., Greengard, P., Science 174, 1346,(1971).

4. Nathanson, J.A., Physiol. Rev., 57, 157, (1977).

5. Bockaert, J., Premont, J., Glowinski, J., Thierry, A.M., Tassin, J.P., Brain Research, 107, 303, (1976).

6. Miller, R.J., McDermed, J. in: The Neurobiology of Dopamine, eus. Horn A.S.,Korf J., Westerink B.H.C.,Academic Press London, 159, (1979).

7. Spano, P.F., Chiara, G.D., Tonon, G.C., Trabucchi, M., J. Neurochem., 27, 1565, (1976).

8. Seeber, U., Kuschinsky, K., Experientia, 32, 1558, (1976).

9. Geffen, L.B., Jessell, T.M., Cuello, A.C., Iversen, L.L., Nature (London), 260, 258, (1976).

10. Korf, J., Zieleman M., Westerink, B.H.C., Nature, Lond., 260, 257, (1976).

11. Von Voigtlander, P.F., Boukma, S.J., Johnson, G.A., Neuropharmacology, 12, 1081, (1973).

12. Mishra, R.K., Gardner, E.C., Katzmann, R., Makman, M., Proc. Nat. Acad. Sci. U.S.A., 71, 3883, (1974).

13. Schwarcz, R., Coyle, J.T., Life Sciences, 20, 431, (1977).

14. Kebabian, J.W., Petzold, G.L., Greengard, P., Proc. Nat. Acad. Sci., U.S.A., 69, 2145,(1972).

15. Creese, I., Burt, D.R., Snyder, S.H.,Life Sci., 17, 1715, (1975b).

16. Clement-Cormier, Y.C., Kebabian, J.W., Petzold, G.L., Greengard, P., Proc. Nat. Acad. Sci. U.S.A., 71, 1113, (1974).

17. Clement-Cormier, Y.C., Parrish, R.G., Petzold, G.L., Kebabian, J.W., Greengard, P.J., Neurochem.25, 143, (1975).

18. Rodbell, M., Lin, M.C., Solomon, V., Londos, C., Harwood, J.P., Martin, B.R., Rendell, M., Berman, M., Advances in Cyclic Nucleotide Research, Raven Press, New York, 3, (1975).

19. Titeler, M., Seeman, Ph., in: The Neurobiology of Dopamine, eds. Horn A.S., Korf J. Westerink B.H.C. Academic Press London, 179, (1979).

20. Creese, I., Burt, D.R., Snyder, S.H. (1975b) Life Sci. 17, 1715

21. Creese, I., Usdin, T., Snyder, S.H., Nature 278, 577 (1979).

22. Hamblin, M., Creese, I., Eur. J. Pharmacol., 65, 119, (1980)

23. Seeman, P., Woodruff, G.N., Poat, J.A., Eur. J. Pharmacol. 55, 137, (1979).

24. Leysen, J.E., Long-term Effects of Neuroleptics, 123, Raven Press, New York, (1980).

25. Nagy, J.I., Lee, T., Seeman, P., Nature 274, 278, (1978).

26. Creese, I., Snyder S.H., Eur. J. Pharmac. 56, 277, (1979).

27. Carlsson, A., in: Pre- and Postsynaptic Receptors, Modern Pharmacology-toxicology, 3, eds. Usdin E., Bunney, Jr., W.E., Marcel Dekker Inc., New York, (1975).

28. Kehr, W., Carlsson, A., Lindqvist, M., Magnusson, T., Atack, C., J. Pharm. Pharmacol., 24, 744, (1972).

29. Christiansen, J., Squires, R.F., J. Pharm. Parmacol., 26, 367, (1974).

30. Farnebo, L.-O., Hamberger, B., Acta physiol. scand., 371, 35, (1971).

31. Starke, K., Reimann, W., Zumstein, A., Hertting, G., Nauyn-Schmiedeberg's Arch. Pharmacol., 305, 27, (1978).

32. Skirboll, L.R., Grace, A.A., Bunney, B.S., Science 206, 80, (1979).

33. Aghajanian, G.K., Bunney, B.S., Frontiers in Catecholamine Research, 643, Pergamon Press, Great Britain (1973)

34. Hjorth, S. Carlsson, A., Wikström, H., Lindberg, P., Sanchez, D., Hacksell, U., Arvidsson, L.-E., Svensson, U., Nilsson, J.L.G. Life Sciences, 28, 1225, (1981)

35. Kebabian, J.W., Cote, T.E., Trends in Pharmacol. Sciences, 69, (March 1981)

36. Thorner, M.O., Clin. Endocrin Metab. 6, 201, (1977).

37. De Camilli P., Spada, A., Giovanelli, M., Meldolesi, S., Faglia, G., Abstracts7th International Congress of Pharmacology, 596, (IUPHAR, Paris, 1978).

38. Laville,C., Margarit, J., C.r.Seanc.Soc.Biol. 162,869, (1968)

39. Mancini A.M., Guitelman, A. Vargas, C.A., Debeljuk K., Aparicio N.J., J.clin. Endocr. Metab., 42, 181, (1976).

40. Elliott, P.N.C., Jenner, P., Huizing, G., Marsden, C.D., Miller, R., Neuropharmacology 16, 333,(1977).

41. Woodruff,G.N., Andrews, C.D., in: Sulpiride and other Benzamides (eds. Spano P.F., Trabucchi M., Corsini G.U. u. Gessa, G.L.), 11, Italian Brain Research Foundation Press, Milan (1979).

42. Laville,C., Lille med. 17, Suppl. 1, 4, (1972).

43. Trabucchi M., Longoni R., Fresia P., Spano P.F., Life Sci. 17, 1551, (1975).

44. Spano P.F., Govoni S., Trabucchi M., in: Dopamine,Adv.Biochem. Psychopharmacol.(eds. Roberts P.J.,Woodruff G.N.,Iversen L.L.), 19, 155, Raven Press, New York, (1978).

45. Woodruff G.N., Freedman, S.B., Neuroscience 3, 407, (1981).

46. Schwarcz,R., Creese,I.,Coyle J.T.,Snyder,S.H., Nature 271, 766, (1978).

47. Lackovic,Z., Neff,N.H., Brain Research 193, 289, (1980).

48. Dinerstein R.J.,Vannice J.,Henderson R.C.,Roth L.J.,Goldberg L.I., Hoffmann P.C., Science 205, 497, (1979).

49. Bell C.,Lang W.J.,Laska F., J.Neurochem. 81, 77, Pergamon Press. (1978).

50. Brown E.M.,Carroll R.J., Aurbach G.D.,Proc.Natl.Acad.Sci U.S.A. 74, 4210, (1977).

51. Goldberg L.I.,Volkman P.H.,Kohli J.D.,Ann.Rev.Pharmacol.Toxicol. 18, 57, (1978)

52. Boucher M.,Lavarenne J.,Duchene-Marullaz P.,in: Advances in the Biosciences 20, eds.Imbs J.L.,Schwartz J.,117, Pergamon P.,(1978).

53. Langer S.Z.,Dubocovich M.L.,in: Advances in the Biosciences 20, eds.Imbs J.L.,Schwartz J., 233, Pergamon Press, (1978).

54. Brown R.A., Brown R.C., O'Connor S.E., Solca A.M., Br.J.Pharmac. 67, 420 (1979)

55. Calne D.B., Trends in Pharmacol. Sciences 1, 412, (1980).

IV. β-ADRENERGIC RECEPTOR

APPLICATION OF NEW CHEMICAL TOOLS FOR BETA-ADRENERGIC RECEPTOR INVESTIGATION

W. Burgermeister and M. Hekman
Department of Physiological Chemistry, University of Würzburg
Koellikerstrasse 2, D-8700 Würzburg

A. Study of Receptor Distribution and Mobility with a Fluorescent Antagonist

The ß-adrenergic receptor is a protein located in the plasma membrane of most vertebrate cells. Interaction of the hormone, epinephrine or a synthetic agonist, e.g. isoproterenol with ß-receptors leads to an increased intracellular concentration of cAMP which acts as a "second messenger" mediating various cellular functions. According to present knowledge, this process of signal transmission involves interaction of three membrane proteins which have been physically separated (1,2): The hormone-receptor complex (R^o) at first activates a guanylnucleotide binding protein (G) by promoting the exchange of bound GDP for GTP. The activated G in turn interacts with the catalytic unit (C) of the adenylate cyclase to form the active enzyme. Since a small fraction of the ß-receptors can activate the entire pool of G and C units (3,4), lateral mobility of at least one of the three components is supposed to be necessary for their effective interaction. Direct measurement of the distribution and lateral mobility in the membrane of the individual components may yield valuable information on the role of diffusional encounters in the activation process.

Using the fluorescent high-affinity ß-adrenergic antagonist, Alp-NBD (Fig. 1), ß-receptors of intact Chang liver cells have been visualized and investigated with the techniques of fluorescence recovery after photobleaching (FRP) (5) and video intensification microscopy (VIM) (6). A detailed account of these experiments has been published (7).

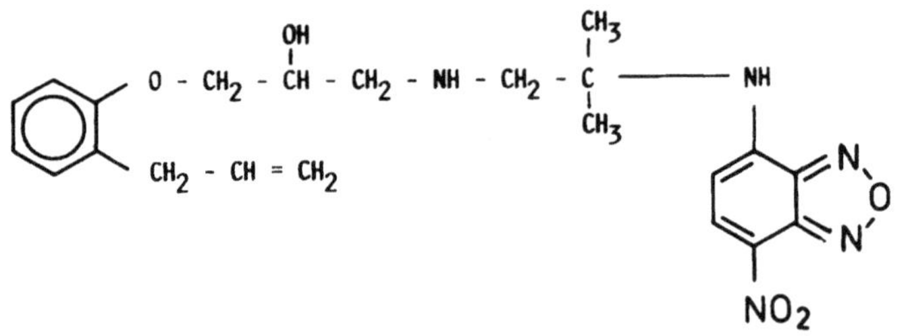

Fig. 1. Structure of alprenolol-NBD (Alp-NBD)

When cells were incubated for 30 s with 4 x 10^{-8}M Alp-NBD at 4°C and washed, the bound fluorescence was mainly in aggregates (Fig. 2A) and remained patchy after 1 hr at 37°C (Fig. 2C). Paraformaldehyde fixation prior to labeling prevented binding of Alp-NBD to cells, presumably due to modification of the ß-receptors (Fig. 2D). The fluorescent patches seen after normal labeling were mostly due to specific labeling of ß-receptors since the nonspecific staining in presence of an excess of nonfluorescent ß-antagonist was much weaker (Fig. 2B). Quantitative measurements revealed that 60 to 75% of the bound fluorescence could be displaced by 10^{-5}M propranolol or carazolol. Specificity was also checked using (+) and (-)pindolol at 5 x 10^{-8}M concentration, respectively. The (-) isomer which binds tightly to ß-receptors displaced 60% of the fluorescence whereas the (+) isomer which has a much lower affinity displaced less than 10%. The observation of fluorescent patches already after brief labeling at 4°C suggests that the ß-receptors are aggregated prior to antagonist binding.

FPR measurements were carried out using an argon ion laser beam (λ = 476.5 nm) focused through the fluorescence microscope on a spot (2.25 um radius) of the cell surface labeled with Alp-NBD (for details see Ref. 7). 50 to 70% of the initial fluorescence was irreversibly bleached by a 40 ms pulse

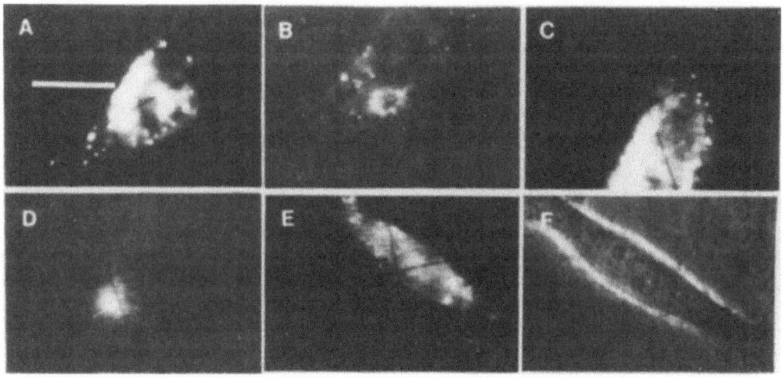

Fig. 2. Distribution of Alp-NBD on Chang liver cells. A, cell labeled with 4 x 10^{-8}M Alp-NBD for 30 s at 4°C. B, cell labeled as in A however in presence of 10^{-5}M propranolol. C, cell labeled as in A, after 1 hr at 37°C. D, Alp-NBD fluorescence on cells fixed with 3% paraformaldehyde prior to labeling. E, Alp-NBD fluorescence on cell preincubated for 30 min with 1.6 x 10^{-5}M (-)isoproterenol at 37°C and then labeled as in A. F, Phase contrast micrograph of E.

of 0.2 mW intensity. The rate and amount of fluorescence recovery in the bleached area due to lateral diffusion of fluorophores was then monitored using the attenuated laser beam. Representative FPR curves are shown in Fig. 3. After a first bleach, fluorescence recovery of cells labeled with 4 x 10^{-8}M Alp-NBD was only (15 ± 4)% (Fig. 3A). This indicates that 85% or more of the bound Alp-NBD is immobile within the examined time period (up to 10 min tested). The small mobile fraction of fluorescence could be attributed to nonspecifically bound label as revealed by control experiments in presence of nonfluorescent competitor (not shown). It can be concluded that most if not all of the Alp-NBD-receptor complexes on Chang liver cells are incapable of lateral motion over um distances. When subsequent bleaches on the same spot were carried out, 100% fluorescence recovery was recorded (Fig. 3B). This is expected since only the mobile fraction of fluorescence is bleached under these conditions.

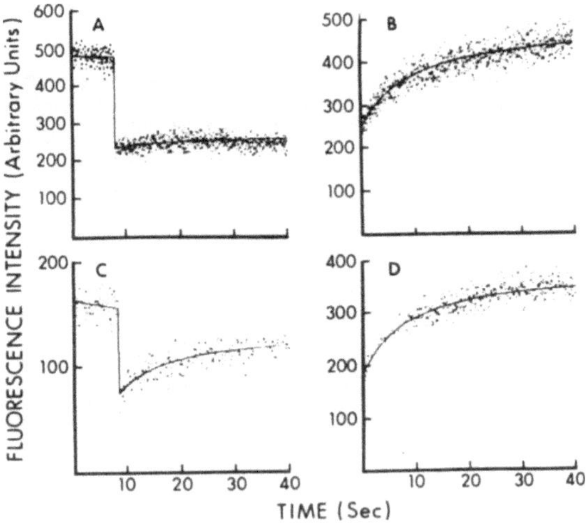

Fig. 3. Representative FPR curves of Alp-NBD on Chang liver cells. Cells were labeled with 4 x 10^{-8}M Alp-NBD for 30 s at 23°C before (A,B) and after (C,D) 30 min preincubation at 37°C with 1.6 x 10^{-5}M (-)isoproterenol. Shown are curves of a first bleach (A,C) and synchronized sums of four successive recovery curves on the same spot (B,D).

Agonists but not antagonists are capable of promoting coupling of the receptor with the G protein, as well as the subsequent steps, adenylate cyclase activation and desensitization (8). It was therefore of interest to study the effect of preincubation with agonist on the lateral mobility and distribution of ß-receptors. Chang liver cells were incubated at 37°C with 1.6 x 10^{-5}M (-)isoproterenol, washed and then labeled with 4 x 10^{-8}M Alp-NBD. This procedure did not alter the specificity of Alp-NBD labeling, as confirmed by control experiments (not shown). Five min preincubation with (-)isoproterenol did not affect the mobility or the fluorescence pattern of Alp-NBD on the cells. However, after 15 to 30 min preincubation two distinct changes were observed: The patchy appearance of the Alp-NBD fluorescence on the cell surface was turned into a more homogeneous pattern (Fig. 2E), and the mobile fraction of ß-receptor-Alp-NBD complexes was markedly increased (Fig. 3C) reaching values of 73 to 91%. The lateral mobility of the lipid probe, NBD-phosphatidylethanolamine was found to be unaffected by the (-)isoproterenol treatment. This rules out increased lateral mobility of membrane lipids as the mechanism of the (-)isoproterenol effect.

The experimental findings indicate that ß-receptors on Chang liver cells are aggregated in patches prior to ligand binding and immobile on the experimental time scale. The slow (15 to 30 min) mobilization of receptors by (-)isoproterenol treatment does not correlate with the activation of adenylate cyclase in Chang liver cells which requires only 2 to 3 min (Bakardjiev, unpublished results). This suggests that macroscopic lateral mobility of receptors is not required for cyclase activation. Mobility of the G protein or/and the C unit may still permit diffusional encounters of these components with the receptor in the activation process. Since receptor mobilization by (-)isoproterenol occurs at a similar rate as adenylate cyclase desensitization (Bakardjiev, unpublished results), the observed dispersal of receptors may be related to receptor transport and loss during desensitization (8). Further experiments using direct labeling with a fluorescent agonist are required to test this hypothesis.

B. New Affinity Chromatography Gels for Receptor Purification

Two types of ß-adrenergic affinity gels have been described so far (9,10). Both contain alprenolol as the immobilized ß-adrenergic ligand, attached via its allyl side chain and a hydrophilic spacerarm to an agarose matrix. Synthesis of these gels requires 6 (9) or 4 (10) reaction steps and is not adaptable to other ß-adrenergic antagonists lacking an allyl group. We have developed a new type of affinity gel (11) which has the following favorable features: (i) The synthesis is accomplished in only 3 analytically controllable steps, (ii) the concentration of immobilized ligand can be predetermined with reasonable accuracy, (iii) most ß-adrenergic antagonists can be immobilized in completely analogous fashion, (iv) due to stable ether and amine bonds between matrix, spacerarm and ligand, respectively, a time-dependent leakage of ligand from the gel is not encountered.

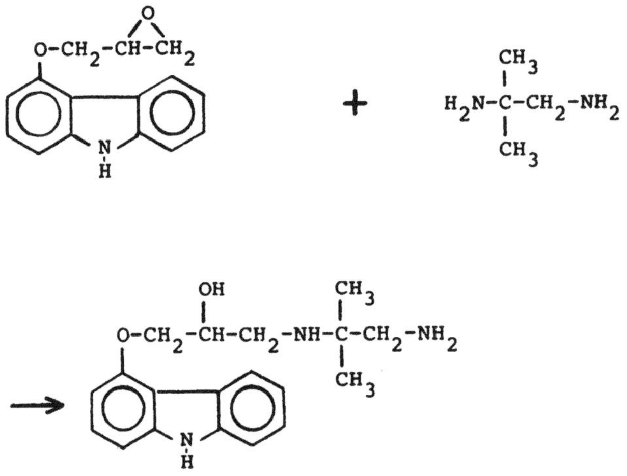

Fig. 4. Synthesis of carazolol-amine.

In the first step, a ß-adrenergic antagonist derivative possessing a primary amino group was synthesized. As an example, synthesis of carazolol-amine is shown in Fig. 4. The 1,2-epoxy-3-(carbazol-4-yloxy)-propane was generously provided by Dr. W. Bartsch, Boehringer Mannheim. Utilizing the analogous epoxide precursors of alprenolol, pindolol and cyanopindolol, amine derivatives of these antagonists have also been prepared. These compounds bind with high affinity to ß-adrenergic receptors of turkey erythrocyte membrane (K_D in the range of 10^{-10} to 10^{-9}M). As shown in Fig. 5, the antagonist amine derivative was reacted with the epoxide group of agarose derivatized with 1,4-bis-(2,3-epoxypropoxy)-butane to yield the affinity gel. The agarose-spacerarm derivative shown is also commercially available (Pharmacia Fine Chemicals). The concentration of

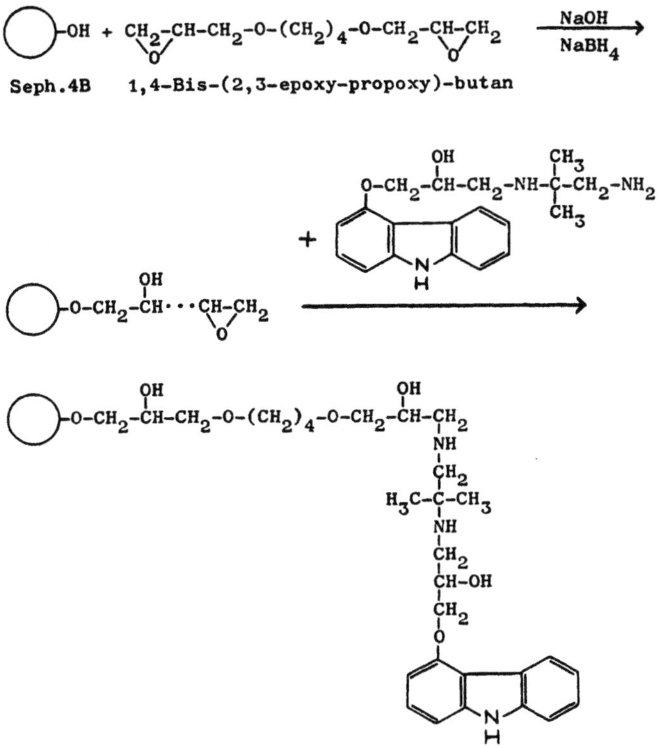

Fig. 5. Synthesis of an affinity gel with immobilized carazolol.

epoxide groups in this derivative can be easily titrated (12). For determination of immobilized ligand concentration, gel samples were made transparent by suspending them in a mixture of polyethyleneglycol (m.w. 6,000)/water (1:1, w/v), and the UV absorption of the ligand was measured directly in the transparent gel sample. The concentration of immobilized ligand could be predetermined; it was found to be proportional to the product of the reacting epoxide and free ligand concentrations at constant reaction time.

We have synthesized affinity gels with immobilized carazolol concentrations in the range of 0.07 to 4.4 µmol/g gel. For a rapid test of these gels with respect to binding and release

of ß-receptors, the following batch procedure was employed.
(1) Incubation of the affinity gel with a digitonin extract from turkey erythrocyte membranes containing solubilized ß-receptors, and separation of the supernatant by filtration.
(2) Washing of the gel with ice-cold buffer to remove nonspecifically adsorbed proteins.
(3) Incubation of the gel with 1 mM alprenolol to release receptors from the gel.
(4) Dialysis of the eluate to dissociate the receptor-alprenolol complex and remove alprenolol.
(5) Determination of receptor concentration by radioligand binding assay.
The recovery of purified receptors was found to be strongly dependent on the immobilized carazolol concentration in the respective gel. Maximal receptor recovery of 30% was obtained at 0.5 µmol carazolol/g gel. At < 0.1 µmol carazolol/g gel and >1 µmol carazolol/g gel, receptor recovery was only 10% or less. At 30% recovery, receptor purification with respect to total protein was up to 70-fold. Purification factors described in the literature don't exceed 100-fold for one cycle of batch affinity chromatography (13). Since the receptors are sufficiently stable, they may be progressively purified by several consecutive cycles of affinity chromatography. Very small amounts of highly purified ß-receptor have recently been isolated in this manner (13). We are now trying to work out an efficient method of receptor isolation using repeated purification cycles on the new ß-adrenergic affinity gels.

C. Photoaffinity Labeling of Receptor Subunits

Two radioactive arylazide derivatives of the potent ß-adrenergic antagonist, iodocyanopindolol (ICYP) have been prepared (14)(Fig. 6). The starting material of the synthesis, 2-cyano-4-(2,3-epoxypropoxy)-indol was a generous gift from Drs. G. Engel and R. Berthold, Sandoz Ltd, Basle, Switzerland. It was reacted with 1,2-diamino-2-methyl-propane to give 3,3-dimethyl-6-hydroxy-7-(2-cyano-indol-4yloxy)-1,4-diazaheptane (for an analogous reaction cf. Fig. 4). This intermediate was reacted either with methyl-4-azido-benzimidate or N-hydroxysuccinimidyl-4-azido-benzoate to give the noniodinated CYP-azide-1 and -2. Both compounds were radioiodinated with the chloramine-T method to theoretical specific radioactivity (2.2 Ci/µmol) and purified as described for $[^{125}I]$ICYP by Engel et al. (15,16).

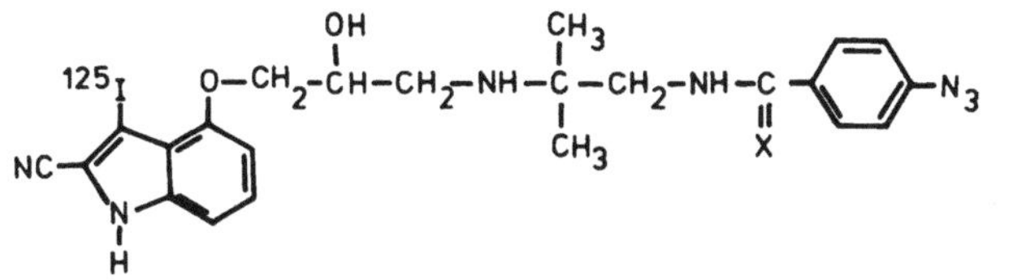

Fig. 6. Structure of two ß-adrenergic photoaffinity labels.

$[^{125}I]$ICYP-azide-1 and -2 bind with very high affinity (K_D = 40 pM) to the same total number of ß-adrenergic sites in turkey erythrocyte membranes as determined with reversible radioligands, e.g. $[^3H]$dihydroalprenolol or $[^{125}I]$iodohydroxybenzylpindolol. When the incubation mixture with membranes and $[^{125}I]$ICYP-azide-1 or -2 was irradiated with UV light (254 nm) for 5 min and subjected to SDS-polyacrylamide gel electrophoresis, part of the ^{125}I-radioactivity was incorporated in two proteins (Fig. 7 c, e - j). Another part of radioactivity migrated with the dye front; this was presumably due to free label or label bound to lipid molecules. No covalent incorporation of radioactivity into proteins occurred when the irradiation step was omitted or when $[^{125}I]$ICYP instead of $[^{125}I]$ICYP-azide was used (not shown). The photochemical reaction is therefore most likely a consequence of the reactivity of the nitrenes formed on photolysis of the aromatic azides. The Coomassie-blue staining profile of membrane proteins (Fig. 7 a, b) was not changed by irradiation, indicating that crosslinking of membrane proteins did not occur during the photolysis.

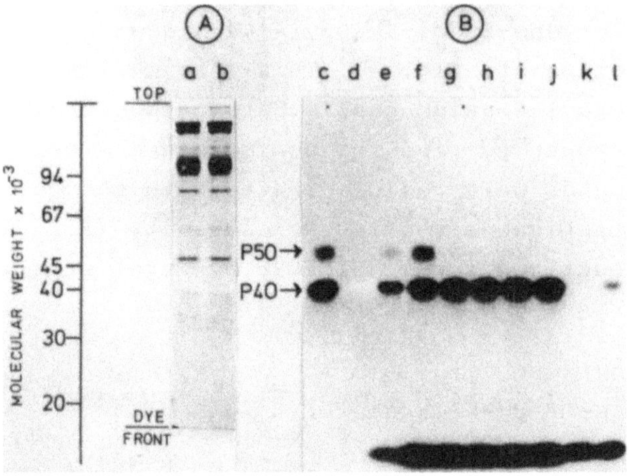

Fig. 7. SDS-polyacrylamide gel electrophoresis of turkey erythrocyte membranes after photoaffinity labeling with [^{125}I]ICYP-azide-1 and -2. A, Coomassie-blue staining profiles of control membranes kept in the dark (a) and UV-irradiated (b). B, Autoradiographs of photolabeled membranes. Concentrations of photoaffinity labels and non-radioactive competitors during the incubations were as follows: [^{125}I]ICYP-azide-2 at 30 pM (c) and at 30 pM in presence of 5 µM (-)alprenolol (d); [^{125}I]ICYP-azide-1 at 10 pM (e), 30 pM (f), 100 pM (g), 200 pM (h), 500 pM (i), 1,000 pM (j), 1,000 pM in presence of 5 µM (-)alprenolol (k), and 500 pM in presence of 20 µM (-)isoproterenol (l). The molecular weight scale given in the ordinate was obtained by using marker proteins (14).

The apparent molecular weight of the two proteins labeled by [^{125}I]ICYP-azides was 40,000 (P40) and 50,000 (P50). Labeling of P40 and P50 was ß-receptor specific because it could be prevented by incubation in presence of the ß-adrenergic antagonist, (-)alprenolol (Fig. 7 d, k) or the ß-adrenergic agonist, (-)isoproterenol (Fig. 7 l). The small residual labeling of P40 even in presence of 20 µM (-)isoproterenol may be explained on the basis of the relatively low receptor affinity of (-)isoproterenol (K_D = 0.34 µM). The two specifically labeled proteins, P40 and P50 may represent subunits of the ß-adrenergic receptor. P40 was under all conditions tested more heavily labeled than P50. Labeling of P40 increased in the range of 10 pM to 100 pM [^{125}I]ICYP-azide, approaching a limiting value at higher label concentrations (Fig. 7 e - j). Since this concentration dependence corresponds to the saturation of specific binding sites by the radioactive probe, it appears likely that P40 contains the ligand binding site of the receptor. Substantial labeling of P50 was only observed at [^{125}I]ICYP-azide concentrations below its K_D value (Fig. 7 c, e, f) whereas at higher probe concentrations, P50 labeling was weak and barely visible in the autoradiographs (Fig. 7 g - j). It appears therefore that higher (>30 pM) concentrations of [^{125}I]ICYP-azides promote a conformational change of the receptor which renders P50 less accessible to photoaffinity labeling. The relationship of the P50 protein to the P40 protein and to a possible ß-receptor subunit structure remains however unclear at present.

For quantitation of photoaffinity labeling, gel tracks were cut into 2 mm slices and counted. In Fig. 8 an autoradiograph and the corresponding histogram are shown resulting from a labeling experiment at 500 pM concentration of [^{125}I]ICYP-azide-2. Specific labeling of P40 is visible as a sharp peak in the histogram. Specific labeling of P50 amounts to only 8.3% of total specific labeling. At low (30 pM) concentration of [^{125}I]ICYP-azide-2, specific labeling of P50 represents 29% of total (not shown). The level of nonspecific labeling in presence of 5 µM (-)alprenolol is very low. When labeling experiments with [^{125}I]ICYP-azide-1 were quantitatively evaluated, very similar histograms as shown in Fig. 8 were obtained. The amount of free unbound radioactive probe migrating with the dye front was however consistently greater with [^{125}I]ICYP-azide-1 than with [^{125}I]ICYP-azide-2 (cf. Fig. 7). Taking into account the amount of ß-receptors in the sample and the specific radioactivity of the probe at the time of the experiment, the yield of specific label incorporation can be calculated.

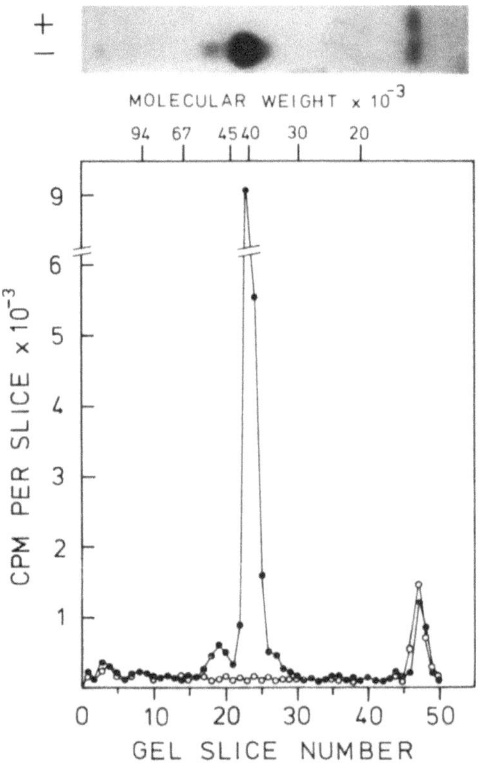

Fig. 8. Distribution of radioactivity in SDS-polyacrylamide gels after photoaffinity labeling of turkey erythrocyte membranes with [^{125}I]ICYP-azide-2. At the top, autoradiographs are shown from gels of membranes photolabeled at 500 pM [^{125}I]ICYP-azide-2 in the absence (-) and presence (+) of 5 µM (-)alprenolol. Below, radioactivity profiles of the same gels are plotted: without (-)alprenolol (●—●), with (-)alprenolol (○—○).

At saturating probe concentration (1 nM), yields of 8.9% and 17.2% were obtained with [^{125}I]ICYP-azide-1 and -2, respectively. These yields are quite satisfactory considering other photolabeling reactions reported in the literature. Since both probes bind reversibly to approximately the same total number of sites, the different yields of covalent incorporation may reflect an influence of structural features on the labeling reaction itself. For instance, the amidine group of [^{125}I]ICYP-azide-1 is protonated at pH 7.4 and therefore has a much higher polarity than the amide group of [^{125}I]ICYP-azide-2. The different polarities of these groups might affect the positioning of the probe at the site of reaction.

Photoaffinity labeling of ß-receptors using [^{125}I]iodoazidobenzylpindolol was recently described (17,18). In turkey erythrocyte membranes a polypeptide of M_r = 43,500 was specifically labeled which corresponds within the limits of error to the P40 labeled in our experiments. In the work cited, variable amounts of alprenolol-displaceable radioactivity were found at the top of the SDS-polyacrylamide gels complicating structural assignment. Furthermore the relative amount of nonspecific labeling was much higher than that in our present study. Molecular weights of ß-receptor proteins have also been determined using a different approach: solubilized receptor preparations were purified by affinity chromatography, radioiodinated and analyzed by SDS-polyacrylamide gel electrophoresis. Molecular weights of 170,000, 33,000 and 30,000 (19) or 70,000, 31,000 and 22,000 (20), respectively were reported for the intact ß-receptor and ß-receptor subunits from turkey erythrocyte membranes. Highly purified ß-adrenergic receptor from frog erythrocytes has a subunit molecular weight of 58,000 (13). Final clarification of ß-receptor subunit structure and composition will require isolation of these proteins in amounts sufficiently large to permit sequence analysis and physical characterization. The photoaffinity labels presented here may aid in identification of the ß-receptor polypeptides at all stages of purification.

References

1 Citri, Y., Schramm, M.: Nature 287, 297-390 (1980).

2. Ross, E.M., Gilman, A.G.: Annu. Rev. Biochem. 49, 553-564 (1980).

3. Tolkovsky, A.M., Levitzki, A.: Biochemistry 17, 3795-3810 (1978).

4. Tolkovsky, A.M., Levitzki, A.: Biochemistry 17, 3811-3817 (1978).

5. Koppel, D.E., Axelrod, D., Schlessinger, J., Elson, E.L., Webb, W.W.: Biophys. J. 16, 1315-1329 (1976).

6. Willingham, M.C., Pastan, I.: Cell 13, 501-507 (1978).

7. Henis, Y.I., Hekman, M., Elson, E.L., Helmreich, E.J.M.: Proc. Natl. Acad. Sci. USA (1981), in press.

8. Lefkowitz, R.J., Wessels, M.R., Stadel, J.M.: Curr. Topics in Cell. Regul. 17, 205-230 (1980).

9. Vauquelin, G., Geynet, P., Hanoune, J., Strosberg, A.D.: Eur. J. Biochem. 98, 543-556 (1979).

10. Caron, M.G., Srinivasan, Y., Pitha, J., Kociolek, K., Lefkowitz, R.J.: J. Biol. Chem. 254, 2923-2927 (1979).

11. Hassauer, M. (1981). Work performed in partial fulfillment of the requirements for Dipl. Chem. of the Faculty of Chemistry and Pharmacy, University of Würzburg.

12. Axên, R., Drevin, H., Carlsson, J.: Acta Chem. Scand. B29, 471-474 (1975).

13. Shorr, R.G.L., Lefkowitz, R.J., Caron, M.G.: J. Biol. Chem. 256, 5820-5826 (1981).

14. Burgermeister, W., Hekman, M., Helmreich, E.J.M.: J. Biol. Chem., submitted for publication.

15. Engel, G.: Triangle (Sandoz Ltd, Basle, Switzerland) 19, 69-76 (1980).

16. Engel, G., Hoyer, D., Berthold, R., Wagner, H.: Naunyn-Schmiedeberg's Arch. Pharmacol. (1981), in press.

17. Rashidbaigi, A., Ruoho, A.E.: Proc. Natl. Acad. Sci. USA 78, 1609-1613 (1981).

18. Rashidbaigi, A., Ruoho, A.E.: Fed. Proc. Fed. Am. Soc. Exp. Biol. 40, 1823 (abstract) (1981).

19. Durieu-Trautmann, O., Delavier-Klutchko, C., Vauquelin, G., Strosberg, A.D.: J. Supramolec. Struct. 13, 411-419 (1980).

20. Fraser, C.M., Venter, J.C.: Proc. Natl. Acad. Sci. USA 77, 7034-7038 (1980).

ROLE OF MEMBRANE LIPID COMPOSITION FOR ß-ADRENERGIC RECEPTOR FUNCTION

A. Bakardjiev
Inst. of Physiological Chemistry, Würzburg University,
Koellikerstraße 2, 8700 Würzburg, FRG

Introduction

Membranous environment may be crucial to hormonal regulation of adenylate cyclase because of its influence on the lateral distribution and association of the protein components. It has received increasing attention in recent years (1-5).

Earlier studies from this laboratory (6) strongly suggested that changes of the physical state of the plasma membrane bilayer influences the number of assayable ß-adrenergic receptors and specific activity of isoproterenol-stimulated adenylate cyclase. Chang liver cells in culture were fused with liposomes prepared from synthetic phospholipids and the plasma membrane was enriched with 20-30 mol% phospholipid. The data indicated that the phase transition, but not the charged group of the incorporated phospholipid was responsible for the changes in receptor number and cyclase activity. It was not clear what happens to receptors not available at 37°C. In this paper we extend our earlier observations by higher enrichment (40-60 mol%) of the plasma membrane of Chang liver cells with DMPC ("fluidizing") and DPPC (not "fluidizing" lipid). The date indicate that "disappearence"

Abbreviations used: DMPC, dimyristoylphosphatidylcholine; DPPC, dipalmitoylphosphatidylcholine; DOPC, dioleoylphosphatidylcholine; PBS, phosphate buffered saline of ß-receptors accompanies the phase transition even in control, not phospholipid enriched cells.

Materials and Methods

Cell material, preparation of liposomes and their fusion with cells as well as plasma membrane preparation were described previously (6). A random distribution of the incorporated phospholipids was ascertained by freeze-etch electron microscopy which was carried out by Dr. W. Haase from the Max-Planck-Institute for Biophysics in Frankfurt/M., FRG.

Measurement of cAMP. cAMP content of the cells and analysis of medium for cAMP was measured after 2 min exposal of the cells in monolayer to 1 x 10^{-5} M isoproterenol and 1 mM 1-methyl-3-isobutylxanthin according to Johnson et al. (7).

Binding Assay. Aliquots of intact cells were incubated with 2-16 nM DL-(^{3}H)carazolol or with 50-250 nM (^{3}H)hydroxybenzyl-isoproterenol in PBS buffer, pH 7.4 at 37°C for 5 min in a total volume of 500 µl. The samples were filtered through a 25 mm Whatman GF/B filter. The filter was washed five times with 5 ml cold 0.15 M NaCl, dried, and counted. Specific binding was defined as the amount of radioligand bound in the absence of competing ligand minus the amount bound in the presence of 5 x 10^{-5} M DL-carazolol. Temperature dependency of binding in the interval 4-37°C was measured with 4 nM DL-(^{3}H)carazolol. Incubation times were 5-30 min depending on incubation temperature. Maximal specific binding obtained under those conditions was ploted against temperature.

Fluorescence Measurements. Freshly harvested cells, suspended in PBS buffer, pH 7.4 were incubated with 5 x 10^{-3} M ethanolic solution of pyrene decanoic acid for 10 min at 37°C. Ethanol concentration was below 1 %. The cells were washed after incubation once with cold PBS buffer, suspended in the same buffer and the lateral mobility of the marker was measured between 10-40°C (8). Concentration of pyrene decanoic acid was 2-3 mol% of the cell lipid. For details see Galla and Sackmann (9) and Galla and Luisetti (10). The lateral diffusion coefficient of the marker (D_{diff}) was estimated according the equation:

$$D_{diff} = \frac{\lambda^2}{4} \cdot n_s \cdot \frac{I'}{I.k} \frac{k_f}{k_f' \tau_o'} \qquad [1]$$

where λ is the average jump length of a marker molecul; n_s is the average step number; I'/I is the experimentally obtained eximer to monomer ratio; k is a proportionality constant between I'/I and the ratio of quantum yields $\emptyset'/\emptyset$; k_f/k_f', the ratio of the transition probabilities for the radiative decay of the excited monomer and excimer; τ_o' is the radiative life time of the eximer, determined experimentally in Chang liver cell membrane with laser flash spectrometer.

The exact marker concentration was determined in each case from a calibration curve of I'/I against mol% label with respect to the total lipid extracted from normal cells. This curve was identical to those obtained with DOPC/DPPC liposomes (1:1) at 37°C. The sample was sonicated prior to this particular measurement.

A detailed description of the application of Montroll model for diffusion collision is given by Galla et al. (11). D_{diff} of pyrenedecanoic acid in control and phospholipid-manipulated cells was related to viscosity by means of the following empirical relationship (12):

$$D_{diff} = (1.0 + 1.07\eta)/(\eta + 0,26\eta^2) \cdot 10^{-5} cm^2 \ sec^{-1} \quad [2]$$

Results

Binding Studies. Incorporation of 20-30 mol% DOPC or DMPC into plasma membranes resulted in about 50% reduction of the number of binding sites per cell at 37°C. The same amount of DPPC had no effect on the receptor number (6). At higher enrichment with DPPC (40-60 mol%) the same loss of ß-receptors at 37°C occured. Comparable incorporation of DMPC (40-60 mol%) did not have additional effect to that already observed at lower incorporation (Fig.1).

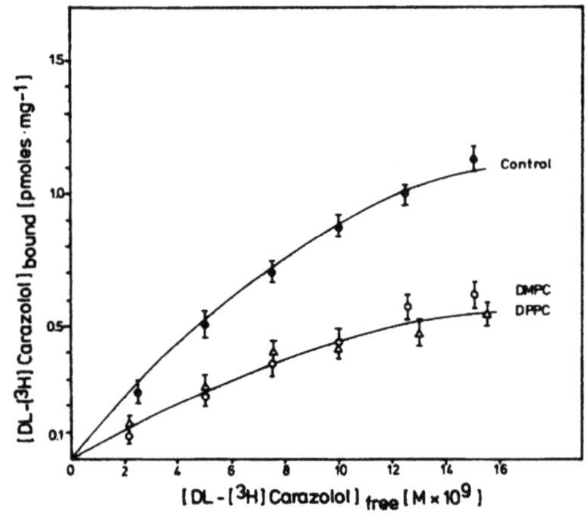

Specific binding of DL- (^{3}H) carazolol to Chang liver cells at 37°C. (● - ●) Control cells; (o - o) DMPC; (Δ - Δ) DPPC. Each point represents the mean of four experiments ± SD, respectively.

We compared some characteristics of control and highly enriched with DMPC or DPPC cells and their changes with the temperature. Antagonist binding component in liposomes separated after cell contact or in the cytosol of liposome-treated cells could not be recovered. It was still possible to consider endocytosis of the receptor, which is trapped in liposomes and not accessible to ligands. We compared the temperature dependency of DL-(^{3}H)carazolol binding to control and manipulated cells between 4 and 37°C. The maximal number of ß-adrenergic binding sites in all three cases was the same, but the positions of the binding maxima were at different temperatures (Fig.2).

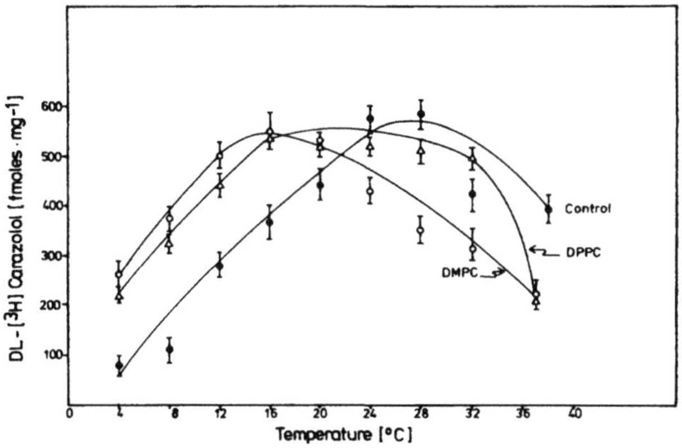

Temperature dependence of DL-(^{3}H)carazolol binding to control and phospholipid-enriched cells. For experimental details, see Materials and Methods. (● - ●) Control cells; (o - o) DMPC; (Δ - Δ) DPPC. The data are representative examples of several experiments. Each point is mean of four determinations ± SD.

A narrow maxima between 24 and 28°C in the control and between 16 and 20°C in DMPC-enriched cells are discernible, as well as a broad maximum between 16 and 32°C in DPPC-treated cells. The binding sites at 37°C compared with those of the corresponding maximum were reduced by 20-25 % in the control and by 60 % in lipid-manipulated cells.

The affinity of the assayable ß-receptors at physiological

temperature for the agonist (^{3}H)hydroxybenzylisoproterenol and for the antagonist, (^{3}H)carazolol was determined by Scatchard analysis of binding data (13). The calculated K_D values for the agonist in control and manipulated cells ranged from 2,2 to 3,1 x 10^{-7} M and for the antagonist - from 1,7 to 2,5 x 10^{-8} M. It indicates that the fraction of the receptors available in the phospholipid-enriched cells at 37°C had unchanged affinity to radioligands.

Adenylate cyclase. The specific agonist-stimulated activity of adenylate cyclase in Chang liver cells is directly proportional to the number of binding sites occupied by agonist (6). L(-)-Isoproterenol-stimulated activity in lipid-treated cells were reduced at 37°C, as expected, but not at 26°C for control and DPPC- and at 17°C for control and DMPC-enriched cells (Fig.3).

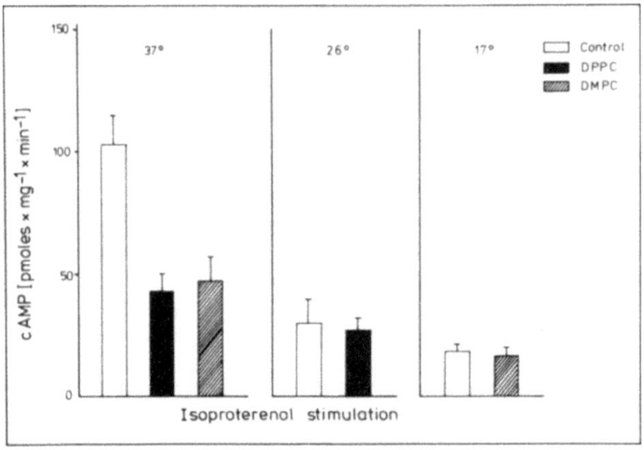

Specific activities of adenylate cyclase in Chang liver cells at different temperatures. Cells were incubated with 1 x 10^{-5}M isoproterenol. cAMP represents a sum of the maximal intracellular amount produced by the cells and the corresponding extracellular cAMP.

<u>Phase transitions and determination of pyrene decanoic acid lateral mobility in the membrane</u>. Whole cells were used for the fluorescence measurements reported below. The transition temperature, as well as the width of the transition, as measured with pyrenedecanoic acid as a probe, agree very well in whole cells, plasma membranes and total lipid extracts. The temperature dependence of the excimer to monomer ratio I'/I was followed up to 40°C (Fig.4).

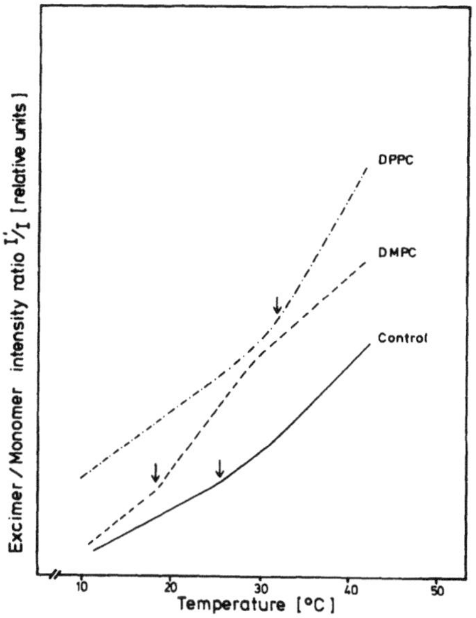

Temperature dependence of the excimer to monomer intensity ratio I'/I of pyrenedecanoic acid incorporated into normal and lipid-manipulated cells. Arrows indicate the beginning of the lipid phase transition. The data are representative examples of several experiments.

A slope change on the curve was interpreted as a beginning of order↔disorder transition of the phospholipids. Increasing the temperature only up to 32-33°C gave reversible curve. Exposure of the probe to a temperature above 40°C for 15 min caused a strong decrease of fluorescence and breakdown of the cells.

Characteristic breaks on the control curve were obtained at 25 and 30°C, suggesting lateral phase separation in this temperature interval. There was no change in the slope between 30 and 50°C in the melting curve of the lipids extracted from normal cells which suggested that above 30°C the lipids were in liquid-crystalline state.

Compared with control curve, the melting curve of DMPC-enriched cells showed discontinuities shifted to lower temperatures: 18° and 29°C. The width of the lateral phase separation was markedly affected (7°C extended to lower temperature). The onset of the phase transition in DPPC-enriched cells was at about 30-31°C. It was not possible to measure exactly the end of the melting process because of membrane decomposition.

Fluorescence studies carried out with lipids extracted from normal cells showed the same melting curve as those with the whole cells with less sharp discontinuities (data not shown). A visible and analogous to the cell-curves changes were obtained by addition of at least 30 mol% synthetic DMPC or DPPC.

Calculation of D_{diff} in control and phospholipid-manipulated cells. Table 1 presents a summary of calculated diffusion coefficients and viscosities in control and phospholipid-treated cells as well as in extracted lipids at 37°C. Two parameters have been taken from the literature: λ = 8 Å is given by the average distance of the lipid lattice and k_f/k_f' = 0,14 is a ratio determined for pyrenedecanoic acid (14). The excimer life time, τ_o' in the plasma membranes of Chang liver cells was $6,9.10^{-9}$ sec and *k* for this fluorescence probe and spectrometer was 0,49. The term n_s, the average step number is given by the equation:

$$n_s = \frac{2}{\pi \cdot X_{La}} \cdot \ln \frac{2}{X_{La}} \qquad [3]$$

where X_{La} is the molar fraction of label molecules with respect to the lipid.

Table 1: Diffusion coefficients of pyrenedecanoic acid and viscosities in membranes and lipid extracts at 37°C

	Cells		Lipid extract	
	D_{diff} ($\times 10^7$ cm^{2}sec^{-1})	η (P)	D_{diff} ($\times 10^7$ cm^{2}sec^{-1})	η (P)
Control	2,41 ± 0,55 (n = 7)	1,67	2,27	1,57
DMPC	2,72 ± 0,54 (n = 6)	1,47	2,30	1,57
DPPC	2,52 ± 0,48 (n = 8)	1,57	2,31	1,57

There is a striking similarity between the values of the lateral diffusion coefficients in plasma membranes and their lipid extracts as well as between control and manipulated cells.

Conclusions

1. The decrease of receptor number at 37°C in phospholipid-enriched cells is not caused by receptor endocytosis because receptor number is restored to normal level by adjusting the temperature to the "optimal" ranges given in Fig. 2.

2. A general fluidization of the membrane by the incorporated phospholipid can be excluded because the lateral diffusion coefficients of pyrenedecanoic acid at 37°C of control and lipid-enriched cells are approximately equal.

3. The decrease of receptor number correlates with the pretransition temperature of the incorporated lipids (Fig.2 and 4).

4. A hypothetical explanation for the reversible modulation of accessible receptor sites can be offered: The incorporated phospholipid is likely to participate in the lipid annulus surrounding the receptor. Above the pretransition temperature, the chain mobility of the incorporated lipid is increased (e.g. trans-gauche isomerization has been measured (15)). This may destabilize the exact orientation of the receptor in the membrane necessary for ligand binding. Lowering the temperature below the pretransition value restores a more rigid lipid annulus and reversibly permits an optimal orientation of the receptor.

5. It is possible that because of irregular distribution of the receptor on the cell surface the incorporated lipid effects association-dissociation process in the protein diluted membrane. The measured binding is lower although the receptor number is constant. The effect is seen above the phase transition temperature of the corresponding membrane,where a motion of the lipids begins.

Acknowledgements

The work was supported by a grant to E.J.M. Helmreich, A. Bakardjiev and W. Burgermeister from the Deutsche Forschungsgemeinschaft (He 22/34).

Literature

1. Rubalcava, B., and Rodbell, M.:J.Biol.Chem., 248, 3831-3837 (1973).
2. Puchwein, G., Pfeuffer, T., and Helmreich, E.J.M.: J.Biol.Chem.,249, 3232-3240 (1974).
3. Orly, J., and Schramm, M.: Proc.Natl.Acad.Sci., USA, 72, 3433-3437 (1975).
4. Houslay, M.D., Hesketh, T.R., Smith, G.A., Warren, G.B., and Metcalfe, J.C.: Biochim.Biophys.Acta,436, 495-504 (1976).
5. Hesketh, T.R., Smith, G.A., Houslay, M.D., McGill, K.A., Birdsall, N.J.M., Metcalfe, J.C., and Warren, O.B.: Biochemistry, 15, 4145-4151 (1976).
6. Bakardjieva, A., Galla, H.-J., and Helmreich, E.J.M.: Biochemistry, 18, 3016-3023 (1979).
7. Johnson, G.L., Wolfe, B.B., Harden, T.K., Molinoff, P.B., and Perkins, J.P.: J.Biol.Chem., 253, 1472-1480 (1978).
8. Freitag, G.: Diplom work, University Würzburg (1981).
9. Galla, H.-J., and Sackmann, E.: Biochim.Biophys.Acta, 339, 103-115 (1974).
10. Galla, H.-J., and Luisetti, J.: Biochim.Biophys.Acta, 596, 108-117 (1980).
11. Galla, H.-J., Hartmann, W., Theilen, U., and Sackmann, E.: J.Membrane Biol., 48, 215-236 (1979).
12. Dembo, M., Glushko, V., Aberlin, M.E., and Sonenberg, M.: Biochim.Biophys.Acta, 522, 201-211 (1979).
13. Scatchard, G.: Ann.N.Y.Acad.Sci., 51, 660-672 (1949).
14. Sackmann, E.: Z.physik.Chem.N.F., 101, 391-416 (1976).
15. Levin, I.W., and Bush, S.F.: Biochim.Biophys.Acta, 640, 760-766 (1981).

V. GLYCINE RECEPTOR
TETRAHYDROCANNABINOL RECEPTOR

PHOTOAFFINITY-LABELLING OF THE GLYCINE RECEPTOR OF RAT SPINAL CORD

D. Graham, F. Pfeiffer, H. Betz
Max-Planck-Institut für Psychiatrie, Abteilung Neurochemie, D-8033 Martinsried

Introduction

The amino acid glycine is a major inhibitory neurotransmitter in mammalian spinal cord (1-3). The binding of glycine molecules to their postsynaptic receptor sites leads to a hyperpolarization of the postsynaptic membrane via an increased conductance of chloride anions. This hyperpolarizing action of glycine has been shown to be antagonized specifically by the alkaloid strychnine. In synaptosomal membrane preparations from rat spinal cord a single class of high-affinity binding sites for the ligand, ^{3}H-strychnine, has been identified (4,5). The high-affinity binding of strychnine can be displaced specifically by glycine (4,5) and also non-competitively by chloride anions (6). ^{3}H-Strychnine thus is used as a probe for the postsynaptic glycine receptor.

Recently, the glycine receptor has been solubilized from rat spinal cord membranes and characterized as a 8.3 S macromolecule with a Stokes radius of 73 Å (4, and this volume). Also, a one-step affinity-chromatographic procedure has succeeded in highly purifying this receptor moiety (this volume). In the present study we were seeking to characterize the high-affinity strychnine binding site of the glycine receptor. ^{3}H-Strychnine was shown to be a natural photoaffinity ligand upon UV-illumination of the ligand in the presence of the receptor. A polypeptide with a molecular weight of 48,000 daltons was identified as the strychnine binding subunit of the postsynaptic glycine receptor.

Table 1. Incorporation of ^{3}H-strychnine into membranes from rat spinal cord upon UV-light illumination in the presence of various ligands.

Ligand	CPM Retained on Filter
^{3}H-strychnine	2423 ± 76 (n = 3)
^{3}H-strychnine (without illum.)	129 ± 20
^{3}H-strychnine + unlabelled strychnine	268 ± 69
^{3}H-strychnine + glycine	654 ± 33
^{3}H-strychnine + GABA	1696 ± 117
^{3}H-strychnine + glutamic acid	2672 ± 118
^{3}H-strychnine + histamine	2587 ± 181

Membranes were incubated for 30 min at 4°C in the presence or absence of the various ligands listed above (final concentrations: ^{3}H-strychnine = 23 nM; unlabelled strychnine = 100 µM; other ligands = 1 mM). After UV-light illumination, an excess of unlabelled strychnine was added to each incubation mixture to chase off ^{3}H-strychnine that was bound reversibly to the membranes. Aliquots of each incubation mixture were filtered through Whatman GF/B glass fibre circles. Each filter was subsequently washed extensively and counted in 7 ml of Aqualuma.

Irreversible UV-induced cross-linking of ^{3}H-strychnine to rat spinal cord membranes

When synaptosomal membranes from rat spinal cord were incubated with ^{3}H-strychnine and then illuminated with UV light, the radioactive ligand became bound irreversibly to these membranes (Table 1). With non-irradiated control samples, ^{3}H-strychnine was not incorporated irreversibly into the membranes. The UV-induced cross-linking of ^{3}H-strychnine to the membranes exhibited a glycinergic specificity: glycine, but not GABA or other neurotransmittory substances, dramatically reduced the irreversible incorporation of radioactive ligand.

Identification of 48K labelled polypeptide

Photoaffinity-labelled membranes were solubilized and then electrophoresed on 10% SDS gels and the gels subjected to fluorography. With the membranes that were exposed to UV-light in the presence of ^{3}H-strychnine, a polypeptide band with an apparent molecular weight of 48,000 $\pm$ 2,000 (n=3) was labelled (Fig. 1). Digestion of these labelled membranes with pronase did not subsequently produce a radioactive band upon fluorography, indicating that the labelled moiety is proteinaceous. The labelling of this polypeptide with ^{3}H-strychnine was inhibited in the presence of either glycine or unlabelled strychnine, but not in the presence of GABA.

Furthermore, solubilization of the postsynaptic glycine receptor from rat spinal cord membranes using non-ionic detergents, and then subsequent photoaffinity-labelling of the solubilized material with ^{3}H-strychnine in the presence of UV-light, also produced a 48,000 dalton labelled polypeptide upon electrophoresis and fluorography.

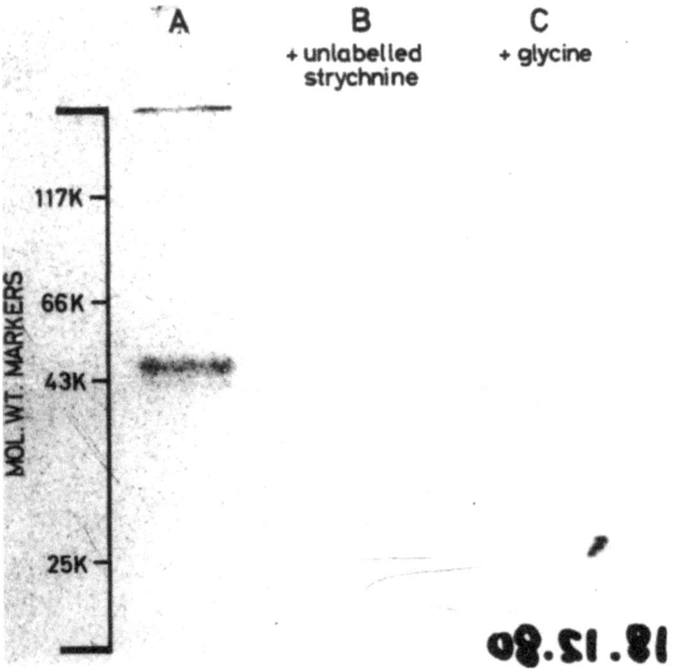

Fig. 1. Fluorogram illustrating irreversible ^{3}H-strychnine binding to rat spinal cord membranes upon UV-illumination. Lane A: membranes illuminted in the presence of ^{3}H-strychnine; Lane B: membranes illuminated in the presence of ^{3}H-strychnine and unlabelled strychnine; Lane C: membranes illuminated in the presence of ^{3}H-strychnine and glycine.

Discussion

The present report demonstrates that strychnine can be bound irreversibly to rat spinal cord membranes upon UV illumination. Under these conditions, strychnine labels a 48,000 M.W. polypeptide moiety. The pharmacological specificity of this labelling indicates that the 48,000 M.W. polypeptide contains the antagonistic binding site of the postsynaptic glycine receptor.

In conclusion, the photoaffinity-labelling procedure, as described here, may offer a valuable tool in the localization and characterization of the postsynaptic glycine receptor.

Acknowledgements

We wish to thank Ms G. Kurth and Ms S. Mayer for expert technical assistance. Also, the help of Ms C. Bauereiss and Ms E. Eichler during the preparation of this manuscript is gratefully appreciated. This work was supported by the Stiftung Volkswagenwerk and the Deutsche Forschungsgemeinschaft. H.B. holds a Heisenberg award from the Deutsche Forschungsgemeinschaft. The provision of laboratory facilities by the Max-Plank-Gesellschaft is gratefully acknowledged.

References

1. Curtis, E.R., Hösli, L., Johnston, G.A.R.: Exp. Brain Res. 6, 1-18 (1968).
2. Curtis, D.R., Hösli, L., Johnston, G.A.R., Johnston, I.H.: Exp. Brain Res. 5, 235-258 (1968).

3. Werman, R., Davidoff, R.A., Aprison, M.H.: Nature 214, 681-683 (1967).

4. Pfeiffer, F., Betz, H.: Brain Res. (in press, 1981).

5. Young, A.B., Synder, S.H.: Proc. nat. Acad. Sci. USA 70, 2832-2836 (1973).

6. Young, A.B., Synder, S.H.: Proc. nat. Acad. Sci. USA 71, 4002-4005 (1974).

SOLUBILIZATION AND PURIFICATION OF THE POSTSYNAPTIC GLYCINE RECEPTOR FROM RAT SPINAL CORD

F. Pfeiffer, D. Graham, H. Betz
Max-Planck-Institut für Psychiatrie, Abteilung Neurochemie, D-8033 Martinsried

1. Introduction

Several lines of evidence indicate that glycine is a major inhibitory neurotransmitter in the spinal cord and other parts of the central nervous system (1-5). The inhibitory action of glycine is caused by an increased chloride conductance of the postsynaptic membrane. Strychnine, an alkaloid from Strychnos nux-vomica, specifically antagonizes the postsynaptic action of glycine and thus causes convulsions (2). High-affinity strychnine binding to spinal cord membranes is glycine-displaceable and therefore is thought to occur at the postsynaptic glycine receptor (6). In an attempt to biochemically characterize the glycine receptor, we have solubilized and purified the high-affinity strychnine binding site from rat spinal cord.

2. Solubilization of the glycine receptor

Spinal cord and brain stem from 150 g Wistar rats were dissected and immediately frozen in liquid nitrogen. Membranes were prepared from the frozen material by differential centrifugation as described (7). The membranes were suspended in 25 mM potassium phosphate buffer, pH 7.4, containing 200 mM KCl, frozen in liquid nitrogen and stored at -70°C. The glycine receptor could be solubilized from these membranes using Triton X-100. Routinely, 1-3 % (w/v) Triton X-100 and KCl-concentrations of 0.2 - 1 M were used. After 1 h at 4°C with repeated homogenization, unsolubilized material was removed by centrifugation for 1 h at 150 000 g. The binding of ^{3}H-strychnine to the supernatant was determined, using a polyethyleneglycol precipitation assay (7). Other detergents, such as Nonidet P-40, cholate, deoxycholate and octylglucoside also solubilized the glycine receptor from spinal cord membranes (F. Pfeiffer, unpublished).

3. Characterization of the glycine receptor

Scatchard analysis of ^{3}H-strychnine binding data showed a single class of binding sites with dissociation constants of 11.3 nM and 20.4 nM for membranes and Triton-extract, respectively. The concentrations of the receptor agonists glycine, β-alanine and taurine required for half maximal displacement of ^{3}H-strychnine binding were similar in both preparations, but GABA had little effect. The glycine receptor thus retained its pharmacological properties upon solubilization.

Sucrose density gradient centrifugation revealed a sedimentation coefficient of 8.3 S for the Triton-solubilized glycine receptor. Upon gel exclusion chromatography, the strychnine binding activity could only be preserved if phospholi-

Table 1: Properties of the solubilized glycine receptor

1) K_D for strychnine binding 20.2 ± 0.7 nM.
2) Strychnine binding inhibited by glycine, β-alanine, taurine.
3) Sedimentation coefficient of 8.3 ± 0.4 S.
4) Stokes radius of 73 ± 3 Å.
5) Phospholipid required for stability.
6) Strychnine binding site located on 48 kD polypeptide.

pids were included in the column buffer (7). The receptor migrated with a Stokes radius of 73 Å. These figures indicate a molecular weight of more than 200 kD for the receptor-detergent micelle. In addition, photoaffinity-labelling of membrane-bound and solubilized glycine receptor with ^3H-strychnine labelled only one polypeptide with 48 kD molecular weight (8, and see this volume). From these results it is concluded that the glycine receptor is a multimeric protein with a 48 kD strychnine binding subunit.

4. Purification

The solubilized glycine receptor was purified more than 1000-fold by one-step affinity chromatography on strychnine-derivatized agarose. In order to minimize non-specific ionic and hydrophobic interactions, the purification was performed in the presence of 1 M KCl and 1 % (w/v) Triton X-100. Pharmacologically specific elution was achieved with glycine. This procedure ensured that only active receptor was eluted, and that even after extensive purification the glycine and strychnine binding sites interacted with each other.

SDS-Polyacrylamide gel electrophoresis of the purified material revealed a simple polypeptide pattern. The major protein had a molecular weight of 48 kD, corresponding to the photoaffinity-labelled polypeptide from spinal cord membranes (8). In order to investigate the receptor specificity of the isolated polypeptides, equal amounts of Triton-extract were adsorbed onto equal amounts of strychnine-derivatized agarose in the presence or absence of strychnine. After elution with glycine and SDS-gelelectrophoresis, the polypeptide patterns of both eluates were compared. As shown in figure 1, a 48 kD and a 92 kD polypeptide were found after absorption in the absence of strychnine only, and thus

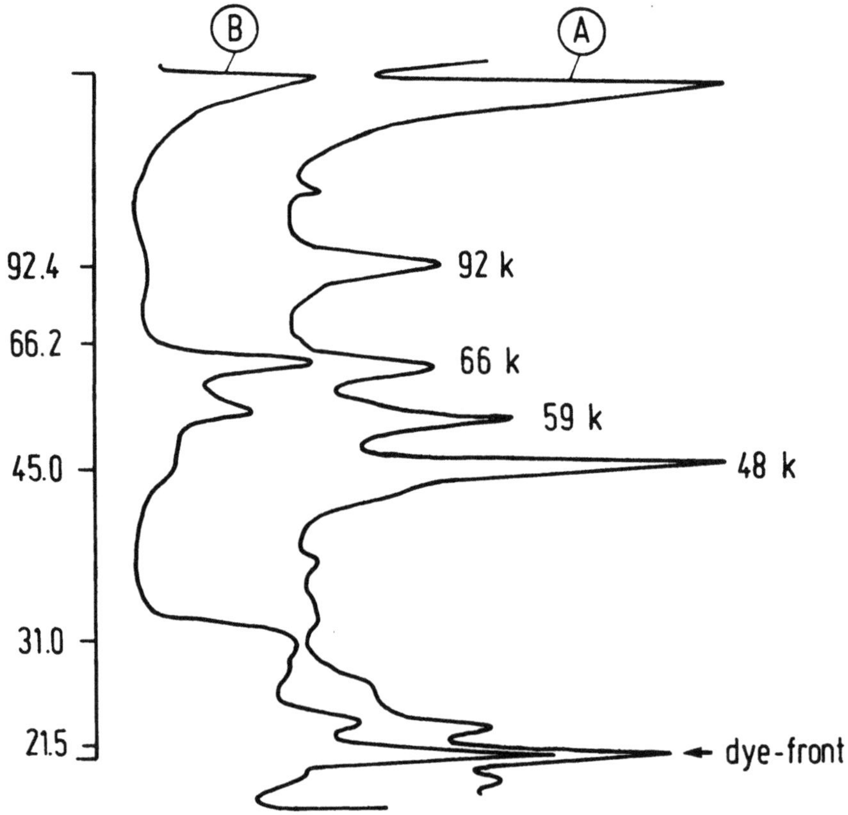

Fig.1. Densitometric tracings of silver-stained SDS-polyacrylamide gels of:
A: The affinity-purified glycine receptor. Triton-solubilized glycine receptor was bound to strychnine-derivatized agarose in the presence of 1% (w/v) Triton X-100 and 1 M KCl. After washing, the receptor was eluted with 200 mM glycine. Using this procedure, the glycine receptor was purified more than 1000-fold.
B: Material unspecifically bound to strychnine-derivatized agarose. Triton-solubilized glycine receptor was incubated with strychnine-derivatized agarose under the same conditions as in A, except that 100 µM strychnine was present in the incubation mixture. Under these conditions, the receptor was not retained and only nonspecifically absorbed material was eluted with glycine.

are considered to be receptor-specific. A 59 kD-band was much fainter in the "nonspecific" eluate, which probably indicates the superposition of a specific and a nonspecific band.

The affinity-purified glycine receptor bound to concanavalin A- and wheat germ agglutinin-sepharose and thus is thought to be a glycoprotein. Chromatography on lectin columns was used to remove glycine from the purified receptor preparation. After elution, the receptor was photoaffinity-labelled with ^{3}H-strychnine and subjected to SDS-gelelectrophoresis. Fluorography as well as gel-slicing showed that the 48 kD polypeptide was labelled.

5. Conclusions

The postsynaptic glycine receptor can be efficiently solubilized by Triton X-100 and other detergents.

Upon solubilization, the receptor retains its pharmacological properties.

The detergent-solubilized glycine receptor exhibits a sedimentation coefficient of 8.3 S and a Stokes radius of 73 Å.

The glycine receptor can be purified more than 1000-fold from membrane extracts by a one-step affinity-chromatographic procedure.

The strychnine-binding subunit of the glycine receptor, a polypeptide of 48 kD as revealed by photoaffinity-labelling, is the major polypeptide in our purified receptor preparation. Additional polypeptides of 59 kD and 92 kD molecular weight also seem to be receptor-associated.

The glycine receptor binds to immobilized lectins and thus is a glycoprotein.

Thus, after the peripheral nicotinic acetylcholine receptor, the glycine receptor may become the second biochemically well characterized neurotransmitter receptor coupled to a chemically gated ion channel.

Acknowledgments

We thank Ms G. Kurth and Ms S. Mayer for technical assistance and Ms E. Eichler and C. Bauereiss for help during the preparation of the manuscript. Work in the authors' laboratory was supported by the Stiftung Volkswagenwerk and by the Deutsche Forschungsgemeinschaft. H.B. holds a Heisenberg award from the Deutsche Forschungsgemeinschaft. The provision of lab space and facilities by the Max-Planck-Gesellschaft is gratefully acknowledged.

References

1. Curtis, D.R., Hösli, L., Johnston, G.A.R.: Exp. Brain Res. 6, 1-18 (1968).
2. Curtis, D.R., Hösli, L., Johnston, G.A.R., Johnston, I.H.: Exp. Brain Res. 5, 235-258 (1968).
3. Werman, R., Davidoff, R.A., Aprison, M.H.: Nature 214, 681-683 (1967).
4. Cunningham, R., Miller, R.F.: Brain Res. 197, 123-138 (1980).
5. Collingridge, G.L., Davies, J.: Brain Res. 212, 345-359 (1981).
6. Young, A.B., Snyder, S.H.: Molec. Pharmacol. 10, 790-809 (1974).
7. Pfeiffer, F., Betz, H.: Brain Res., in press.
8. Graham, D., Pfeiffer, F., Betz, H.: Biochem. Biophys. Res. Comm., in press.

IS THERE A THC RECEPTOR?
CURRENT PERSPECTIVES AND APPROACHES TO THE ELUCIDATION OF THE MOLECULAR MECHANISM OF ACTION OF THE PSYCHOTROPIC CONSTITUENTS OF CANNABIS SATIVA L.

Michael Binder and Ingo Franke

Institut für Physiologische Chemie der
Ruhr-Universität Bochum
Postfach 10 21 48, D-4630 Bochum 1
Federal Republic of Germany

Summary

(3R,4R)-Δ^1-Tetrahydrocannabinol (=Δ^1-THC) is the major psychoactive constituent of the drugs hashish and marihuana derived from the indian hemp, cannabis sativa L. In spite of the widespread use of the drug, scientific research sofar has offered little information on the molecular mechanism of action of Δ^1-THC. This paper discusses the current hypotheses including some evidence that Δ^1-THC acts on a specific neuronal receptor of its own. It further describes our work on cannabinoid model compounds and the synthesis of cannabinoid affinity gels.

Introduction

The drugs hashish and marihuana derived from the indian hemp, cannabis sativa, have a long history of use by men, dating back to the old vedic scriptures of 1200 B.C. Only some 15 years ago the structure of its psychotropic principle (3R,4R)-Δ^1-tetrahydrocannabinol (=Δ^1-THC) (s. Fig. 1) was elucidated, followed by several stereospecific syntheses of this compound and for the last ten years a lot of work has been devoted to biochemical, pharmacological and psychological investigations. Sofar neither pharmacologists nor neurochemists have provided really conclusive evidence concerning the molecular mechanism of action of THC.

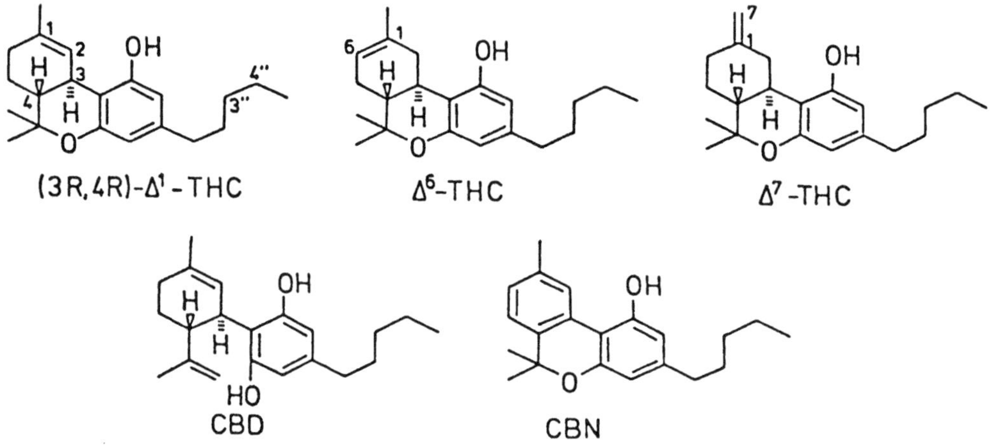

Fig. 1 Structures of the natural cannabinoids Δ^1-THC, Δ^6-THC, CBD and CBN.
Δ^7-THC was prepared by synthesis from Δ^6-THC.

Let us briefly review why Δ^1-THC is a candidate for interactions on the neuronal level:

Δ^1-THC exerts its psychotropic activity at concentrations in the nano to micromolar range, comparable to physiological neurotransmitter levels. The action of the drug is stereospecific, the enantiomeric (3S,4S)-Δ^1-THC being practically inactive. Structure-activity relationships (8) like this demonstrate that very little may be changed about the molecule without causing complete loss of psychotropic activity. The phenolic hydroxyl group of Δ^1-THC should be free or, if derivatized, easily hydrolysable. The double bond in the isoprenoid part of the molecule enjoys a certain degree of freedom. The $\Delta^{1(2)}$ (=Δ^1-THC) and the $\Delta^{1(6)}$ (=Δ^6-THC) isomers are psychotropically active, shifting the double bond to the 1(7) (=Δ^7-THC) position abolishes activity. Carbons No. 3 and 4 must be in the R-configuration. The aliphatic pentyl side chain may be shortened, lengthened or branched to some extent.

These structural features are prerequisites for the interaction of Δ^1- or Δ^6-THC with a specific receptor, a lock to which this molecular key fits tightly. Below, some speculations on the topography of this lock, the hypothetical THC receptor will be offered.

The hydrophobicity of Δ^1-THC leads to serious difficulties: detergents or organic solvents must be used in receptor assays which might give rise to experimental artefacts. A comparison of the structure of Δ^1-THC to those of the well established neurotransmitters reveals no similarities, in fact the molecule not even contains nitrogen - this would be expected of any reasonable psychotropic drug - and, therefore, is unsuited for ionic interactions.

Hypothetical mechanisms of action of Δ^1-THC.

Three hypotheses on the action of Δ^1-THC are discussed at present.

First, Δ^1-THC interacts with the lipid phase of the neuronal membrane by changing its fluidity and (or) permeability, thus posing as a general anaesthetic.

Second, Δ^1-THC acts on one or several of the known neurotransmitter-receptor systems influencing availability, reuptake or turnover of the transmitters or interacting with the corresponding receptors.

Third, Δ^1-THC acts on a receptor of its own, implicating the existence of a physiological THC agonist.

The latter hypothesis seems the most attractive one. It might lead to the discovery of something like the enkephalins and, therefrom, to therapeutically interesting compounds.

The membrane hypothesis

Based on a certain structural resemblance of Δ^1-THC to steroids and on experiments with spin-labeled liposomes it was concluded that Δ^1-THC behaved to some extent like alfaxalone, a steroid anaesthetic, fluidizing the neuronal membrane and mimicking the action of general anaesthetics. This action of Δ^1-THC was compared to the psychotropically inactive cannabinoids cannabidiol (CBD) and cannabinol (CBN) and a differential effect was claimed (4).

The structure-activity considerations discussed above and the investigation of the psychotropically inactive Δ^7-THC (1) which closely resembles Δ^1-THC in its physicochemical properties indicate that the rather specific psychotropic effects of Δ^1-THC could not be explained by such rather unspecific interactions with membranes.

The transmitter hypothesis

Early investigations on the influence of Δ^1-THC on biogenic amines were controversial, the in vitro experiments with synaptosomal preparations indicating a reduced uptake of radioactively labeled transmitters or their precursors. In a typical in vitro experiment Δ^1-THC was shown to inhibit the uptake of ^{3}H-trypthophane and ^{3}H-choline in a crude mouse brain synaptosomal preparation at 30 µmol/l while pretreatment of the mice with up to 100 mg Δ^1-THC/kg (!) did not influence the uptake characteristics of synaptosomes prepared from these impregnated brains.

A reduction in hippocampal turnover of acetylcholine accompanied by a twofold increase in GABA turnover after Δ^1-THC was interpreted as a GABAmimetic action of the cannabinoid (10).

The most promising results come from experiments with "in vivo labeled" synaptosomes prepared after intravenous injection of cannabinoids in mice (e.g. 10 mg Δ^1-THC/kg). These synaptosomes showed an increased uptake of dopamine (DA), norepinephrine (NE), 5-hydroxytryptamine (5-HT) and especially GABA. This increase was specific for Δ^1-THC. A much smaller effect was observed with CBD and (3S,4S)-Δ^6-THC gave no effect at all. The increase in DA uptake was more pronounced in cortical synaptosomes compared to a striatal preparation and Δ^1-THC blocked stereotyped behaviour induced by tail pinch (like haloperidol) but not stereotyped behaviour induced by amphetamines and apomorphine (unlike haloperidol). It was, however, suggested that Δ^1-THC might act as a DA antagonist in the cortex, thereby stimulating the activity of several neurotransmitter systems (6).

Recently it was demonstrated that Δ^1- and Δ^6-THC had a biphasic effect on transmitter uptake: low concentrations (10^{-8} - 10^{-7} mol/l) stimulated DA and NE uptake, larger concentrations (10^{-5} - 10^{-4} mol/l) inhibited uptake. CBD and CBN led only to inhibition of uptake (9).

There is some specific, high affinity, displaceable binding of Δ^6-THC to the crude nuclear fraction from hepatoma cells and some displaceable but not saturable binding to rat brain homogenates. The latter type of binding was stereospecific: no displacement of Δ^6-THC was obtained with (3S,4S)-Δ^1-THC at 37°C. The action of Δ^6-THC (and Δ^1-THC) on steroid receptors was implicated (5). This may hold for a number of "steroidal" actions of Δ^6-THC, not discussed in this review, but seems rather unlikely concerning the psychotropic action of Δ^1- and Δ^6-THC which has a quick onset in the range of a few minutes.

To sum up, in spite of many hints, there is at present no clearcut evidence for the specific interaction of Δ^1-THC with one of the known neurotransmitter-receptor systems.

The THC receptor hypothesis

The idea that Δ^1-THC acts on a specific receptor of its own is more or less the consequence of the inconclusive results discussed above. It was formulated first by Edery and others in 1971 (2) and we believe to have some more, still indirect evidence for the existence of this receptor. Δ^7-THC was conceived on the base of molecular model considerations as the THC isomer being closest to the psychotropically active Δ^1- and Δ^6-THC's (1). In fact, the only actual difference is a steric one: in its energetically most favourable conformation, the exocyclic methylidene group (C-7) of Δ^7-THC which has replaced the methyl group of Δ^1- and Δ^6-THC lies only 0.1 nm above the plane of the aromatic ring of the molecule compared to the 0.2 nm of the methyl group (C-7) in Δ^1- and Δ^6-THC. To illustrate this, steric formulas of Δ^1- and Δ^7-THC are given in Fig. 2.

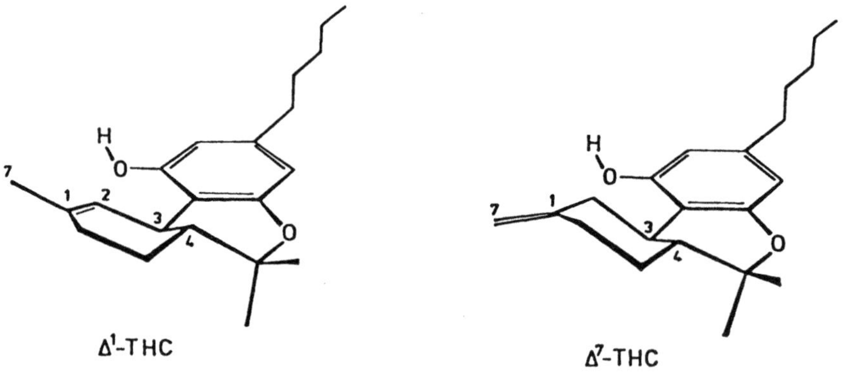

Fig. 2 Steric formulas of Δ^1-THC and Δ^7-THC. Note that in Δ^7-THC C(7) is closer to the plane of the aromatic ring than in Δ^1-THC.

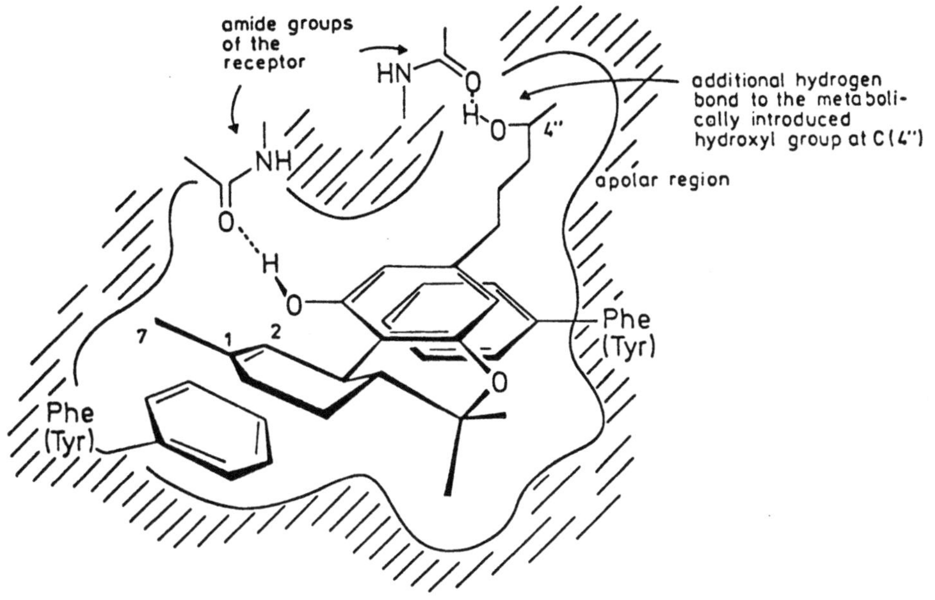

Fig. 3 Δ^1-THC on its hypothetical receptor. Close contact is achieved between carbons (1), (2), (6) and (7) and an aromatic residue (Phe or Tyr) of the receptor.

Thus the molecule has become somewhat flatter. This difference, nothing else having been changed, is sufficient to prevent the binding of Δ^7-THC to the receptor. In the rhesus monkey Δ^7-THC in doses up to 100 times the threshold dose of Δ^1-THC required to elicit behavioural changes, is completely devoid of psychotropic activity. This observation defines the topography of the THC receptor more strictly and we dare draw a picture of the receptor (Fig. 3). Supposing the receptor to be a protein or lipoprotein there should be an aromatic nucleus at the THC binding site, able to interact with the π electrons of the double bond in 1(2), 1(6) or 1(7) position. The phenolic hydroxyl group forms a hydrogen bond to an amide group of the protein, and an apolar region on the receptor interacts with the aliphatic side chain of the THC's.

Metabolites of Δ^1-THC bearing hydroxyl groups at C-7, C-3" or C-4" are of slightly higher psychotropic potency than the parent compound, probably because these hydroxyl groups can form additional hydrogen bonds to the receptor. Now, in Δ^7-THC the van der Waals interaction of the methylidene group C-7 with the receptor "surface" prevents the formation of the phenolic hydrogen bond and the binding of Δ^7-THC to the receptor causing thus the psychotropic inactivity of Δ^7-THC.

Though this picture is still speculative, Δ^7-THC remains an essential tool to differentiate between unspecific effects of Δ^1- and Δ^6-THC caused by their similarity to steroids or their lipophilicity and their specific effects on the "psychotropic" THC receptor. Any effect of Δ^1-THC that can be mimicked by Δ^7-THC does not relate to the mechanism of the psychotropic action of Δ^1-THC.

How to isolate the THC receptor?

Based on the evidence for the existence of the THC receptor resulting from our work with Δ^7-THC, we have devised an affinity chromatography approach to isolate THC binding macromolecules. As mentioned above 3"-hydroxy- and 4"-hydroxy-$\Delta^{1(6)}$-THC are strongly psychotropic indicating that in these positions of the pentyl side chain some space is left for a substituent without inhibiting the binding to the receptor (cf. Fig. 3). Therefore we synthesized two affinity ligands, (3R,4R)-$\Delta^{1(6)}$-THC-5"-oic acid (13a) and 4"(R,S)-methyl-(3R,4R)-$\Delta^{1(6)}$-THC-5"-oic acid (13b) via the substituted resorcinols 10a and 10b resp.. The experimental details for the syntheses of 10a and 10b have been published (3). This synthesis is outlined in Figs. 4 and 5. Both acids 13a and 13b were coupled to AH-Sepharose 4B using 1-ethyl-3-(3'-dimethylaminopropyl)-carbodiimide (EDC) leading to the affinity gels 14a and 14b. The yields of coupled ligands, calculated on the NH_2 group density of the sepharose (24 -40 mol/g gel) ranged from 25 to 50 %.

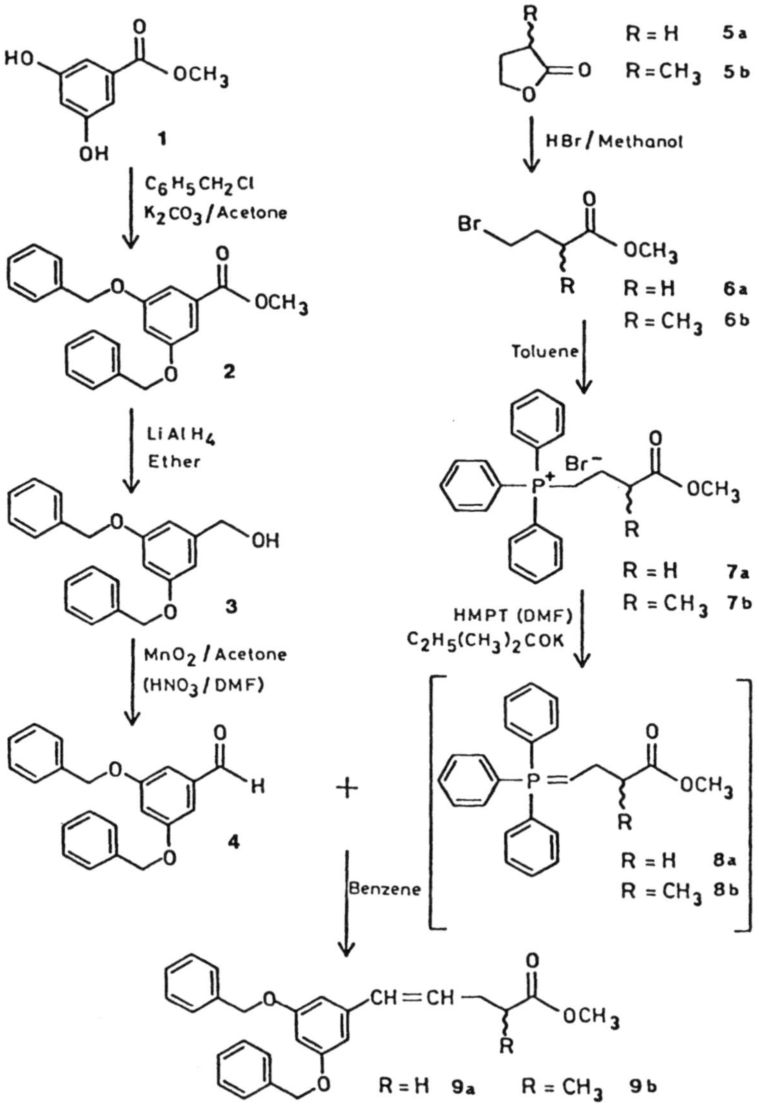

Fig. 4 Syntheses of the affinity gels.

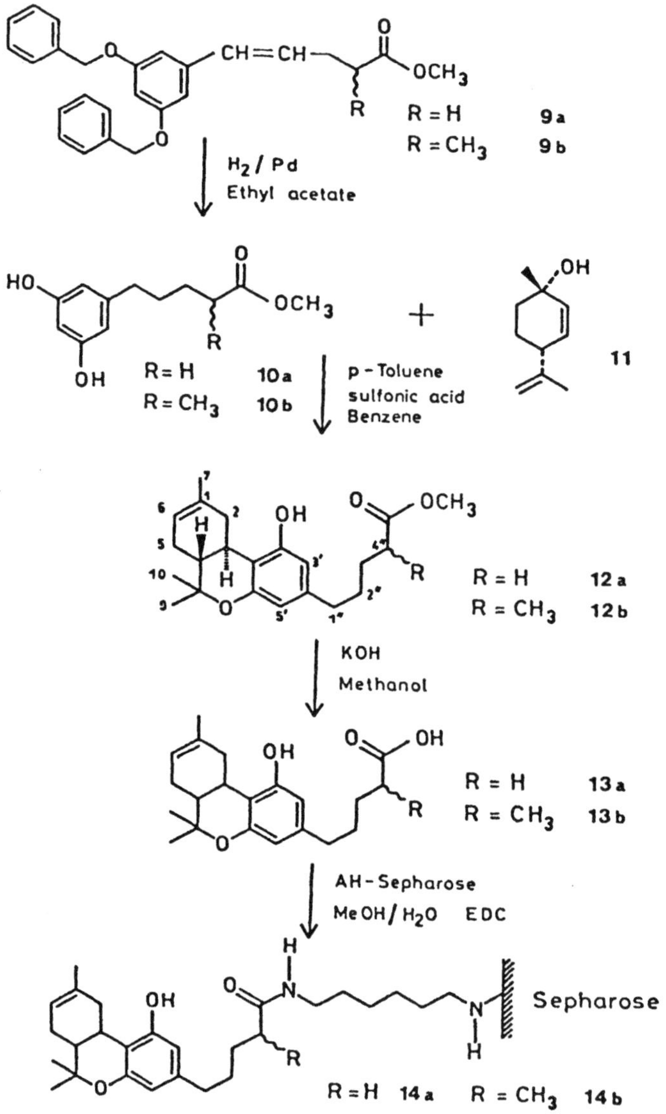

Fig. 5 Syntheses of the affinity gels (continued).

Work on the isolation and characterisation of THC binding macromolecules is in progress.

The authors thank the Deutsche Forschungsgemeinschaft for financial support of the syntheses of the affinity gels.

References

1. Binder, M., Edery, H., Porath, G.: In: G.G. Nahas, W.D.M. Paton (Eds.), Advances in the Biosciences, Vols. 22 & 23, "Marihuana: Biological Effects", Pergamon Press, Oxford and New York, 71 - 80 (1979).
2. Edery, H., Grunfeld, Y., Ben-Zvi, Z., Mechoulam, R.: Ann. N.Y. Acad. Sci. 191, 40 - 50 (1971).
3. Franke, I., Binder, M.: Helv. chim. acta 63, 2508 - 2514 (1980).
4. Gill, E.W., Jones, G., Lawrence, D.K.: Biochem. Pharmacol. 22, 175 - 184 (1973).
5. Harris, L.S., Carchman, R.A., Martin, B.R.: Life Sci. 22, 1131 - 1138 (1978).
6. Hershkowitz, M., Szechtman, H.: Eur. J. Pharmacol. 59, 267 - 276 (1979).
7. Johnson, K.M., Dewey, W.L.: Psychopharmacology 17, 83 - 87 (1978).
8. Mechoulam, R., Edery, H.: In: R. Mechoulam (Ed.) "Marijuana", Academic Press, New York, 101 - 136 (1973).
9. Poddar, M.K., Dewey, W.L.: J. Pharm. Exp. Ther. 214, 63 - 67 (1980).
10. Revuelta, A.V., Cheney, D.L., Wood, P.L., Costa, E.: Neuropharmacology 18, 525 - 530 (1979).

VI. ACETYLCHOLINE RECEPTOR (central and muscarinic)

CHARACTERIZATION OF A PUTATIVE NICOTINIC ACETYLCHOLINE RECEPTOR IN CHICK RETINA

Heinrich Betz and Hubert Rehm
Max-Planck-Institute for Psychiatry, Department of Neurochemistry, 8033 Martinsried, Germany

1. Introduction

Snake venom α-toxins bind with high affinity to the agonist recognition sites of the nicotinic acetylcholine receptor (AChR) in fish electric organ and skeletal muscle and thus block cholinergic receptor function in these excitable tissues (1-3). One of these basic polypeptides, α-bungarotoxin (α-Btx) from Bungarus multicinctus, has become an important tool for characterizing and purifying AChR from muscle and related sources (see this volume).

Binding sites for α-Btx having nicotinic cholinergic specificity are also found in the peripheral and central nervous systems of vertebrates and invertebrates (4,5). Though often referred to as nicotinic AChR, the nature of these toxin sites has been a matter of considerable debate since α-Btx is unable to antagonize the nicotinic cholinergic response of various types of neurons (4,5). Here, we summarize studies on the α-Btx binding protein of chick retina. It is suggested that this protein may be tentatively identified as a neuronal nicotinic AChR.

2. Distribution, ontogenesis and regulation of the α-Btx binding protein in chick retina

In 1976, Vogel and Nirenberg showed that chick retina contains high affinity binding sites for [^{125}I]α-Btx (6). In the adult animal, these sites are located at synapses in the inner plexiform layer (7). On embryonic retinal neurons in tissue culture, however, α-Btx receptors are distributed over the entire cell surface (6; see fig. 1). Synaptogenesis in the retina thus involves a redistribution of the toxin binding component on the neuronal cell surface, i.e. receptor concentration in the synaptic membrane. Similar localization processes in the developing motor endplate have been extensively documented for muscle AChR (3,8).

Fig. 1. Autoradiograph of a [^{125}I] α-Btx labeled neuron from chick embryo retina in tissue culture.

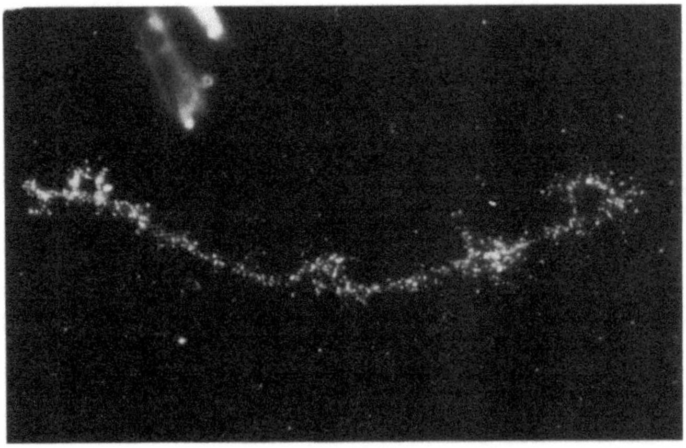

In addition to its synaptic localization in vivo, the ontogenesis and regulation in tissue culture of the retinal α-Btx binding site are also consistent with the hypothesis that this toxin receptor is associated with a neuronal nicotinic AChR:

i) the α-Btx receptor content of developing retina shows a peak at hatching, i.e. after most of the synapses have been formed, and declines thereafter (9). A similar developmental pattern is found with muscle AChR and reflects the degradation of excess extrasynaptic receptor molecules after innervation (10-12); ii) in primary cultures of chick neural retina, the accumulation of α-Btx binding sites can be modulated by membrane depolarizing agents and cyclic nucleotides in a fashion analogous to that found with AChR in embryonic muscle cell cultures (8, 13-15).

3. Properties of the retinal α-Btx binding site

The major pharmacological and biochemical properties of the α-Btx binding site of chick retinal neurons are listed in table 1 (for data see ref. 16). Both the kinetics of the toxin binding reaction and its inhibition by drugs acting on

Table 1: Properties of the retinal α-Btx binding site

1) High affinity for α-Btx (K_D = 0.57 nM, K_{+1} = 1.76 x 10^5 $M^{-1}sec^{-1}$, K_{-1} = 1.15 x $10^{-4}sec^{-1}$).

2) Toxin binding inhibited by nicotinic cholinergic ligands, local anaesthetics, histrionicotoxin.

3) Sedimentation coefficient of detergent-solubilized toxin binding site 10.5 - 11.0 S.

4) Is a glycoprotein.

5) Exposure to nicotinic cholinergic agonists (but not antagonists) produces a time-dependent increase in agonist affinity.

6) Crossreacts with antibodies to AChR from *Torpedo marmorata*.

the peripheral AChR are compatible with the α-Btx binding glycoprotein being a nicotinic cholinergic receptor. Agonist-induced changes in ligand affinity and an immunological cross-reactivity with antibodies against AChR from Torpedo marmorata further support this interpretation. The major argument against identifying the toxin binding sites as AChR comes from electrophysiological and Na^+-flux studies. With neither method, an antagonism of nicotinic-cholinergic responses by α-Btx could be detected (16,17).

In order to explain the discrepancy between the physiological and the biochemical and binding data, it has been proposed that only a part of the cholinergic agonist binding sites of the neuronal AChR may be occupied by α-Btx (4,16). For fish and muscle AChR, the existence of two agonist sites per receptor molecule which both bind α-toxin has been documented in detail (2,18). If one assumes that neuronal AChR also contains two or more functional agonist binding sites of which only one is accessible to α-toxins, a simple model for explaining the inefficiency of α-Btx in blocking neuronal nicotinic-cholinergic transmission can be designed (fig. 2).

Fig. 2. Models for α-Btx binding to peripheral and central AChR.

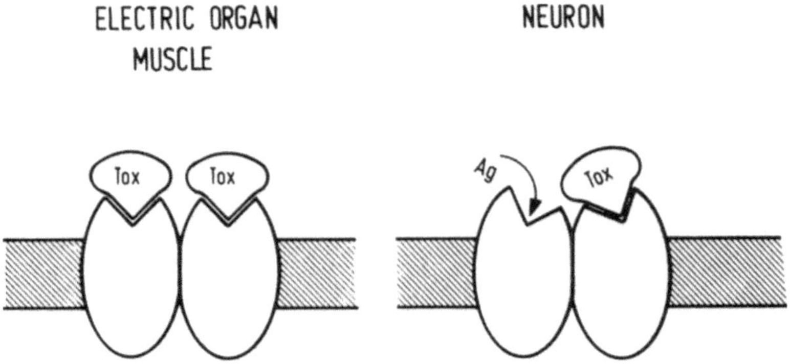

Recently, we have provided evidence for the existence of cryptic α-Btx binding sites in neuronal membranes. Both phospholipase C treatment and detergent extraction were found to double the absolute number of high affinity binding sites for [^{125}I]α-Btx in retinal membrane fractions (fig. 3; 19). Interestingly, the unmasked toxin binding sites can be distinguished from the preexisting ones by a different sensitivity to the divalent cation Co^{2+} (19).

Fig. 3. Scatchard plots of [^{125}I]α-Btx binding to phospholipase C-treated (o) and control (x) membrane fractions from chick retina.

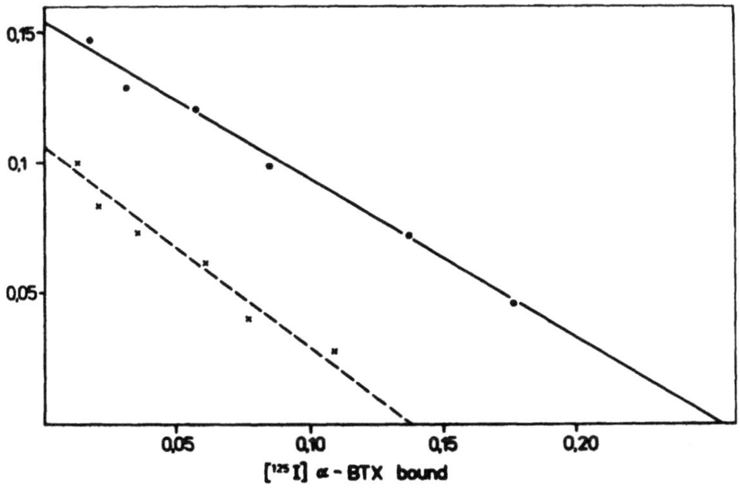

The subunit structure of the neuronal α-Btx binding protein is not yet well explored. Preliminary crosslinking studies with [^{125}I]α-Btx and affinity purification from [^{35}S]methionine-labelled retina cultures suggest that the major polypeptide involved in toxin binding has an apparent molecular weight of 55K. In addition, polypeptides of 38K and 26K may be located close to the α-Btx binding domain (20).

4. Conclusions

The synaptic localization, the metabolism and the immunological and pharmacological properties of the α-Btx binding protein in chick retina suggest that this protein is identical to or associated with a neuronal nicotinic AChR. Both the toxin binding affinity and the currently available data on the subunit structure of the retinal receptor distinguish it from the peripheral AChR in skeletal muscle or electric organ. These differences may be the result of a different evolution of a common ancestor AChR polypeptide (21).

Acknowledgments

We thank Ms U. Müller for expert technical assistance, Ms E. Eichler and C. Bauereiss for help during the preparation of the manuscript, and Drs. D. Graham and F. Pfeiffer for a critical reading. Work in the authors' laboratory was supported by the Deutsche Forschungsgemeinschaft (grant Be 718/5,6 and Heisenberg award to H.B.). The provision of lab space and facilities by the Max-Planck-Gesellschaft is gratefully acknowledged.

References

1. Chang, C.C., Lee, C.Y.: Arch. Int. Pharmadyn. Ther. 144, 241-257 (1963).
2. Heidmann, T., Changeux, J.P.: Ann. Rev. Biochem. 47, 317-357 (1978).
3. Fambrough, D.: Physiol. Rev. 59, 165-227 (1979).

4. Morley, B.J., Kemp, G.E.: Brain Res. Rev. 3, 81-104 (1981).

5. Oswald, R.E., Freeman, J.A.: Neuroscience 6, 1-14 (1981).

6. Vogel, Z., Daniels, M.P., Nirenberg, M.: Proc. Natl. Acad. Sci. USA 73, 2370-2374 (1976).

7. Vogel, Z., Maloney, G.J., Ling, A., Daniels, M.P.: Proc. Natl. Acad. Sci. USA 74, 3268-3272 (1977).

8. Betz, H. and Rehm, H.: In Biological Chemistry of Organelle Formation (Bücher, T., Sebald, W., Weiss, H., eds.) pp. 175-186, Springer Verlag, Berlin-Heidelberg-New York (1980).

9. Wang, G.K., Schmidt, J.: Brain Res. 114, 524-529 (1976).

10. Betz, H., Bourgeois, J.P., Changeux, J.P.: FEBS Lett. 77, 219-224 (1977).

11. Burden, S.: Devel. Biol. 61, 79-85 (1977).

12. Betz, H., Bourgeois, J.P., Changeux, J.P.: J. Physiol. 302, 197-218 (1980).

13. Betz, H.: Adv. Physiol. Sci. 36, 313-322 (1981).

14. Betz, H., Rehm, H.: Soc. Neurosci. Abstr., Vol.6, p.253 (1980).

15. Betz, H., Changeux, J.P.: Nature 278, 749-752 (1979).

16. Betz, H.: Eur. J. Biochem. 117, 131-139 (1981).

17. Masland, R.H., Ames, A.: J. Neurophysiol. 32, 424-442 (1976), and personal communication.

18. Colquhoun, D.: in The Receptors (O'Brien, R.D. ed.) Vol. 1, pp. 93-142, Plenum Press, New York-London (1979).

19. Rehm, H., Betz, H.: Biochem. Biophys. Res. Comm., in press (1981).

20. Betz, H., Graham, D., Rehm, H.: in preparation.

21. Tsartos, S.J., Lindstrom, J.M.: Proc. Natl. Acad. Sci. USA 77, 755-759 (1980).

PHARMACOLOGICAL CHARACTERIZATION OF SOME PROPERTIES OF THE MUSCARINIC RECEPTOR OF SMOOTH MUSCLE CELLS

D. Kuhnen-Clausen

Fraunhofer-Institut für Toxikologie und Aerosolforschung
D 5948 Schmallenberg-Grafschaft

Introduction

Long before clearcut biochemical investigations could be done with purified receptor protein, pharmacological characterisations of receptors have been done with isolated organs of smooth muscle cells (e.g. 1,2). By the analysis of structure-activity relationships, attempts were made to describe the surface of muscarinic receptors (3-5). Further studies are still limited to the in situ receptor because purification procedures gave unstable preparations with low yields (6). From binding studies to homogenates of brain or of ileum muscle cells results were obtained which often differ from the pharmacological dates with respect to the homogenity of the receptor type, to affinity constants and to the mechanisms of agonism and antagonism (7,8).

Pharmacological characterization of properties of the muscarinic receptor are based on the dose response relationship to receptor activation, keeping in mind, that this relationship is not necessarily linked by a linear proportionality. A chain of events is coupled with receptor activation, which finally leads to the specific response of the effector cell. Nevertheless, respecting this statement, some informations can be obtained with the investigation of drug receptor interactions. This paper presents results of the last ten years and discusses questions of structure activity relationship of different pyridinium compounds with the muscarinic receptor, of the significance of reactive disulfide bonds or sulfhydryl groups for the receptor activation, and the significance of the use of alkylating agents for the demonstration of reserve receptors.

Methods and Materials

Longitudinal muscle strips, isolated from the guinea pig ileum according to (2) were suspended in an organ bath at 37 ^{o}C, containing Tyrode solution of the following composition (mM): NaCl 137, KCl 3.7, $CaCl_2$ 1.8, $MgCl_2$ 1.05, NaH_2PO_4 0.2, $NaHCO_3$ 11.9, glucose 5.5 and hexamethonium chloride 0.01. The bath was gassed with 5 % CO_2 in O_2, the pH was 7.4. Isotonic contractions were recorded on a kymograph with a magnification von 1 : 8. The load of the lever was 150 mg.

Cumulative dose response curves to acetyl-ß-methylcholine (MeCh) were performed as described recently (9). The activity of antagonists were defined as pA_2-values according to (10): pA_2 is the negative logarithm of the antagonist concentration in M that requires a doubling of the dose of the agonist to compensate for the action of the antagonist. As a reference compound for competitive antagnism Lachesine (benzylate ester of ethyldimethyl(2-hydroxymethyl)ammonium chloride) was chosen because of its structural relationship to acetylcholine or MeCh. For further detail see text.

Results and Discussions

A. Structure-activity relationship of pyridinium salts to the muscarinic receptor.

A large series of pyridinium salts was synthesized in a systematical search for drugs with antidotal properties against organophosphorus poisoning (11-14). Because organophosphorous compounds inhibit acetylcholinesterase (AChE, E.3.1.1.7.), the antidotal effects should not only protect or reactivate the enzyme but also protect nicotinic and muscarinic receptors against endogenous AChE, released in excess after AChE-inhibition. The antimuscarinic activity was found to depend on substituents and their position in the pyridinium ring (15). The most active substances were those which bear hydrophobic groups (16,17). Kinetical analyses of the antagonism of mono- and bisquaternary pyridines against muscarinic agonists lead to the supposition that the mechanism of action was not allways a classical competitive one (18-20).

To answer the question, whether a pyridinium ring binds to the same site where the onium group of acetylcholine (ACh) or MeCh can be attached, N-(ß-Acetoxyethyl)pyridinium salts were synthesized and tested for muscarinic receptor interactions (19). Agonist activity indicates that receptor binding is substantially retained when the ammonium group of ACh is formally replaced by a pyridinium ring. The introduction of alkyl groups in position 4 of the ring yields antagonists. A tert.-butylpyridinium derivative (HB 6, Fig. 1) is proved to have an antimuscarinic activity superior to that of the methyl pyridinium salt.

The agonistic action of the unsubstituted pyridinium salt is very similar to that of MeCh. Dose response curves have the same shapes and maxima, they display the same intrinsic activity. However, 250 fold higher concentrations of the pyridinium salt than of MeCh are needed to induce equivalent respondes. This is thought to originate in the low degree of complementarity between the pyridinium ring and the onium binding site. A conformational analysis (21) showes a crowded conformation of the pyridinium salt related to intramolecular interactions of the anionic and cationic heads, which are more effective than in ACh due to the reduced spherical screening around the nitrogen atom. Also the charges of the pyridinium salt are quite different from those of ACh. The charges of polar groups and the cationic head of the pyridinium compound are lower than in ACh. These differences decrease the apparent affinity of the pyridinium compound but not the intrinsic activity, when compared with ACh of MeCh. Seemingly, the introduction of the tert.-butylgroup into the pyridinium ring affects both conformation and charges, abolishes the intrinsic activity and transforms the parent compound from an agonist to an antagonist, which acts on muscarinic receptors by a competitive mechanism (19).

Bisquaternary pyridinium salts (Tab. 1) display also antimuscarinic activities. Their affinities are influenced by the substituents in both rings and increase with increasing hydrophobicity of the molecules. Therefore it was assumed that a nonpolar area is located in the direct vicinity of the anionic centre of the muscarinic receptor. Such a nonpolar site has been postulated in former studies (22). On the other hand, with accessory

TABLE 1. Bisquaternary pyridinium salts with antimuscarinic properties. Their affinities (pA_2-values) depend on the substituents in the rings.

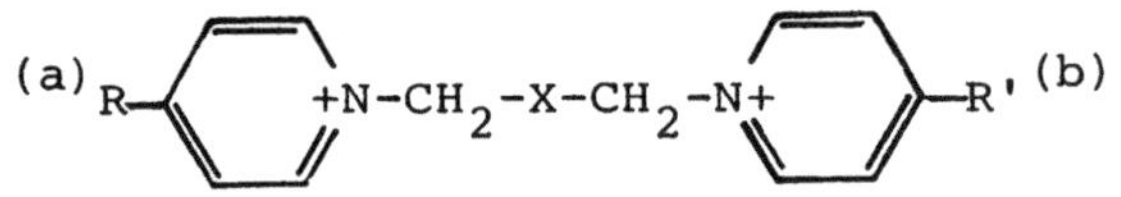

compound	R	a	R'	b	X	
TMB-4	-CH=N-OH	4	-CH=N-OH	4	$-CH_2-$	4.7
Toxogonin	-CH=N-OH	4	-CH=N-OH	4	-O-	4.2
SAD 128+	$-C(CH_3)_3$	4	$-C(CH_3)_3$	4	-O-	5.3
HY 10	$-CH=N-O-C(CH_3)_3$	4	$-CH=N-O-C(CH_3)_3$	4	-O-	5.1
HY 39	$-NH-CO-C(CH_3)_3$	4	$-NH-CO-C(CH_3)_3$	4	-O-	5.8
HGG 42	-CH=N-OH	2	$-CO-C_6H_{11}$	3	-O-	5.3
HGG 12	-CH=N-OH	2	$-CO-C_6H_5$	3	-O-	5.8

+ref 11 and 12

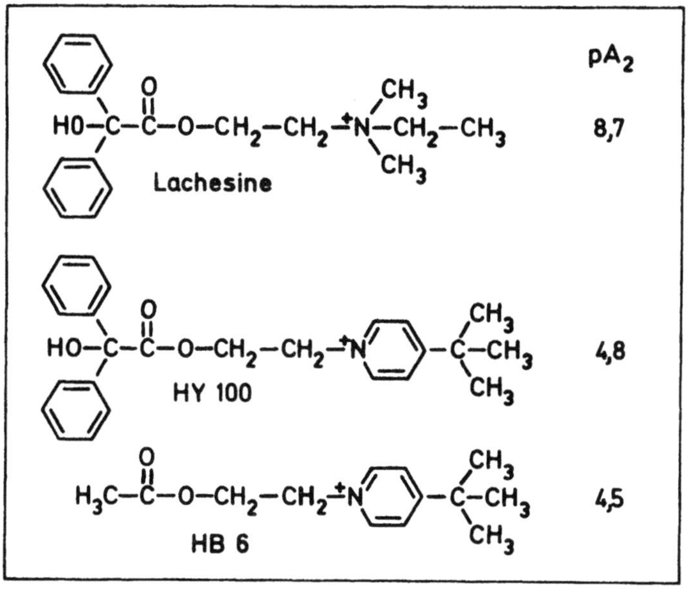

Figure 1. Structural analogues of acetylcholine with hydrophophobic moieties and ring structures either at the ester site or the ammonium site. Note the influence of the substituents on the affinity (pA_2-value) of the antimuscarinic compounds.

binding areas near the ester binding site, to which bulky ring structures as in Benzilylcholine or Lachesine (Fig. 1) bind, the antagonistic effect of such molecules has been described (23). The increased affinities of symmetrically substituted pyridinium salts like SAD 128 or HY 10 or HY 39, when compared with the oxime substituted compound TMB-4 or Toxogonin (Tab. 1), possibly may be interpreted by a binding to both postulated areas. There is some evidence for this hypothesis, as shows Fig. 1. As metioned above, in the pyridinium analogue of ACh with antimuscarinic properties, the compound with the tert.-butylgroup is the more active antagonist than that with a methyl group in the ring. Fig. 1, however, shows, that both nonpolar areas are not independent, their simultaneous occupation is less favourable than the occupation of the nonpolar area near the ester binding site.

The results, represented here, lend support to the supposition, that the symmetrically substituted compound of Tabl. 1 bind only with one of the pyridinium rings to the ACh recognition site of the muscarinic receptor. Further evidence will be presented in the following chapters.

B. The significance of disulfide bonds and sulfhydryl groups in muscarinic receptor activation

Intact disulfide bonds and sulfhydryl groups have been shown to be essential for the capacity of brain muscarinic receptors to bind agonists and antagonists (6,8). For smooth muscles some evidence could be demonstrated for an inhibitory effect of -SH group blockade but not of S-S bond reduction (24). Further experiments on this problem shall be presented here.

Ileal muscle strips were exposed for 10 min to 1 mM of dithioerythriotol (DTE), a disulfide reducing reagent. The treatment caused a slight sensitization to MeCh with no significant changes in maximum contraction or n_H values of the Hill plot, constructed with the dose response curves to MeCh. The effect is irreversible by washing. The same effect will be obtained, when histamine is the spasmogene for the muscle strips, and is regarded therefore as a nonspezific action of DTE. S-S- bonds seem to play a negligible role with respect to muscarinic receptor activation.

On the other hand, -SH groups seem to be essential for the induction of contractions of smooth muscles by MeCh. When the muscle strips are exposed to 15 μM of p-chloromercurybenzoate (PCMB), a mercaptide-formating agent, for 10 min and then rinsed extensively, dose response curves of MeCh are shifted to higher concentrations of the agonist. The shift increases with time and comes up to an apparent steady state after 50-60 min. The shift is accompagnied by a moderate decrease of the maximum contraction and an increase in the n_H values of the respective Hill plot. These effects resemble the desensitization of the muscle preparation after a treatment with high doses of MeCh. The desensitizing effect of PCMB can be prevented by a pre-treatment of the muscle strips with 1 mM DTE.

For inhibitors that are supposed to produce their effects on a specific receptor, more definite arguments are obtained from protection experiments with specific ligands like the agonist proper or its competitive antagonists. Such experiments have been done with MeCh, Lachesine and two bisquaternary pyridines, Toxogonin and HY 10 (Tab. 1). The compounds were added to the organ bath 2 min prior to the addition of PCMB for 10 min. Then the preparations were rinsed, and after a resting time of 5 min four subsequent dose response curves to MeCh were constructed with a time intervall of 15 min. From these curves the ratios of MeCh concentrations, necessary to produce 10 % maximum contraction after and before the treatment with PCMB, were determined. A plot of the reciprocal of the dose ratios (1/DR) versus post-incubation time reflects the loss of sensitivity of the ileal muscles for the agonist.

Fig. 2 shows protection experiments with MeCh and Lachesine, in the concentrations of 80 nM and 10 nM respectively. The dose of the agonist MeCh produces in the untreatened muscle preparation of about 40 % maximum contraction but no desensitization. The dose of the antagonist Lachesine induces a dose ration of MeCh of about 5. Both compounds display in no way any protecting effect. In contrast, they enhance the onset of the desensitization of the ileal muscle by PCMB. However, protection can be achieved by the application of the pyridinium compounds HY 10 or Toxogonin in the concentraions of 50 μM and 0.1 mM, respectively. These doses are equieffective to the dose of Lachesine. The results are presented in Fig. 3.

According to these results, reactive -SH groups are involved in muscarinic receptor activation and its sensitivity to the

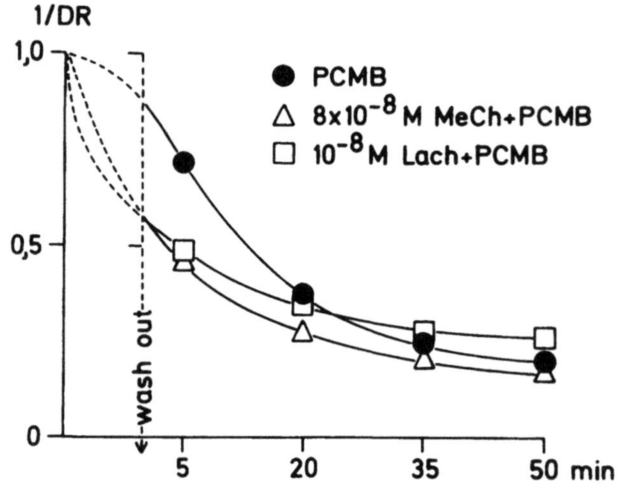

Figure 2. Protection experiments with the agonist acetyl-ß-methylcholine (MeCh) or the antagonist Lachesine (Lach) against -SH blockade by p-chloromercurybenzoate (PCMB). Ordinate: relative sensitivity; abszissa: time after incubation (10 min). (Further details see text).
In the presence of the specific ligands, the desensitizing effect of PCMB is accelerated

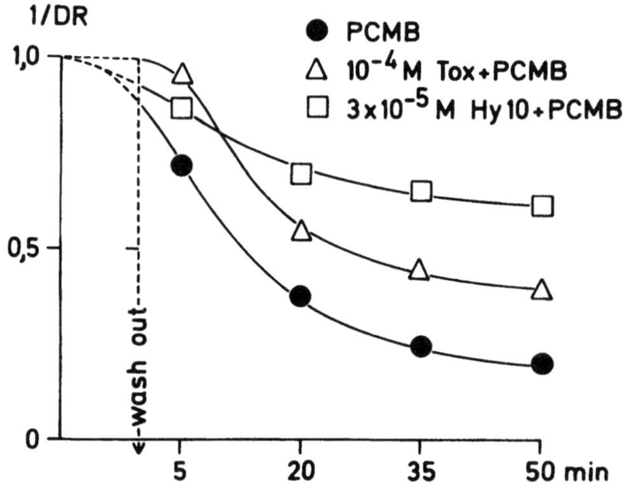

Figure 3. Protection experiments with two bisquaternary pyridines with antagonistic properties against -SH blockade by p-chloromercurybenzoate (PCMB). Ordinate and abszissa like in Fig. 2.
The presence of the antagonists, with a relative low affinity (Tab. 1) inhibits the desensitizing effect of PCMB

agonist MeCh. Seemingly, in the resting receptor the sulfhydryl groups are "burried" within the receptor molecule and PCMB need to cross a diffusion barrier before mercaptide-formation can occur. The occupation of the receptor by specific ligands like the activator MeCh oder the specific antagonist Lachesine exposes the -SH groups thus increasing the velocity of the mercaptide-formation. Weaker antagonists, structurally different from specific muscarinic ligands with respect to the CO-O-C-C- chain, stabilize the receptor conformation or its environment with the "burried" -SH groups and, therefore, protect the sulfhydryl groups against reduction. The highly protective effect of HY 10 is assumed to stem from the binding to hydrophobic areas near the muscarinic receptor through the tert.-butyl groups of this compound (Tab. 1).

C. The problem of Dibenamine and the receptor reserve

The concept of the receptor reserve is based on the assumption that potent agonists need to occupy only a small fraction of the total receptor concentration to generate maximum response of the effector cell. This assumption is founded in attemps to reduce the concentration of particular ligang receptors by the mean of irreversible blocking agents. The alkylating compound Dibenamine ($(C_6H_5CH_2)_2NCH_2CH_2Cl$) produces with potent agonists an initial parallel shift of the dose response curves prior to the reduction of maximum response, thus blocking different receptor types like those of muscarin, catecholamines, histamine and others (3, 25-28). It was supposed that Dibenamine alkylates exclusively a given specific receptor and that the reduction in maximum response occurs when all reserve receptors are occupied by the irreversible antagonist. The specificity of the effect of Dibenamine has been studied by means of protection experiments with potent competitive antagonists of the respective receptor-specific agonist. Also cross protection experiments have shown, that acetylcholine but not catecholamines or histamine protects muscarinic receptors and vice versa (27).

In studies on the parasympatholytic effects of quaternary pyridines on the isolated guinea pig ileum (9), a treatment with Dibenamine changed the activities of some of these compounds. This observation is not consistent with the simple elimination of a fraction of muscarinic receptors, but is linked to the assumption that alkylation may modulate the binding sites for the pyridines and/or the specific receptor activation. Another doubt arises on the direct interaction of Dibenamine with muscarinic receptors from protection experiments with the agonist MeCh proper. Normally very high concentrations are used to overcome the irreversible effect of Dibenamine. However, very poor protecting effects have been observed (4). Possibly, desensitization of the muscarinic receptor by such high agonist doses may interfere in the reaction of Dibenamine with the receptor. In order to get a better insight into the problem, a series of protection experiments with different ligands were made. Some of the results are presented in this paper.

The experimental procedure was as follows: The muscle strips were incubated with 10 µM Dibenamine for 20 min, which was eliminated subsequently from the organ bath by rinsing. Two dose response curves to MeCh were constructed, the second was used for calculating the remaining sensitivity to the agonist as a measure of the protective effect. Preleminary experiments have shown, that further dose response curves to MeCh do not differ from this second curve with respect to maximum response, slope and position. Each experiment was carried out twice with one muscle preparation. For protection experiments, the ileal muscles were incubated with the respective compound 2 min before Dibenamine was added to the organ bath. Both compounds were eliminated after 20 min by rinsing. From the dose response curves to MeCh dose ratios were evaluated from equieffictive concentrations generating 10 % maximum contraction. The remaining sensitivity, compared as the percentage of that of the control curve, was estimated with the formula: (1/DR)x100. The results of some of such experiments are presented in Tab. 2.

From Tab. 2 it can be seen that the protective effect of the agonist MeCh is very poor and, with one exception, independent on the concentration applied, when the first treatment will be regarded. The smallest concentration, 0.64 µM, induces in the

TABLE 2. Protection experiments against the irreversible blockade of muscarinic receptors of longitudinal muscles from the ileum of guinea pigs by Dibenamine. The table contains the remaining sensitivity (%) after two subsequent incubation of the preparations. It gives also the maximum effect E_m of high doses of Acetyl-ß-methylcholin as percentage of the maximum effect on the untreated ileal muscles. For experimental details see text.

Protect. compound	1st treatment remaining sensitivity %	1st treatment E_m	2nd treatment remaining sensitivity %	2nd treatment E_m
none	15.2	96	1.6	50
MEcH				
0.64 M	15.0	99	1.5	39
1.28 M	23.2	99	5.5	71
2.56 M	22.2	98	4.6	82
5.12 M	24.3	97	7.4	82
10.24 M	20.8	95	9.5	83
630.00 M	19.5+			
Lachesine				
0.01 M	22.2	94	1.8	39
0.10 M	58.9	97	23.8	44
1.00	55.6	91	22.7	34
TMB-4				
0.1 mM	58.9	98	17.7	60
1.0	143.0	99	76.9	74
Gallamine				
0.1 mM	20.8	97	1.6	24
d-Tubocurarine				
0.1 mM	50.0	98	6.9	51

+data from Furchgott (1954) (27)

control curves 75-80 % contraction and has no protective effect. All other doses, including that of Furchgott (27) used, of 0.63 mM, has only a very feeble protective effect. Neither the remaining sensitivity nor the maximum response are impressively greater than after the treatment with Dibenamine alone. A somewhat stronger effect occurs with the second treatment, accompagnied by a certain dependence on the dose of MeCh applied.

Tab. 2 containes data derived from protection experiments with two muscarinic and two nicotinic antagonists. It is of special interest to compare the effects of the two lower doses of Lachesine with those of TMB-4. Both compounds have in these concentrations equieffective antimuscarinic properties. However, only the weak antagonist TMB-4 give in the concentration of 1 mM satisfying protection against the effect of Dibenamine in both treatments with respect to the sensitivity and to the maximum response. The very specific antagonist Lachesine is less effective with respect to the remaining sensitivity and has none (first treatment) or an enhancing effect (second treatment) on the depression of the maximum response produced by Dibenamine.

From the experiments, carried out with both nicotinic antagonists no protection against the alkylation of muscarinic receptors by Dibenamine was expected. This holds for Gallamine but not for d-Tubocurarine, which preserves the sensitivity in the first treatment to a comparable degree as does the same concentration of TMB-4. However, both compounds differ clearly when applied in the second treatment. The concentration of d-Tubocurarin, shown in Tab. 2, has only a very weak and noncompetitive antimuscarinic effect.

The phenomena reported here are measured by means and methods, agreeing with those, on which the receptor theory is based (27,28). However, the data obtained with various concentrations of the agonist MeCh and the relatively weak or nonspecific antagonists TMB-4 and d-Tubocurarine lead to a different interpretation. According to the findings, it is rather unlikely that Dibenamine alkylates the cholinergic binding site proper of the muscarinic agonist or competitive antagonist. It is assumed that Dibenamine binds to more or less nonspecific sites in the vicinity of the receptor and modulates indirectly the receptor activation by the agonist or the binding of agonists and antagonists on the receptor. The latter assumption is evidenced from the second treatment with Dibenamine and protecting ligands from Tab. 2.

Conclusions

The statements which will be given here, are certainly somewhat speculative because of the lack of appropriate biochemical studies. However, they will be done in the hope that more sophisticated experiments will corraborate or contradict the ideas, presented here, in the near future.

From the investigation of the structure activity relationship some evidence was found for a tentative model of the surface of the muscarinic receptor with two nonpolar areas in the vicinity of the ionic binding sites of the muscarinic receptors. Mono- and bisquaternary pyridiniumsalts are throught to bind with one pyridinium ring to the onium group binding site. Hydrophobic substituents in the ring, which interact with the nonpolar area near the onium binding site possibly counteract the binding of bulky aromatic groups on the accessory area near the ester binding site (Fig. 1).

For bisquaternary pyridines there is some evidence that the second ring binds to an additional site sensitive for quaternary nitrogene-bearing structures, thus shielding suflhydryl groups near the anionic binding site and preventing mercaptide-formation by PCMB by a conformational stabilization of the muscarinic receptor. A conformational change of the receptor is assumed to stem from the interaction with specific ligands which bear a CO-O-C-C-N- chain in their molecule.

The binding of the "second ring" of bisquaternary molecules to an additional site also prevents the alkylation of the muscarinic receptor by Dibenamine. The results from protection experiments against Dibenamine are not consistent with a mere physical competition of Dibenamine and the protecting ligands at the level of the receptor. Different conformational states of the receptor protein, stabilized by the protecting ligands, are supposed to be responsible for the protecting effects.

The results, derived from the experiments with Dibenamine, do not at all rule out the presence of a receptor reserve for potent muscarinic agonists. However, the alkylating agent and the different protection experiments, reported here and elsewhere, are not suitable to test the respective theory.

Summarizing the results for a tentative, albeit speculative model of the receptor surface, it is assumed that the specific area, which binds cholinergic ligands like ACh or MECh, is neighbored by nonpolar environments. These sites regulate the activity of antagonists. Reactive -SH groups, essential for receptor activation, are located near the ammonium group binding site. An additional site in its vicinity can be regarded as a regulatory site, beeing susceptible for alkylating agents and for one pyridinium moiety of bisquaternary pyridinium salts.

Acknowledgement: I wish to thank Mr. F. Brüggemann for his skillfull assistence and cooperation.

References

1. Clark, A.J.: Quart. J. Exptl. Physiol., 26, 374 (1937)
2. Paton, W.D.M., Rang, H.P.: Proc. R. Soc. London, Ser. B, 163, 1 (1964)
3. Ariens, E.J., Simonis, A.M., van Rossum J.M.: in "Molecular Pharmacology" (Ariens, E.J. ed.) Academic Press, New York and London, Vol. I, 408 (1964)
4. Triggle, D.J.: "Neurotransmittor-Receptor Interactions" Academic Press, London, New York, 339 (1971)
5. Triggle, D.J., Triggle, C.R.: Chemical Pharmacology of the Synapse", Academic Press London, New York, San Francisco, 182 (1976)

6. Hedlund, B., Bartfai, Th.: Mol. Pharmacol., 15, 531 (1979)

7. Kloog, Y., Egozi, Y., Sokolovsky, M.: Mol. Pharmacol., 15, 545 (1979)

8. Arostam, R.S., Triggle, D.J., Eldefrwi, M.E.: Mol. Pharmacol. 15, 227 (1979)

9. Kuhnen-Clausen, D.: Toxicol. Appl. Pharmacol., 23, 443 (1972)

10. Arunlakshana, O., Schild, H.O.: Brit. J. Pharmacol., 14 48 (1959)

11. Dirks, E., Scherer, A., Schmidt, M., Zimmer, G.: Arzneimittel-Forsch. (Drug-Res.), 20, 55 (1970)

12. Dirks, E., Scherer, A., Schmidt, M., Zimmer, G.: Arzneimittel-Forsch, (Drug-Res.), 20, 197 (1970)

13. Hagedorn, I., Gündel, W.H., Hoose, J., Jenter, Chr.: Arzneimittel-Forsch. (Drug-Res.) 26, 1273 (1976)

14. Hagedorn, I. Hohler, W.: Arzneimittel-Forsch. (Drug-Res.) 26, 1515 (2+76)

15. Oldiges, H., Schoene, K.: Arch. Int. Pharmacodyn. Ther., 204, 110 (1973)

16. Schoene, K.: Monogr. Neurol. Sci. (Karger-Basel) 7, 85 (1980)

17. Gross, G.: Thesis, University of Freiburg i. Br, FRA (1980)

18. Kuhnen-Clausen, D.: FEBS Lett., 39, 61 (1974)

19. Kuhnen-Clausen, D., Hagedorn, I., Bill, R.: J. Med. Chem., 22, 177 (1979)

20. Kuhnen-Clausen, D., Brüggemann, F.: Zweites deutsch-niederländisches Symposium "Schutz vor hochtoxischen Substanzen", TNO Rijswijk, NL, 91 (1981)

21. Barone, V., Lelj, F., Russo, N.: Mol. Pharmacol., 18, 331 (1980)

22. Moran, J.F., Triggle, D.J.: in "Cholinergic Ligand Interactions" (Triggle, D.J., Moran, J.F., Barnard, E.A., eds) Academic Press, New York and London, 119 (1971)

23. Ariens, E.J., Simonis, A.M.: Ann. N.Y. Acad. Sci., 144, 842 (1967)

24. Kuhnen-Clausen, D.: Croat. Chem. Acta, 47, 465 (1975)

25. Nickerson, M.: Nature 178, 697 (1956)

26. Stephenson, R.P.: Brit. J. Pharmacol., 11, 379 (1956)

27. Furchgott, R.F.: J. Pharmacol., 111, 265 (1954)

28. Furchgott, R.F., Bursztyn, P.: Ann. N.Y. Acad. Sci., 144, 812 (1967)

ERYTHROCYTE MEMBRANES DO NOT CONTAIN A MUSCARINIC ACETYL-CHOLINE RECEPTOR

H. Prinz and A. Maelicke
Max-Planck-Institut für Ernährungsphysiologie,
Rheinlanddamm 201, D-4600 Dortmund

Summary

Direct binding studies and stopped-flow kinetics of the uptake and release of oxygen by erythrocytes both show that these cells do not have muscarinic acetylcholine receptors in their membranes. Previous claims in this direction appear to be caused by experimental artefacts.

Introduction

It has been claimed that red blood cells contain in their membranes muscarinic acetylcholine receptors (1,2). This claim which was derived from spin label studies of erythrocyte membranes had been supported by a binding study with [^{3}H]-quinuclidinyl benzilate and erythrocyte membranes (3). We therefore began this work in the hope of finding an ideal source for the isolation of a muscarinic receptor. However, we found no indication for such a receptor in our erythrocyte preparations and concluded that the indications from spin label studies cannot be supported by direct binding studies.

Materials and Methods

[^{3}H]-quinuclidinyl benzilate was obtained from Amersham England lot No. TRK.506 Batch 3 with a specific activity of 8.4 Ci/mmol. [^{3}H]-atropine sulphate was obtained from IRE, Fleurus Belgium Batch IO9OI7 with a specific activity of 0.15Ci/mmole. Fresh blood for the binding assays was taken from cattle or pigs immediately after killing and was collected in a vessel containing heparin to prevent clotting. All blood samples were used within 8 hrs after collection and without further treatment. For most of the binding studies the erythrocytes were purified in the following way: The whole blood was centrifuged at 1000 x g for 10 min. All layers on top of the erythrocytes were removed and the sample was diluted 1:5 with a physiological buffer containing 150 mM NaCl, 5 mM KCl, 2 mM $CaCl_2$ 20 mM HEPES, pH 7.4. The centrifugation and subsequent dilution was repeated twice before the sample was used for the measurements.

Membrane fragments were prepared from erythrocytes by adding 6 volumes of destilled water (hypoosmotic shock) followed by centrifugation at 10.000 x g for 30 minutes. The supernatant was discarded and the pellet resuspended into 10 volumes of H_2O. After centrifugation was repeated, the pellet was resuspended in physiological buffer and centrifuged again. The final pellet of densely packed membrane fragments had about 1%-5% of the original blood volume. This pellet was resuspended in physiological buffer (1:1) for binding studies. For stopped flow experiments blood samples were taken from human volunteers, rabbits or cats and were diluted 100-fold with the physiological buffer. Human blood was diluted immediately after extraction. All other samples were heparinized first. The experiments were performed within 3 hours after the samples were taken.

Radioactive assay: The samples (whole blood, erythrocytes or membrane fragments) were first incubated with the non-radioactive ligands for five minutes, then the radioactive ligands were added. After 1 hour of incubation samples were centrifuged in a Heraeus Mikro Haematokrit bench centrifuge for 6 minutes. Reference measurements were done with physiological buffer (or, when binding to whole blood samples was studied with blood serum) using the same procedures.

To determine the volume of the erythrocytes, $[^3H]$-ATP was added to solutions with and without red blood cells and an aliquot of the supernatant was counted after centrifugation.

The concentrations of free ligand (C_F) and bound ligand (C_B) were derived using the following equations:

$$(1) \quad C_F = CPM \times C_o/CPM_o$$

$$(2) \quad C_B = C_o - C_F$$

where C_o is the total concentration of radioactive sample, CPM is the radioactivity in the supernatant and CPM_o is the radioactivity which would correspond to C_o. It was derived from the radioactivity in the reference CPM_R and the quotient of the radioactivity of $[^3H]$-ATP, ATP_S in the supernatant and ATP_R in the reference:

$$CPM_o = CPM_R \times ATP_S/ATP_R$$

The uptake and release of oxygen to and from erythrocytes was monitored spectrophotometrically using the absorbance at 578nm of the oxygen saturated haemoglobin. The signal noise which was mainly caused by light scattering of the erythrocytes was compensated by recording the difference in absorbance $\Delta A = A_{578}-A_{548}$ (the absorbance at 548 nm is not sensitive to the oxygen content of haemoglobin). Furthermore, ΔA does not contain any contributions from scattering light. To obtain such absorbance differences in stopped-flow experiments the dual-wavelength stopped-flow of Hess et al. (4) was used. The settling of erythrocytes in the syringes was compensated by stirring with a magnetic stirrer.

The oxygen partial pressure of the erythrocytes was monitored with an oxygen sensitive electrode between sample syringe and reservoir syringe. To measure oxygen uptake the blood samples were evacuated and then flushed with argon. The process was repeated until no further change in haemoglobin absorption at 578 nm could be detected. Avoiding any contact with air, this sample was transferred into the reservoir syringe of the stopped flow apparatus (4). The other syringe was filled with ligand dissolved in physiological buffer.

To measure the oxygen release of erythrocytes the blood samples were evacuated and flushed with argon until an oxygen partial pressure between 20 and 30 Torr was reached (monitored with an oxygen electrode). The other syringe contained ligand and 8 g/l $Na_2S_2O_4$ in oxygen-free physiological buffer. The presence of $S_2O_4^{2-}$ had the purpose to react with any remaining or developed oxygen during the experiment (5). Prior to each experiment the pH was readjusted to 7.4 (5).

Results

In order to get some information about the concentration of muscarinic acetylcholine receptors in red blood cells (RBC) we first did equilibrium binding studies. For this we used the centrifugation assay described in methods. Fig. 1 shows an equilibrium binding curve of [^{3}H]-quinuclidinyl benzilate to bovine blood in presence and absence of 10^{-4}M atropine. From the same sample erythrocytes were separated and washed. The equilibrium binding to these is shown in Fig. 2.

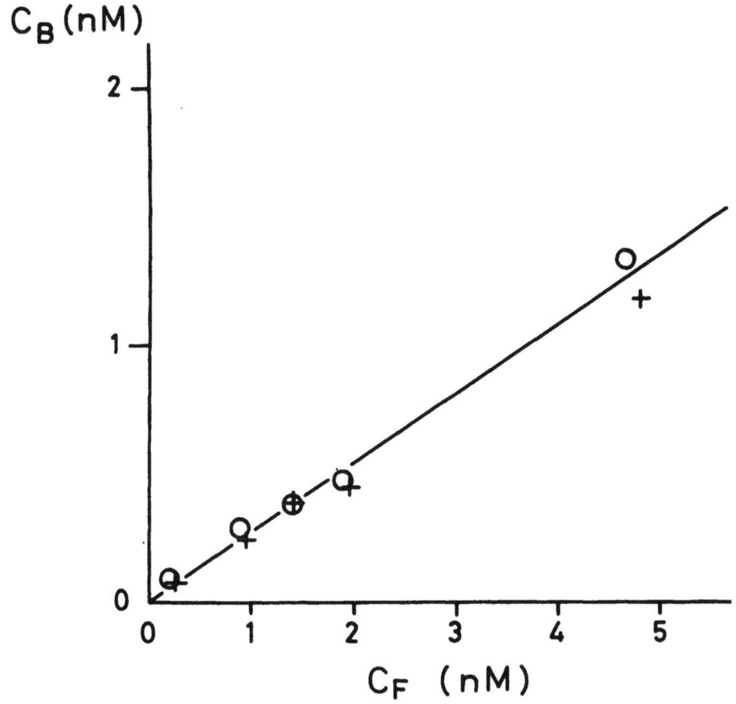

Fig. 1. Equilibrium binding of [^{3}H]-quinuclidinyl benzilate to samples of bovine (♀) blood
+ binding in absence of competing ligand
o binding in presence of 10^{-4} M atropine

Most noticable the binding curves were straight and gave no indication for saturable binding. The reference and calibration measurements (see Methods) were made separately for each ligand concentrations. Errors in these measurements caused errors in the binding curves. The measurements with and without atropine were evaluated with the same reference measurements. Their relative errors therefore were smaller than the absolute errors in the binding curves (Figs. 1 and 2). The main conclusions which can be drawn from these binding studies with [^{3}H]-quinuclidinyl benzilate are: (i) binding is not saturable in the concentration range tested, (ii) atropine does not affect this binding.

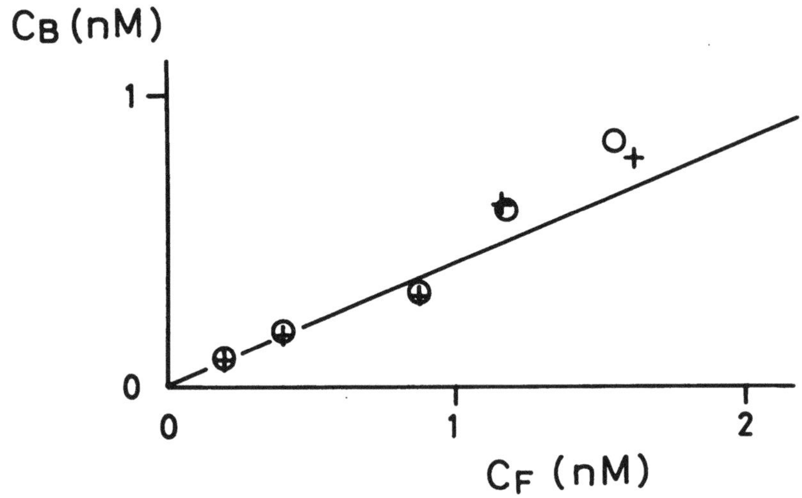

Fig. 2. Equilibrium binding of [^{3}H]-quinuclidinyl benzilate to washed bovine (♀) erythrocytes
\+ binding in absence of competing ligand
o binding in presence of 10^{-4}M atropine

Thus, quinuclidinyl benzilate and atropine do not compete for the same binding site. The experiment was repeated with the following radioactive ligands: muscarine (10^{-6}M and 10^{-8}M) arecoline (10^{-6}M and 10^{-8}M) carbamylcholine (10^{-4}M and 10^{-8}M) acetylcholine (10^{-4}M) and tubocurarine (10^{-6}M). None of these ligands changed the binding pattern of [^{3}H]-quinuclidinyl benzilate to the washed erythrocytes. Furthermore, when binding of [^{3}H]-atropine to whole blood samples and washed RBC was measured, again no saturable binding was observed. None of the competing ligands listed above did modify these curves.

In particular did 10^{-4}M atropine not inhibit the binding of 10^{-7}M [^{3}H]-atropine to the erythrocytes. In no case did the sequence of addition of the ligands to the erythrocytes change the results. We concluded: (i) The binding of none of the ligands applied was saturable. (ii) There was no competition by other ligands to these non-saturable sites. Consequently the binding was totally non-specific in nature. The simplest explanation of these effects is partition of the ligand between particulate (hydrophobic) and solute (hydrophilic) phase.

It could be argued that even though phase partition may be responsible for most of the observed binding, a small contribution of specific binding may have escaped detection.

In this case the fraction of specifically bound ligand would have been detected by atropine displacing a small fraction of bound ligand. Such a case never was detected in our studies. The error with which the deviation of the binding curve in presence of atropine from the curve in absence of competing ligand could be detected was less than 0.1 nM bound ligand ([^{3}H]-quinuclidinyl benzilate) for 1 nM free ligand. If we assume an equilibrium dissociation constant of about 1 nM (3) for the specific binding of [^{3}H]-quinuclidinyl benzilate, this error would correspond to 0.2 nM of available receptor in blood. With blood of 5 x 10^{-6} erythrocytes per μl this corresponds to 24 receptor molecules per erythrocyte. We therefore conclude that specific binding of [^{3}H]-quinuclidinyl benzilate to erythrocytes might not have been detected if the erythrocytes had contained less than 24 specific receptors per erythrocyte. To further limit this range of uncertainty, the concentration of binding sites had to be increased. This was achieved by using washed RBC membranes (Fig. 3) instead of whole cells. Although such preparations were 20-100 fold more concentrated than whole blood, again (i) no saturable binding was observed and (ii) competing ligands had no effect on the binding of the radioactive ligand (Fig. 3).

We felt that these results could in principle not be dramatically changed by additional binding experiments. It was therefore necessary to develop an assay by which the function of a possible cholinergic receptor on erythrocytes might be detected.

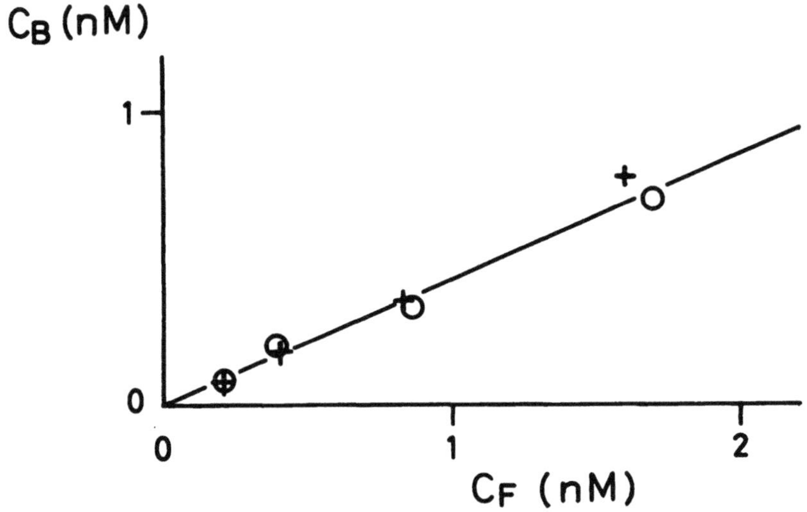

Fig. 3. Equilibrium binding of [^{3}H]-quinuclidinyl benzilate to membrane fragments from bovine (♀) blood
+ binding in absence of competing ligand
o binding in presence of 10^{-4}M atropine

2. Stopped Flow Experiments

The most prominent function of erythrocytes is the transport of oxygen. The most obvious speculation for the function of a muscarinic receptor on erythrocytes would therefore concern the uptake or release of oxygen by these cells. Since these reactions are one order of magnitude slower for erythrocytes than they are for solubilised haemoglobin (6), we speculated that a cholinergic system on erythrocytes might increase the rates of one of these reactions. Fig. 4 shows that the rate of oxygen uptake to erythrocytes was not affected by carbamylcholine.

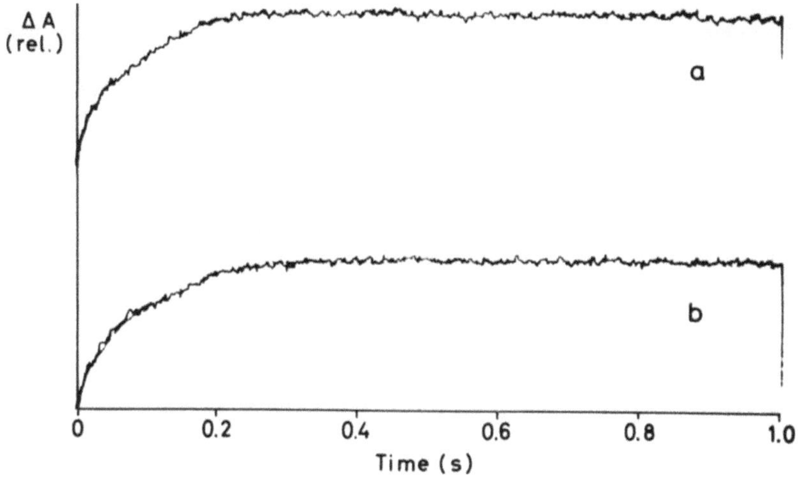

Fig. 4. Absorbance change ΔA (see Methods) measured with feline blood upon oxygen uptake at 15.5°C. (a) stopped flow trace without additional ligand, (b) stopped flow trace obtained with simultaneous addition of 10^{-4}M carbamylcholine to the erythrocytes.

Similar experiments were performed with acetylcholine, atropine, prostaglandine E_2, and arterenol in the concentrations of 10^{-4}M, 10^{-6}M and 10^{-8}M and at the temperatures of 15.5°C, 18.7°C or 37°C. No influence of these ligands on the rates of oxygen uptake was observed although a small increase (7%) of the signal amplitude could not be ruled out.

The oxygen release was measured by mixing a suspension of rabbit erythrocytes with 8 g/l $Na_2S_2O_4$ and various concentrations of cholinergic ligands (see Methods). Fig. 5 shows the oxygen release in the presence and absence of 10^{-5}M carbamylcholine. Again the rate of the reaction was not influenced by the cholinergic ligand although a small (3%) increase of the amplitude may exist. Similar experiments at 37°C in the presence of 10^{-6}M and 10^{-8}M muscarine, tubocurarine or atropine yielded the same results.

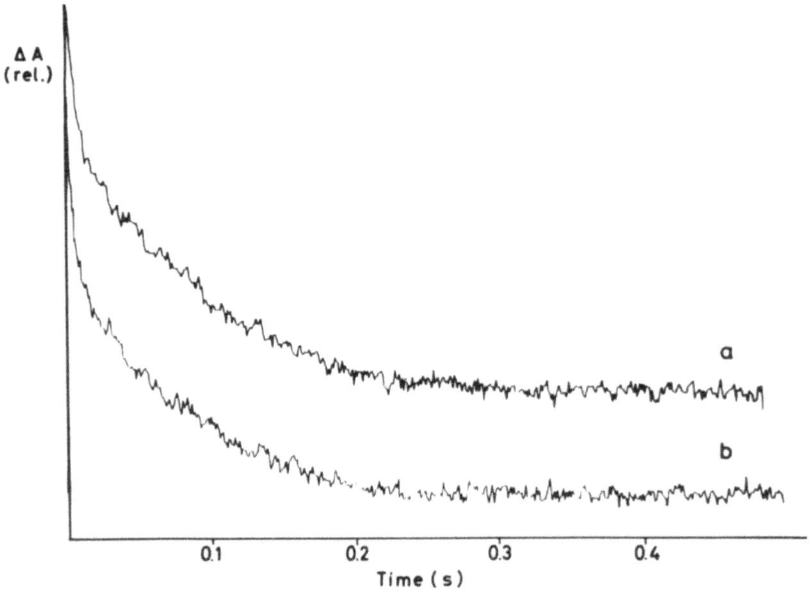

Fig. 5. Absorbance change ΔA (see Methods) measured with rabbit blood upon oxygen release at 37°C, (a) stopped flow trace without additional ligand, (b) stopped flow trace obtained with simultaneous addition of 10^{-5}M carbamylcholine to the erythrocytes.

Discussion

None of the results described in this paper indicate the existence of a muscarinic acetylcholine receptor on erythrocytes. This is in contrast with previous studies (1-3) if we do not assume a significant difference between human blood on the one side and porcine or bovine blood on the other. How can we then explain these discrepancies in finding? In view of our finding that there is a high (20-30%) degree of non-specific incorporation of muscarinic ligands into the erythrocyte membrane, the immobilisation of the spin label (1,2) may have been caused by the non-specifically incorporated ligands. This view is supported by an independent spin label study (7) which pointed out that erythrocyte membranes contain fluid and solid phases which have been neglected in the studies by Huestis (1,2). It is not so easy, however, to find an explanation for the discrepancy to the binding studies by Aronstam et al. (3). This group has used a filtration assay in order to determine the amount of bound [^{3}H]-quinuclidinyl benzilate. This would in principle give too low values for the bound ligand since only the slowly dissociating ligands would be detected, but the substrate specificity should be the same. Unfortunately this study (3) did not quantify the amount of non-specific binding so that a direct comparison of the results is impossible. The binding study (3) was performed with membrane fragments whose concentration had been calibrated with the protein content by an unreferenced method which may have been unreliable in presence of membranes. We therefore could not relate their receptor concentration to the receptor concentration in blood and again could not compared results. The main conclusion, however, can be compared. If there is a high affinity receptor (K_D = 1.3 nM) located in the erythrocyte membranes (3) there is a contradiction: In our study a muscarinic receptor only would have escaped detection if (i) its affinity would be low ($K_D \gg 1$ nM) or (ii) if there were less than 24 receptors per erythrocyte and if in this case the receptor had not been co-purified with our membrane preparation.

In conclusion, the immobilisation of a spin-label by carbamylcholine and the reversal of this effect by atropine (1,2) may have been coincidence. These results cannot be interpreted as proof for a muscarinic receptor on erythrocytes. We do not understand why another group (3) had claimed to have obtained such a proof.

References

1. Huestis, W.H., McConnell, H.M.: Biochem. Biophys. Res. Commun. 57, 726-732 (1974).

2. Huestis, W.H.: Journal of Supramolecular Structure 4, 355-365 (1976).

3. Aronstam, R.S., Abood, L.G., MacNeil, M.K.: Life Sciences 20, 1175-1180 (1977).

4. Hess, B., Kleinhans, H., Schlüter, H.: Hoppe-Seyler's Z. f. Physiol. Chem. 351, 515-531 (1970).

5. Legge, J.W., Roughton, F.J.W.: Biochem. J. 47, 43-52 (1950).

6. Gibson, Q.H., Kreuzer, F., Meda, E., Roughton, F.J.W.: J. Physiol. 129, 65-89 (1955).

7. Shiga, T., Suda, T., Maeda, N.: Biochem. Biophys. Acta 466, 231-244 (1977).

VII. ACETYLCHOLINE RECEPTOR
(nicotinic)

EMBRYOLOGICAL DEVELOPMENT OF THE ELECTRIC ORGAN OF *TORPEDO MARMORATA*: ACETYLCHOLINE RECEPTOR AND ACETYLCHOLINESTERASE

V. Witzemann and V.P. Whittaker
Abteilung Neurochemie, Max-Planck-Institut für Biophysikalische Chemie, D-3400 Göttingen, FRG

Introduction

Differentiation of synapses during development is governed by complex interactions between the cells of the target tissue and between these and the innervating nerve cells. Such interactions may well be mediated not only by trophic factors, but agents passing in both directions across the synapse or diffusing laterally along pre- or postsynaptic cells. Most of our present information concerning the changes that occur in development and the possible interactions which coordinate these was obtained from studies on the neuromuscular junction in rat, chick or frog (for reviews and references see 1-4) and from studies of synapse formation in cell and tissue culture.

In recent years the electromotor system of the electric rays such as *Torpedo marmorata* has been widely used as a source material and as a model for the study of cholinergic transmission. We have followed as a function of embryological development morphological (5,6), physiological and biochemical changes (7). The correlation of the observed changes in these parameters should yield basic information about the mechanisms of differentiation and synaptogenesis in this system. The principle focus here is on the biochemical characterization of the nicotinic acetylcholine receptor (AChR) and the various molecular forms of acetylcholinesterase (AChE, E.C. 3.1.1.7) at different stages of embryonic development. In the electric organ of adult *Torpedo marmorata* both of these proteins are present in exceptionally high concentrations which facilitate biochemical investigation. The understanding of the molecular events leading to the acquisition of function by these two components will help to elucidate aspects of development, such as their possible role in synaptogenesis and interactions between nerve and muscle.

Morphological Aspects

Torpedo marmorata is a wild, ovoviviparous species that is not currently bred in captivity. The development of the electromotor system takes place over virtually the entire period of embryogenesis, during which the body length of the embryo increases steadily from 10 to 120 mm, then levels off to slower growth rates (8) at birth and thereafter. Recent electron-microscopic investigations (5,6,9) confirm the earlier findings with light microscopy (10,11) that the cells of the electric organ are derived from embryonic muscle cells. During the "myogenic phase" (5) vertically oriented myoblasts fuse to form columns of true myotubes. Axons of the electromotor neurones grow between these columns but do not make synaptic contact. At about 40 mm of embryo length the "electrogenic phase" (6) is characterized by a cell shape transformation. The appearance of a postsynaptic membrane and a basal lamina signals the differentiation of the myotubes into electrocytes. At the end of this period the differentiated electrocytes have flattened horizontally and are packed in stacks. Between 50 and 60 mm embryo length the axons begin to branch and invade the intercellular space between the electrocytes. Synaptic contacts are established and the number of mature synapses increases exponentially up to 120 mm of embryo length (7). At about 130 mm of embryo length birth occurs. Since the entire period of embryogenesis takes as long as one year a high resolution can be achieved in the sequencing of morphological and functional events throughout development.

Acetylcholine Receptor

AChR is certainly the most extensively described component of the developing junction. A convenient measure of its concentration is made possible by the fact that neurotoxins bind to it with high affinity and specificity (for review and reference see 12). We have used α-bungarotoxin, a component of the venom of the snake <u>Bungarus multicinctus</u>, which was radiolabelled with ^{125}I. AChR is detectable in the organs of 28 mm embryos. The concentration represents about 1 to 2% of the adult values. Until 50 mm embryo length the level remains at $\leq$ 5% and then begins to rise steeply between 50 and 60 mm. Maximum values are reached at 110 - 130 mm embryo length and are 10 - 20% higher than those of adults.

Morphological observations show that during the "myogenic phase" the AChR molecules are diffusely distributed over the myotube surface. When the cells undergo the transformation from vertically oriented myotubes to horizontally flattened electrocytes the ventral membrane becomes a region of high AChR density relative to the dorsal membrane, a process which occurs prior to the ingrowth of axons (13). The molecular mechanisms leading to this ventral localization of AChR are still unknown. Results suggest however that neural contact may not be necessary for the developing electrocytes of <u>Torpedo marmorata</u>. On the other hand a regulative influence of the nerve terminal on the postsynaptic cell appears to cause the accumulation of receptors in the junctional area at the beginning of the "synaptogenetic phase".

The question whether the receptor protein itself plays an instructive role during innervation cannot be answered definitively but several lines of evidence (for review see 4) argue against this possibility. The results from *Torpedo* show that the AChR molecules become mainly located in the ventral membrane of the electrocyte, the future attachment sites for electromotor nerves. Since a basal lamina exists along the entire ventral surface prior to innervation (6) it is difficult to envision how axonal growth cones could interact with the membrane-bound AChR.

The AChR has biological and physiological properties that change during development. At mature neuromuscular junctions the AChRs were found to have a long half-life in the membrane (~ 11 days) whereas extrajunctional receptors have a much faster turnover rate of about 20 hours (2,3 and references therein). Whether this difference in metabolic stability is the mechanism whereby receptor accumulates at the junctional sites needs further investigation. For *Torpedo* no data are available concerning the turnover rates of the AChR of the electrocytes. However, denervation had no effect on receptor levels (14), and no extrajunctional receptors were formed.

With muscle, the most notable change during development is that the mean opening time in response to neurotransmitter of embryonic ion channels associated with the AChR appears to be relatively long in comparison to mature channels (see O. Hamill, this volume). Furthermore it was found that the physiological response to d-tubocurarine and its affinity for AChR changes with development (15,16,17). There is also some evidence that the isoelectric points and therefore possibly the state of phosphorylation of AChR undergo developmental changes (17). Receptor from Torpedo embryos of 65 to 130 mm body length was compared with adult receptor with regard to its toxin binding capacity and its affinity for d-tubocurarine. In both cases no significant differences could be detected. A rate of $14 \pm 1\ mM^{-1}\ S^{-1}$ was measured for ^{125}I α-bungarotoxin binding and the apparent dissociation constant for d-tubocurarine was

1.4 x 10^{-7} M. When Triton X-100 solubilized [^{125}I-α-bungarotoxin-AChR] -complexes were analyzed on isoelectrofocusing gradient polyacrylamide gels a single, rather broad [receptor-toxin] band was obtained. The peak fraction focuses at pH 5.3 ± 0.1. These results suggest that the bulk of the AChR has similar isoelectric points during the whole period of development investigated (64 mm - 110 mm embryo length).

The polypeptide composition of the adult AChR from Torpedo has been a matter of controversy for the past 10 years (for review see 14,18). There is now general agreement that the receptor from Torpedo marmorata consists of four polypeptides of approximately Mr 40 000, 50 000, 57 000 and 65 000 in a ratio of 2 : 1 : 1 : 1 (18). Affinity chromatography of detergent-extracted embryonic receptor (75 - 110 mm embryo length) on α-bungarotoxin-Sepharose columns revealed the existence of the same number of polypeptide chains with identical molecular weights and in a similar molar ratio.

We have recently shown that crossed immunoelectrophoresis is a very sensitive technique for studying the multisubunit nature of the AChR and to detect structural changes (19). A slight variation, tandem immunoelectrophoresis (20), allows the direct comparison of antigens. We used adult and embryonic AChR (64 mm - 120 mm embryo length) in detergent-solubilized form as antigens. The antiserum used was raised to affinity purified AChR complex (19). The immunoprecipitation lines of the two antigens showed complete fusion indicating that the immunochemical properties are largely identical using antibodies raised to the 'native' AChR complex. However, differences of primary structure undetected by denaturing gel electrophoresis, isoelectric focusing or crossed-immunoelectrophoresis, might still exist between adult and embryonic AChR.

Acetylcholinesterase

Acetylcholinesterase (AChE) has a widespread distribution and is most abundant in nervous tissue and muscles. It is also present in serum, erythrocytes, placenta and other tissues. But only the function at neuromuscular junctions is relatively well established (12). There the enzyme rapidly hydrolysis acetylcholine into acetate and choline thus terminating the action of transmitter released by the nerve and providing choline molecules for resynthesis of ACh after uptake into nerve terminals.

Studies on the purified enzyme isolated mainly from the electric organ of electric fish indicate that the catalytic subunits are arranged in multimers, which can be distinguished by velocity sedimentation on sucrose density gradients as multiple molecular forms (see review 21). The major molecular AChE forms which appear during the development of Torpedo marmorata electric organ have apparent sedimentation coefficients of 17 S, 13 S, 11 S and 6 S. Clear structural homologies exist between the various forms throughout the range of vertebrates (22,23). There is evidence that the slowly sedimenting forms serve as precursors of the heavier ones (24,25), and that the rapidly sedimenting forms are predominantly located in the endplate regions strongly associated with the basal lamina (for review see 21).

AChE was not detectable histochemically in embryos smaller than 55 mm (13). The reaction product obtained at 55 mm of embryo length is confined to regions of the nuclear envelope, elements of smooth endoplasmatic reticulum, the ventral plasma membrane and the basal lamina. However AChE can be identified biochemically in 28 mm embryos in amounts of about 0.1% of the adult value. The total amount of esterase activity remains at this rather low level until 50 mm embryo length. From then on a steady rise follows throughout embryogenesis. The adult values are 10 to 20% lower than those of 120 - 130 mm embryos.

During the development of the electric organ the distribution of the multiple AChE forms changes dramatically. The "myogenic phase" is characterized by the predominance of 6 S and 11 S forms. Comparison with findings on the molecular forms in other embryonic tissues (23,26) reveals a striking similarity in that in these cases also the slowly sedimenting forms are the most abundant. This suggests that early embryonic regulation of AChE molecular forms is similar in different cholinergic tissues. With differentiation and maturation however, different tissue-specific mechanisms influence the regulation of AChE forms.

As already mentioned the mechanisms responsible for electrocyte differentiation are as yet unknown, but occurring concomitantly with cellular transformation is the appearance of a basal lamina on the ventral surface. During that time both 6 S and 11 S forms decrease and the 13 S and 17 S forms become predominant. It is therefore tempting to assume that the pools of 6 S and 11 S AChE are related to pools of other molecular forms via a dynamic equilibrium. Association and dissociation of the various AChE molecular components would then be regulated by specific cellular events. In our case differentiation of the postsynaptic membrane would induce a shift in the AChE molecular forms, which occurs ahead of the formation of nerve-electrocyte contacts. Whether trophic factors are involved at that stage and whether the newly synthesized fast sedimenting forms are immediately associated with the developing basal lamina and support the formation of nerve contacts by guiding the subsequently developing neurites is not known.

A second remarkable change in the distribution of the AChE molecular forms coincides with the onset of synaptogenesis. A transient increase in 13 S AChE around 55 mm embryo length is followed by constantly rising amounts of 17 S forms. Again, this could indicate that the 13 S form is the intermediate precursor for the faster sedimenting AChE. The observed alterations in enzyme pattern at that stage appeared to be induced by the establishment of synaptic contacts suggesting that neuronal elements may regulate the accumulation of 17 S AChE in junctional areas. Denervation studies on the other hand had little or no effect on the distribution of esterase forms in the adult organ (unpublished results). Thus, the nerve appears to be unnecessary for the maintenance of AChE in the electric organ. A number of findings using developing embryos of warm blooded species suggest that initial accumulation and the subsequent maintenance of junctional AChE requires muscle activity (27,28).

Bioelectric maturation of the electric organ and onset of function starts very slowly at 60 - 70 mm embryo length but increases exponentially to reach adult levels at birth (7). The development of functional synapses is paralleled by increasing amounts of 6 S AChE. This fraction appears as a homogeneous band upon sucrose density centrifugation, but represents at least two different types of molecules: one which is soluble in the absence of salt or detergent and another of hydrophobic nature and extracted only in the presence of detergent (29). Little is known about the structural relationship between these forms. Preliminary results suggest that the 6 S form increasingly synthesized during the later "synaptic phase" (80 - 90 mm onwards) is of hydrophobic nature and might play an important role in neurotransmission. The "low salt soluble" 6 S form together with the 11 S form, both present at early stages of development, could represent a stable pool of precursor molecules that are transformed into more complex structures such as the fast sedimenting 17 S and 13 S (basal lamina associated) forms or progressively integrated into membranes as "hydrophobic" forms. Some of these results are summarized in a schematic diagram in Figure 1.

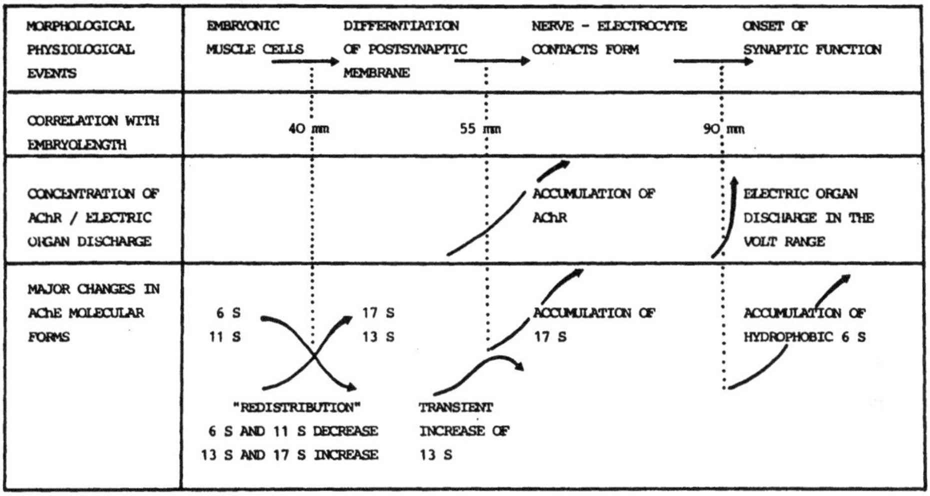

FIGURE 1: Schematic presentation of morphological,physiological and biochemical events occuring during the embryological development of *Torpedo marmorata*.

Conclusion

Certain common features exist between AChR and AChE during embryogenesis. In each case local interactions with the embryonic cells occur at very early stages of development which determine the spatial distribution of the molecules and which seem not to depend on established nerve-electrocyte contacts. Interaction of nerve and electrocytes seem to cause the accumulation of both proteins in the synaptic area. Clearly further studies are needed to characterize these proteins on a molecular level. These "marker" proteins thus provide a means for describing at the cellular level events in cell development, cell-cell interactions, and mechanisms that regulate these events.

References

1. Fambrough, D.M.: In "Neuronal Recognition" ed. Barondes, S., Bloom, F.E., pp. 25-67, New York, Plenum (1976).
2. Edwards, C.: Neuroscience 4, 565-584 (1979).
3. Fambrough, D.M.: Physiol. Rev. 54, 165-227 (1979).
4. Dennis, M.J.: Ann. Rev. Neurosci. 4, 43-68 (1981).
5. Fox, G.Q., Richardson, G.P.: J. comp. Neurol. 179, 677-698 (1978).
6. Fox, G.Q., Richardson, G.P.: J. comp. Neurol. 185, 293-316 (1979).
7. Krenz, W.-D., Tashiro, T., Wächtler, K., Whittaker, V.P., Witzemann, V.: Neuroscience 5, 617-624 (1980).
8. Richardson, G.P., Krenz, W.-D., Kirk, C., Fox, G.Q.: Neuroscience 6, 1181-1200 (1981).
9. Mellinger, J., Belbenoit, P., Ravaille, M., Szabo, T.: Dev. Biol. 67, 167-188 (1978).
10. Fritsch, G.: "Die elektrischen Fische" von Veit, Leipzig (1890).
11. Ogneff, J.: Arch. Anat. Physiol. Abt. pp. 270-304 (1897).
12. Arch. Cytopharmacol.: Vol. 3, "Neurotoxins: Tools in Neurobiology". Ceccarelli, B., Clementi, F. eds. Raven Press (1979).
13. Richardson, G.P.: Dissertation, Sussex University (1980).
14. Clementi, F., Conti-Tronconi, B., Peluchetti, D., Morgutti, M.: Brain Res. 90, 133-138 (1975).
15. Beranek, R., Vyskocil, F.: J. Physiol. London, 188, 53-66 (1967).
16. Chin, T.H., Lapa, A.J., Barnard, E.A., Albuquerque, E.X.: Exp. Neurol. 43, 399-413 (1974).
17. Brockes, J.P., Hall, Z.: Biochemistry 14, 2100-2106 (1975).
18. Raftery, M.A., Hunkapiller, M.W., Strader, C.D., Hood, L.E.: Science 208, 1454-1457 (1980).
19. Witzemann, V., Walker, J.-H.: In "Cholinergic Mechanisms: Phylogenetic Aspects, Central and Peripheral Synapses, and Clinical Significance, pp 653-658, Pepen, G., Landinsky, H. eds. Plenum Press (1981).
20. Axelsen, N.H., Bock, E., Krøll, J.: In "Quantitative Immunoelectrophoresis" pp. 91-94, Axelsen, N.H., Krøll, J., Weeke, B., eds. Universitetsforlaget Oslo-Bergen-Tromsø (1973).

21. Massoulié, J.: Trends Biochem. Sci. 160-164 (1980).

22. Bon, S., Vigny, M., Massoulié, J.: Proc. Natl. Acad. Sci., USA 76, 2546-2550 (1979).

23. Rotundo, R.L., Fambrough, D.M.: J. Biol. Chem. 254, 4790-4799 (1979).

24. Wilson, B.W., Walker, C.R.: Proc. Natl. Acad. Sci., USA 71, 3194-3198 (1974).

25. Cisson, C.M., McQuarrie, C.H., Sketely, J., McNamee, M., Wilson, B.W.: Dev. Neurosci. 4, 157-164 (1981).

26. Lyles, J.M., Silman, I., Barnard, E.: J. Neurochem. 33, 727-738 (1979).

27. Rubin, L.L., Schuetze, S.M., Weill, C.L., Fischbach, G.D.: Nature 283, 264-267 (1980).

28. Lomø, T., Slater, C.R.: J. Physiol. 303, 191-202 (1980).

29. Witzemann, V.: Neuroscience Lett. 20, 277-282 (1980).

EMBRYOLOGICAL DEVELOPMENT OF THE ELECTRIC ORGAN OF TORPEDO MARMORATA: IN VITRO TRANSLATION OF EMBRYONIC mRNA

V. Witzemann and D. Schmid

Abteilung Neurochemie, Max-Planck-Institut für Biophysikalische Chemie, D-3400 Göttingen, FRG

Introduction

The electromotor system of the electric ray Torpedo marmorata represents an ideal model cholinergic system to study the formation and function of cholinergic synapses (V. Witzemann and V.P. Whittaker, this volume and 1,2).

Because of the long gestation period, which can be as long as one year, morphological and functional events can be sequenced with great resolution throughout development. The correlation between morphological and functional events allows some conclusions about mechanisms which regulate the dynamics of development. In the preceeding paper we have attempted to investigate possible developmental changes of biochemical properties of two proteins, the nicotinic acetylcholine receptor (AChR) and acetylcholinesterase (AChE), which are directly involved in neurotransmission. However, it seems very likely that there are other proteins that are also important for development and establishment of synaptic function. One approach to search for such components would be to follow differential genetic expression in the embryonic electric organ.

Proteins of the Developing Electric Organ

Electric organ of different embryonic stages is homogenized

and solubilized by adding sodium dodecylsulphate and Triton X-100. Analysis of such treated samples on sodium dodecyl-sulphate polyacrylamide gels is shown in Fig. 1. At a first glance one would not expect to get too much information from such complex polypeptide patterns, which are visualized after Coomassie Brilliant Blue staining. But surprisingly there is a marked difference comparing the polypeptides from the electric organ of a 55 mm embryo and of the adult fish: Two polypeptides of apparent Mr 43 000 and 45 000 change their relative abundance to each other. At 55 mm embryo length the Mr 45 000 component is predominant with only trace amounts of the Mr 43 000. In the adult organ the Mr 43 000 polypeptide has become the major component. One of the components comigrates with actin (Mr 45 000) and the other with a Mr 43 000 polypeptide which appears to be localized mainly at the postsynaptic membrane (3).

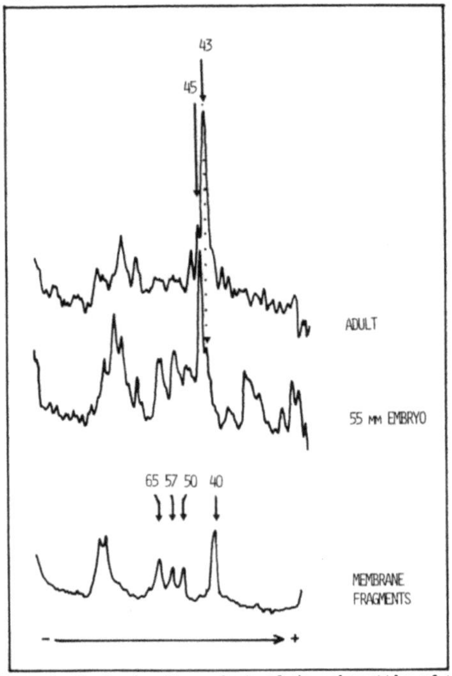

Figure 1: Electrophoretic analysis of the polypeptides of the electric organ of *Torpedo marmorata*. The polyacrylamide gel scans show Coomassie Brilliant Blue stained polypeptides of adult electric organ and electric organ of 55 mm embryos. For comparison pH 11 treated AChR-enriched membranes of the adult electric organ are included. Numbers and arrows indicate the apparent Mr x 10^{-3}.

In Vitro Translation

The rate of synthesis of proteins during development may be controlled either by changes in the amounts of the corresponding mRNAs, or by the activation of preexisting mRNAs, or both.

In a cell-free system one would expect to detect the existence of mRNA which is in a translatable form. We have isolated poly-A containing mRNA, as described in (4), from electric organs of embryos ranging from 50 - 130 mm embryo length. During that period of development, the "synaptogenic phase", a dramatic rise in the concentration of "synapse specific" proteins such as the nicotinic AChR and the AChE (1) is observed and as described above characteristic changes can be detected in the polypeptide composition. Although little is known about the translational control during the differentiation of specialized cell types one might expect a close correlation between the amount of translatable mRNAs and the synthesis of the corresponding proteins. For *in vitro* translation we used a reticulocyte derived, nuclease treated system (5). The translation products were analysed electrophoretically by sodium dodecylsulphate polyacrylamide gel and by two dimensional gel electrophoresis. It is found that the amount of translatable mRNA is significantly higher at stages between 80 - 120 mm embryo length than at earlier stages, around 50 - 60 mm, or in the adult tissue.

In Fig. 2 the ^{35}S-labelled translation products obtained with mRNA isolated at different embryonic stages are visualized by fluorography. Endogenous activity of the translation system gives rise to one polypeptide of apparent Mr 47 000. At 52 mm embryo length significant amounts of a Mr 45 000 component are synthesized and minor amounts of other polypeptides are detectable. The number of newly synthesized proteins increases using mRNA from later embryonic stages. One prominent feature is, however, that the amount of a Mr 43 000 component increases

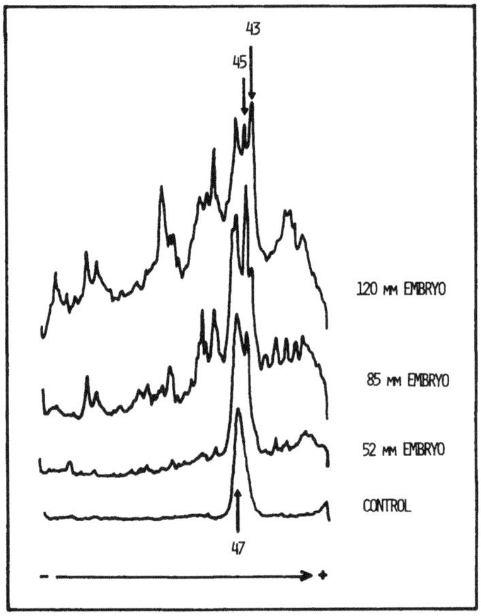

Figure 2: Electrophoretic analysis of polypeptides synthesized in a cell free system. Poly (A) mRNA extracted from the electric organs of Torpedo marmorata at various stages of development (the body length of the embryos used is given) was translated in a nuclease-treated rabbit reticulocyte lysate in the presence of ^{35}S-methionine. Scans of the fluorograms obtained after sodium dodecylsulphate gel electrophoresis are shown. The control shows the pclypeptide synthesized by the endogenous activity of the translation system. Numbers and arrows indicate apparent Mr x 10^{-3}.

steadily to become the most abundant polypeptide at 120 mm embryo length. Analysis of these in vitro synthesized products on two dimensional gel electrophoresis reveals that the major component at Mr 45 000 comigrates with actin. Further experiments will be needed to clarify whether the newly synthesized Mr 43 000 polypeptide corresponds to the protein which is thought to be associated with postsynaptic plasma membranes (3) and whether it plays an important role in synaptogenesis and receptor function. The changes seen in number and relative abundance of the in vitro synthesized polypeptides using embryonic mRNAs appear to reflect changes which are obtained comparing at various embryonic stages the in vivo synthesized polypeptides (Fig. 1). These results support the notion that there is indeed a close correlation between the rate of synthesis of some proteins and the in vitro translatable amounts of mRNAs coding for these proteins. Further characterization of the in vitro synthesized proteins could help to detect synapse specific proteins, which might be synthesized at increased rates during the synaptogenic phase of development.

The importance of the AChR for synaptic function gives special significance to the understanding of mechanisms by which gene expression of this protein is regulated during development. We therefore investigated whether AChR polypeptides are translated in the cell-free system used in our experiments. Electric organ of 120 mm embryos served as source of the mRNA for *in vitro* translation. The ^{35}S-labelled translation products are then incubated with AChR-specific antiserum. Antibody-antigen complexes are absorbed by protein-A-agarose. After extensive washing steps bound material can be recovered and analysed by sodium dodecylsulphate gel electrophoresis. Preliminary results indicate that probably all four receptor polypeptides are synthesized although some discrepancy exists with regard to the molecular weights of the immunoprecipitated polypeptides and the native subunits of AChR. In our experiments a polypeptide of apparent Mr 40 000 $\pm$ 1000 has been identified as a receptor component as follows: Anti-AChR-antiserum was preincubated with saturating amounts of purified Mr 40 000 AChR subunit to react with all the antibodies which are directed towards this polypeptide. This "absorbed" antiserum is then used in parallel with "native" antiserum for immunoprecipitation. Comparing the immunoprecipitated ^{35}S-labelled polypeptides one finds that in case of the "absorbed" anti-AChR-antiserum only the polypeptide of apparent Mr 40 000 is missing and is therefore immunochemically identical with the AChR subunit used to absorb the "native" antiserum. Further experiments will be needed to demonstrate the identity of the other immunoprecipitated translation products as AChR components.

Recently is has been shown by several authors (6,7,8) that the AChR polypeptides can be synthesized *in vitro*. These experiments provide new means to investigate fundamental aspects of gene regulation and their relevance for regulation of AChR synthesis.

References

1. Krenz, W.-D., Tashiro, T., Wächtler, K., Whittaker, V.P., Witzemann, V.: Neuroscience 5, 617-624 (1980).

2. Whittaker, V.P.: in "Cell Compartmentation and Metabolic Channeling", pp 509-523, Nover, L., Lynen, F., Mothes, K. (eds.), VEB Gustav Fischer Verlag, Jena (GDR) and Elsevier/ North-Holland Biomedical Press, Amsterdam (NL), (1980).

3. Froehner, S.C., Gulbrandsen, V., Hyman, C., Yeng, A.Y., Neubig, R.R., Cohen, J.B.: Proc. Natl. Acad. Sci. USA 78, 5230-5234 (1981).

4. Schmid, D., Stadler, H., Whittaker, V.P.: (submitted).

5. Pelham, H.R.B., Jackson, R.T.: Eur. J. Biochem. 67, 247-256 (1976).

6. Anderson, D.J., Blobel, G.: Proc. Natl. Acad. Sci. USA 78, 5598-5602 (1981).

7. Merlie, J.P., Hofler, J.G., Sebbane, R.: J. Biol. Chem. 256, 6995-6999 (1981).

8. Sumikawa, K., Houghton, M., Emtage, J.S., Richards, B.M., Barnard, E.A.: Nature 292, 862-864 (1981).

FLUX AMPLITUDE ANALYSIS AS A TOOL IN RECEPTOR RESEARCH

Julius Bernhardt and Eberhard Neumann
Max-Planck-Institut für Biochemie, D-8033 Martinsried
bei München, Germany

Introduction

Tracer ion flux experiments have been used extensively to study ion flow gating by neuroreceptors in excitable membranes. In these experiments the change in the overall tracer content of closed membrane structures (CMS), due to tracer flux through receptor controlled channels, is measured. Examples of CMS that have been employed in flux studies are: (a) "nicotinic" acetylcholine receptor containing isolated muscle cells (1,2), sealed membrane fragments derived from fish electric organs (3-6), and reconstituted vesicles (7-11), (b) "muscarinic" acetylcholine receptor containing isolated rat parotid acinar cells (12), and (c) ß-adrenergic receptor containing erythrocytes (13).

Two modes of measurement are feasible: flux of tracer from the CMS into a large bath initially containing no tracer (efflux), and flux of tracer from a large bath into CMS initially containing no tracer (influx). In either case flux will persist until equilibration of the bath and the CMS internal tracer ion concentrations takes place. The net amount of tracer transported from or into the CMS when flux is able to reach completion constitutes the maximum flux amplitude ΔX_{max}, given by $\Delta X_{max} = X(0)$ (efflux) and $X_{max} = X(\infty)$ (influx), where $X(0)$ and $X(\infty)$ are, respectively, the initial and the final equilibrium tracer content of the CMS (e.g., amount of tracer ions in the CMS expressed as cpm of a radioactive tracer species, or as fluorescence intensity of a tracer ion sensitive dye).

In practice, attainment of a time-invariant, finite overall tracer content, reflecting a cessation of flux, need not imply that flux has reached completion. In flux experiments using acetylcholine receptor (AcChR) containing CMS, apparent flux amplitudes less than ΔX_{max} have been observed, when: (a) the CMS are exposed to a bath containing neuroactivator (5,6), and (b) the CMS are incubated with snake toxins prior to exposure to neuroactivator (14,15). In both cases there is an apparent cessation of flux prior to a complete equilibration of the bath and the CMS internal tracer concentrations. The resulting flux amplitudes depend on the concentration of the neuroactivator, and/or the amount of snake toxin used in the incubation. The measured amplitudes decrease steadily with decreasing activator ligand concentrations, and/or with increasing amounts of toxin. Figure 1 shows the time independent flux amplitudes resulting for Li^+ efflux from Torpedo marmorata membrane fragments, induced by varying concentrations of carbamoylcholine (CbCh).

A detailed analysis of ligand concentration dependent flux amplitudes has recently been developed (6,16). It was proposed that the observed cessation of flux prior to complete tracer equilibration is due to neuroactivator ligand induced receptor inactivation ('desensitization'), and inhibition of receptors by toxin. A subfraction of CMS having all receptors inactivated or inhibited, will thereby be generated. These CMS can no longer contribute to flux, and thus give rise to less than maximum amplitudes.

Using a variety of experimental techniques based on the filter assay method of flux measurement (3), it was possible to determine the CMS size distribution, the distribution in receptor content per CMS, and the ratio of the effective rate constants for flux and receptor inactivation, from flux amplitudes for AcChR controlled flux (16). These results show

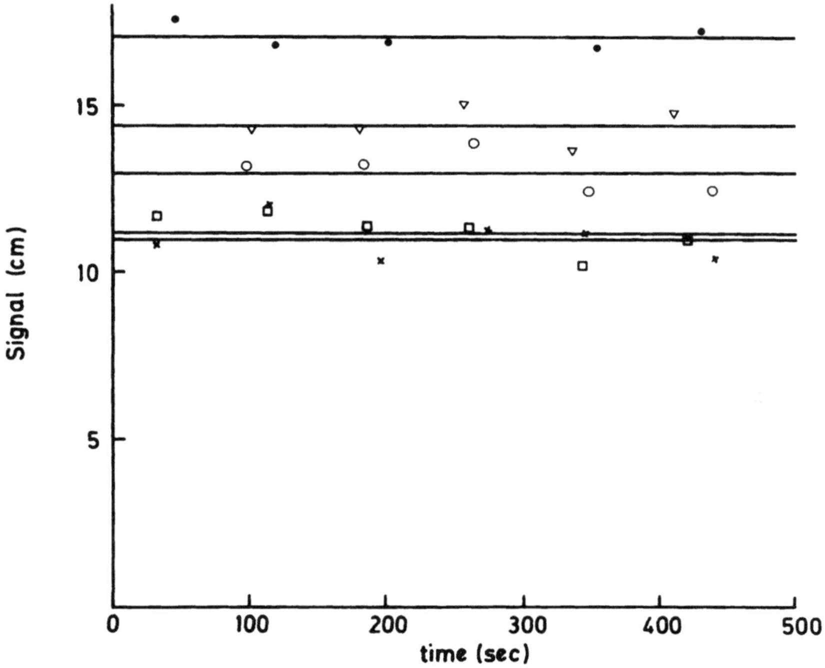

Figure 1: Flux amplitudes resulting for acetylcholine receptor controlled Li^+ efflux from sealed Torpedo membrane fragments. Flux was induced by carbymoylcholine at following concentrations: 0μM(•), 5.2μM (▽), 9.0μM (c), 30.0μM (□), and 480μM (x).

that flux amplitude measurements can be employed (a) to uniquely characterize all factors connected with a suspension of CMS that may vary with the methods of preparation, and (b) to determine the time scale on which flux occurs.

In this article a general procedure for systematically carrying out flux amplitude measurements, and a scheme for analysing the resulting data, is presented.

A. Channel Gating by Receptors and Flux

Physiologically relevant receptor processes occuring under *in vivo* conditions generally involve a series of characteristic reaction steps. Initially receptors are predominantly in the closed channel resting state. Binding of a neurotransmitter ligand leads to an increased population of the active receptor state, and a concomitant increase in the number of open channels. Removal of the transmitter ligand, through diffusion, uptake or enzymatic degradation, leads to a return to the resting state, and thus to net channel closing. Frequently, when receptors are exposed to neuractivator ligands for prolonged periods under *in vitro* conditions, the initial activation phase is followed by one or more inactivation phases, leading to net channel closing ('desensitization'). Most receptors contain binding sites for inhibitory ligands. Occupancy of these sites inhibits activation, and thus also promotes net channel closing. Receptor functional states can thus be divided into open channel states (i.e., active states), and closed channel states (e.g., the resting activatable state and the inactive, inhibited states).

Receptor reaction processes consist of elementary steps in which there is either an increase, or a decrease, in the fraction α, of receptors in closed channel states. When transient reaction processes reach equilibrium or a steady state, α will be invariant with time. Since receptors are localized on the CMS, a mixture of fractionally populated CMS must be considered. A given CMS with a total number of receptors n, will have m receptors in the closed channel state, where $0 \leq m \leq n$. The probability $\mu_m^{(n)}$, that a CMS with n receptors has m receptors in the closed channel state, follows a binomial law (17,18). In particular, the fraction of CMS having all receptors in the closed channel state (i.e., m=n) is given by the simple power low expression $\mu_n^{(n)} = \alpha^n$.

The ion transport properties of a channel can be expressed in terms of the intrinsic flux rate constant k, in units tracer ions transported per unit time. The flux process, for flux through a single open channel on a CMS, will therefore take place on the time scale of the flux time constant k^{-1}. Due to the receptor process controlling channel opening and closing, individual receptors will execute transitions between open channel and closed channel states. A given receptor will spend a mean time k_c^{-1} in a closed channel state before reverting to an open channel state, where k_c is the effective forward rate constant for the channel closing process.

Two limiting situations may arise:

(1) The receptor transitions occur on a time scale much more rapid than flux, i.e., $k_c^{-1} \gg k^{-1}$. Receptors will then fluctuate rapidly between open channel and closed channel states. It is therefore possible to express the mean transport properties of a given channel by the effective flux rate constant $k_{eff} = (1-\alpha)\cdot k$, where $1-\alpha$ is the fraction of receptors in an open channel state. The effect of the gating reaction on flux will thus be to reduce the mean rate of ion transport through all channels on the CMS by the same factor. Flux from or into all CMS will therefore be able to reach completion, and the flux amplitude ΔX_{max} will result.

(2) The mean life-time of a closed channel state is very long on the time scale of flux, i.e., $k^{-1} \gg k_c^{-1}$. This implies that once a receptor executes a transition to a closed channel state, it will remain in that state during the entire period of flux measurement, i.e., channel closing is effectively an irreversible process. A fraction α of receptors will then be in a closed channel state; flux through channels controlled by the remaining $1-\alpha$ receptors will occur with the flux rate constant k. The fraction

$\mu_n^{(n)}$, of CMS having all receptors in a closed channel state, will not contribute to flux, and thus give rise to flux amplitudes less than ΔX_{max}. Examples for long-lived closed channel states are the inactivated state resulting when the neuroactivator induced reaction of AcChR reaches equilibrium, and the inhibited receptor state resulting from snake toxin binding to AcChR. A steady decrease in flux amplitudes with increasing neuroactivator ligand concentrations (as in figure 1) arises when the binding constant for neuroactivator binding to inactive states is greater than the binding constant for binding to active states. At high neuroactivator ligand concentrations both activation and inactivation will occur, while at low concentrations inactivation alone will occur.

B. Methods of Measurement

While flux amplitudes could, in principle, be measured by a variety of techniques, filter assay procedures for measuring efflux amplitudes have proven particularly useful because of their broad range of application (3). Independent of the nature of the CMS used, and of the type of receptors present on the CMS, the following experimental steps are required: (a) filling of the CMS with tracer under conditions leading to an identical concentration of tracer in all CMS; (b) injection of aliquots of a CMS suspension into a dilution bath under vigorous stirring; (c) application of aliquots of the diluted CMS suspension to membrane filters; (d) suction filtration followed by several washings to remove all CMS external tracer; (e) determination of the tracer content of the filters.

Incubation of CMS in a bath containing tracer and neuroactivator ligand, leads to a selective filling of CMS containing functional receptors (4,19). Since leakage flux is generally much slower than flux through receptor controlled channels, nonfunctional CMS will thereby be filled to a lesser extent than functional CMS.

The following filtration measurements can then be made (16):

(1) Determination of the combined total tracer content, X_T, of functional and non-functional CMS. Tracer filled CMS are injected into a dilution bath containing only buffered medium, filtered, and the filters washed with buffered medium.

(2) Determination of the total tracer content X_{NF}, of the nonfunctional CMS, and of ΔX_{max}. Tracer filled CMS are diluted as above, filtered, and the filters washed with successive aliquots of concentrated neuroactivator solution in buffered medium, and buffer medium containing no neuroactivator. The washings must be continued until there is no further change in the tracer content of the filters. This procedure circumvents the possible cessation of flux due to receptor inactivation, and thus leads to a complete efflux of tracer from functional CMS (19). The tracer content of the filters will thus reflect X_{NF}. ΔX_{max} is then given by $\Delta X_{max} = X_T - X_{NF}$.

(3) Determination of the neuroactivator ligand concentration dependence of flux amplitudes. Tracer filled CMS are injected into a dilution bath containing neuractivator solution in buffered medium, filtered, and the filters washed with buffered medium. Subtracting the resulting tracer content of the filters from X_T yields the flux amplitude corresponding to a given bath neuroactivator concentration. Flux amplitudes less than ΔX_{max} imply that both receptor activation and inactivation processes occur.

(4) Determination of flux amplitudes resulting upon effectively irreversible inhibition of receptors.

(a) Tracer filled CMS are incubated with inhibitory ligand and then injected into a bath containing buffered medium, filtered, and washed with successive aliquots of buffered medium and concentrated neuractivator solution in buffered medium. Subtracting the resulting tracer content of the filters from X_T yields the tracer content of the fraction $\mu_n^{(n)}$, of CMS having all receptors inhibited.

(b) Alternatively, the CMS can be injected into a bath containing neuroactivator solution upon inhibition, and the washings carried out using buffered medium. Substracting the resulting tracer content of the filters from X_T then yields the tracer content of the CMS having all receptors either inhibited or inactivated.

C. Flux Amplitude Analysis

The flux amplitudes resulting for the methods of measurement outlined in the preceding section can be analysed to yield (16):

(1) The distribution in CMS internal volumes. Flux measurements to determine ΔX_{max} (preceding section, methods 1 and 2), are carried out using filters of different pore size. The ΔX_{max} for a given type of filter then represents the tracer content of all CMS with a diameter larger than the pore diameter, plus the tracer content of absorbed CMS. ΔX_{max} can be expressed as an integral over the normalized distribution function Q(v), representing the probability that a given CMS has an internal volume v. Numerical curve fitting of this expression for ΔX_{max} to the measured data can be used to determine Q(v). Knowledge of Q(v) then permits evaluation of the mean internal volume $\bar{v}$, and the mean surface area $\bar{s}$, of a CMS.

(2) The distribution in the number of receptors per CMS. The dependence of flux amplitudes $\Delta X(\alpha)$ on the fraction α, of total toxin sites occupied by an inhibitory ligand, is determined using method 4a of the preceding section. For equivalent and independent inhibitor sites, $\Delta X(\alpha)$ is then given by

$$\Delta X(\alpha)=\Delta X_{max} \sum_n P_n \left[1-(1-\alpha)^l\right]^n \qquad (1)$$

where P_n is the fractional internal volume of all CMS with n receptors per CMS, and where l is the number of inhibitor sites per receptor (gating unit). Least squares curve fitting of this equation to the measured $\Delta X(\alpha)$ values permits determination of the P_n, and of l. Knowledge of Q(v), and of the P_n suffices to evaluate (a) the fractions ξ_n representing the probability that a given CMS has n receptors, (b) the mean number $\bar{n}$ of receptors per CMS, and (c) the mean surface density $\bar{\varrho}$ of receptors on the CMS.

(3) The relative time scales of flux and receptor inactivation. Flux amplitude measurements using method 4b of the preceding section permit determination of $\Delta X(\alpha)$, when both inhibition, and neuroactivator induced inactivation of receptors occurs. $\Delta X(\alpha)$ was then found to be given by

$$\Delta X(\alpha) = \Delta X_{max} \sum_n P_n \left[\{ 1-(1-\alpha)^l \cdot (1-\langle e^{-kt}\rangle_\infty^r)\}^n\right]_v \qquad (2)$$

where P_n and l are defined as above, and where inhibition of a single receptor leads to cessation of flux through r associated channels. The outer square brackets denote a volume average of the enclosed expression. The volume dependent mean single channel flux amplitude contribution $\langle e^{-kt}\rangle_\infty$ is given by

$$\left\langle e^{-kt} \right\rangle_\infty = \frac{v}{v+(k'_{eff}/k_c)} \tag{3}$$

where k'_{eff} is the effective flux rate constant for flux through a single channel on a CMS with unit volume, and k_c is the effective forward rate constant for receptor inactivation. Numerical least squares fitting of equation (2) to the measured $\Delta X(\alpha)$ values, assuming prior knowledge of the P_n, l and Q(v), permits determination of the rate constant ratio (k'_{eff}/k_c) and r. Both k'_{eff} and k_c may implicitely depend on the concentration of activator ligand. In the limit of high activator ligand concentrations k'_{eff} and k_c will assume their maximum values. The magnitude of (k'_{eff}/k_c) reflects the relative rates of flux and inactivation.

D. Results

Flux amplitudes for AcChR controlled Li^+ efflux from sealed Torpedo membrane fragments, induced by CbCh, were determined (26); α-Bungarotoxin was used as an inhibitory ligand. A flux amplitude analysis of the data was carried out, as outlined in the preceding section. The characteristic parameters for the CMS suspension used in these measurements were found to be (16) $\bar{v}=0.15\ \mu m^3$, $\bar{s}=1.3\ \mu m^2$, $3.1\leq\bar{n}\leq 4.7$, $2.3\ \mu m^{-2} \leq \bar{\xi} \leq 3.5\ \mu m^{-2}$, and $Q(v)=a^2 \cdot v \cdot \exp(-a\,v)$, with $a=13.7\ \mu m^{-3}$. An optimum fit to the data was obtained for the case l=2, i.e., there are two toxin sites per receptor (gating unit).

The rate constant ratio at high CbCh concentrations was found to fall in the range $0.1 \leq (k_{eff}/k_i) \leq 0.5$, where k_{eff} is the effective flux rate constant for flux through a single channel on a CMS with volume 1 μm^3, and where k_i is the effective forward rate constant for the slowest inactivation mode of the AcChR. Since k_i is of the order 1 sec^{-1}, k_{eff} is presumably much smaller than the flux rate constant k for flux through a permanently open channel. This indicates that the equilibrium fraction of receptors in open channel states is small, for flux measured on the time scale of the slow receptor inactivation process.

E. Conclusions

Analysis of flux amplitudes for receptor controlled tracer flux from or into a collection of CMS permits determination of the distribution of CMS size and receptor content, and of the relative time scales of flux and receptor inactivation processes. The experimental techniques required to measure flux amplitudes are considerably simpler than those required to measure the time course of flux on the millisecond to second time range (15,20). While less information about receptor and flux process is obtained from flux amplitude measurements, it has recently been shown (16) that quantitative analysis of time-dependent flux requires prior knowledge of the parameters P_n and Q(v), which can be determined from flux amplitude data. Flux amplitude analysis is therefore a broadly applicable, simple technique for obtaining information about receptor gating of ion channels.

Acknowledgement

We gratefully acknowledge financial support by the Deutsche Forschungsgemeinschaft, grant Ne 227.

References

1. Sine, S.M., Taylor, P.: J. Biol. Chem. 255, 10144 (1980).
2. Sine, S.M., Taylor, P.: J. Biol. Chem. 256, 6692 (1981).
3. Kasai, M., Changeux, J.-P.: J. Membr. Biol. 6, 1 (1971).
4. Hess, G., Andrews, J.P., Stuve, G.F., Coombs, S.E.: Proc. Natl. Acad. Sci. USA 72, 4371 (1975).
5. Miller, D.A., Moore, H.-P., Hartig, P., Raftery, M.A.: Biochem. Biophys. Res. Commun. 85, 632 (1978).
6. Bernhardt, J., Neumann, E.: Proc. Natl. Acad. Sci. USA 75, 3756 (1978).
7. Epstein, M., Racker, E.: J. Biol. Chem. 253, 6660 (1978).
8. Wu , W. C.-S., Raftery, M.A.: Biochem. Biophys. Res. Commun. 89, 26 (1979).
9. Heidmann, T., Sobel, A., Popot, J.-L., Changeux, J.-P.: Eur. J. Biochem. 110, 35 (1980).
10. Lindstrom, J., Anholt, R., Einarson, B., Engel, A., Osame, M., Montal, M.: J. Biol. Chem. 255, 8340 (1980).
11. Schiebler, W., Bandini, G., Hucho, F.: Neurochem. Internatl. 2, 281 (1980).
12. Landis, C.A., Putney jr., J.W.: J. Physiol. London 297, 369 (1979).
13. Rudolph, S.A., Greengard, P.: J. Biol. Chem. 255, 8534 (1980).
14. Moore, H.P., Hartig, P.R., Raftery, M.A.: Proc. Natl, Acad. Sci. USA 76, 6265 (1979).
15. Neubig, R.R., Cohen, J.B.: Biochemistry 19, 2770 (1980).
16. Bernhardt, J., Neumann, E.: Biophys. Chem. (1982) in press.
17. Bernhardt, J., Neumann, E.: J. theor. Biol. 86, 649 (1980).
18. Bernhardt, J., Neumann, E.: Neurochem. Internatl. 2, 243 (1980).
19. Bernhardt, J., Moss, K.M., Luckinger, R.M., Neumann, E.: FEBS Lett. (1981), in press.
20. Hess, G.P., Derek, J., Aoshima, H.: Nature 292, 329 (1979).

ACETYLCHOLINE RECEPTOR CHANNELS

O.P. Hamill

Max-Planck-Institut für biophysikalische Chemie, Am Faßberg
Göttingen, F.R.G.

Introduction

Acetylcholine (ACh) binds to receptors in the muscle membrane and transiently opens cation selective channels. Over the last 10 years there has been intense interest in the kinetics of this process and the underlying molecular components. From noise analysis of ACh-induced current fluctuations (1,2) and single channel current measurements (3,4) a simple kinetic model of the ACh receptor (AChR) channel has developed (2,5). In this model it is assumed that a conformational change in a membrane protein is the rate-limiting step in channel kinetics and that the channel fluctuates between two conductance states, open or closed, according to a first order reaction scheme

$$\text{closed} \underset{\alpha}{\overset{\beta}{\rightleftharpoons}} \text{open} \qquad \text{SCHEME I}$$

Recently, a number of observations have indicated deviations from this simple scheme. This chapter briefly reviews the nature of such complications and their molecular implications.

A. Multiple Closed States of the AChR Channel

One prediction of scheme I is that the distribution of both closed times and open times of single channels should be described by single exponentials. Recently, three different classes of channel phenomena have been observed in which the

Neuroreceptors

distribution of closed times is not a single exponential as predicted. Each of these phenomena, to be considered below, can be explained by kinetic schemes that involve multiple closed (or non-conducting) states of the AChR channel.

(1) Ion block of the open channel.

A general assumption of scheme I is that channel kinetics are independent of the charge movement through the channel. In other words ion movements are assumed not to influence the transitions between channel states but be merely modulated by this transition. However, recent evidence indicates that both cations that block AChR channels and cations that permeate the channel alter channel kinetics. For example, in the case of certain cationic drugs, most noteably the quaternary amine local anaesthetics, it has been demonstrated (6,7,8,9) that their kinetic effects on ACh induced currents can best be described by a sequential scheme

$$\text{closed} \underset{\alpha}{\overset{\beta}{\rightleftharpoons}} \text{open} \underset{x}{\overset{u(Q)}{\rightleftharpoons}} \text{blocked}_{(B)} \qquad \text{SCHEME II}$$

in which the blocking drug Q enters the open channel and binds to a channel site. In this scheme because there is no direct pathway between closed and blocked states the channel must reopen before it closes. The forward rate constant U incorporates Q concentration and the reverse rate constant is inversely related to the tightness of Q binding. For such a scheme three types of blocking behaviour may arise. (i) If the blocking ion binds tightly so that the blocked state is long lived with respect to the normal open state (i.e. $x \ll \alpha$) single channel currents will display faster kinetics but single channel conductance will be unaltered. (ii) If the blocked state is short lived but in the same time range as the average duration of the unblocked channel ($x \cong \alpha$) then the blocking ion should generate flickering or fast bursts during a single opening (see ref. 9). Again channel conductance should be unaffected. (iii) If the blocked state is very brief (x >> α) and beyond the resolution of the recording system, the channel will appear longer in duration and smaller in conductance with the measured conductance being an average between the true open and blocked conductances.

From consideration of the last case it follows that different permeating cations may also have blocking effects on AChR channels if they bind for longer durations inside the channel and the channel is unable to close normally while occupied by an ion. Such a mechanism has been used to explain the effects of permeant cations on the kinetics and conductance of AChR channels (10,11,12,13). In this model AChR channel kinetics are not independent of ion movement through the channel since they will reflect at least in part the lifetime of the ion-bound states of the channel.

(2) Multiple gating of single AChR channels.

In scheme I it is implied that the agonist binding reaction is rapid with respect to the reactions determining channel opening and closing. The alternative is that agonist binding is slow or comparable to the rate of channel closure so that two or more openings may occur during the time the receptor remains occupied by the agonist (14). Such a model essentially proposes two closed states according to scheme II

$$\text{closed}_2 \underset{k_{-1}}{\overset{k_1}{\rightleftharpoons}} \text{closed}_1 \underset{\alpha}{\overset{\beta}{\rightleftharpoons}} \text{open} \qquad \text{SCHEME III}$$

with one closed state in rapid equilibrium with the open state. In such a scheme one would expect interruptions or gaps during a single channel opening. Such gaps have been observed in suberyldicholine-activated channels in cultured chick muscle (15) and frog end-plate (16). Colquhoun and Sakmann (ref. 16) assumed that the gaps they observed represented brief but complete channel closure and demonstrated that the distribution of closed times was fitted by the sum of two exponentials; one representing the intervals between independent channel activation and the other, gaps within a burst. A simple prediction of scheme III is that the number of gaps per burst should increase with the tightness of agonist binding (14,16).

(3) Desensitization of AChR channels.

In the continued presence of ACh an end-plate current declines to an equilibrium value with a time constant of several seconds. Following removal of ACh complete recovery of the responsiveness takes up to minutes. This process is referred to as desensitization (17). In studies of this phenomenon at the single channel level it has been observed (18) that following the addition of agonist at high concentration there is an initial high current activity representing many overlapping channels. With time this activity decreases as the number of channels drop out due to desensitization. Finally the base line recovers to the resting level but is interrupted by brief bursts of activity. It was demonstrated (18) that the individual pulses within such bursts had similar average lifetimes and conductance properties as those channels recorded at low agonist concentration. This burst behaviour was interpreted as reflecting the channel temporarily moving from the desensitized state (D) into the normal functional closed state (N) as represented in scheme IV

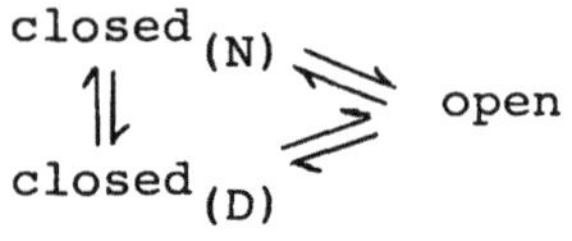

SCHEME IV

Summary The three phenomena, channel block, multiple gating and desensitization share similarities in their basic phenomenology (i.e. current bursts) and under certain kinetic conditions, one process could be interpreted or confused with another. However, distinction is possible on the basis of differences in the changes in their burst kinetics that occur with changes in agonist or blocker concentration. These qualitative differences are described in table 1.

	Phenomenon	Average closed time between bursts	Average closed time within bursts	Average open time	Burst duration
Increasing blocker concentration	CHANNEL BLOCK	no effect	no effect	decrease	increase
Increasing agonist concentration	MULTIPLE GATING	decrease	no effect	no effect	no effect
	DESENSITI-ZATION	increase	decrease	no effect	decrease

Table 1. Comparison of the predicted effects of increasing agonist or channel blocker concentration on the kinetics of bursts caused by channel block, multiple gating or desensitization.

B. Multiple-Open States of the AChR Channel.

In the two state model it is assumed that AChR channels make up a homogeneous population of channels which display the same single channel conductance. In denervated and embryonic muscles neither of these assumptions apply. The nature of the deviations are described below.

(1) Heterogeneity in AChR channel properties.

In denervated adult frog muscle fluctuation analysis has indicated that the extrajunctional channels, that appear over the whole membrane surface, have slower kinetics and a smaller conductance than the junctional channels located at the end-plate region (1,19,20,21). In neonatal rat muscle during the initial stages of synapse formation the kinetics of AChR channels are similar to those of extrajunctional channels but at later stages AChR channels are converted to the junctional class. At intermediate stages both classes of channels coexist (22,23,24,25). Single channel current recordings from the same patch of denervated frog muscle membrane reveal two classes of channels, a major class with extrajunctional properties and a minor class with junctional properties (18, 26). In cultured rat embryonic muscle, before innervation, two classes of channels with extrajunctional and junctional properties are also observed (27,28,29). The two classes display a similar reversal potential (0 mV) and have a similar selectivity for alkali cations with the conductance sequence K>Cs>Na>Li. The receptors of both channel classes also appear similar since they are blocked by α-bungarotoxin, activated by the same variety of agonists and desensitize at similar high agonist concentrations.

(2) Conductance substates of the AChR channel.

In rat embryonic muscle the majority of elementary events from the two different classes show behaviour consistent with two-state channels. However, it was observed at low temperatures (29) that a small proportion of events (<10%) from both classes display more complex behaviour. These complex currents after stepping to one of the two main levels step to a sublevel for a variable duration, then either step back to the original main level or to the resting level. A smaller propertion of events (<1%) show repetitive fluctuation between the main level and the sublevel. At low channel activity, histograms of current levels display three distinct peaks. Two major peaks corresponding to the junctional and extrajunctional class current levels and a minor peak corresponding to the sublevel. Although both main classes display a sublevel of similar amplitude the sublevel associated with the extrajunctional class is always on average longer in duration than the junctional sublevel. Some other properties of the three current levels are summarized below (see ref. 29).

1. The amplitude histograms of all three levels are fitted by gaussian distributions.
2. All three current levels display ohmic behaviour.
3. The conductance of each level is weakly temperature dependent ($Q_{10} \cong 1.2$) whereas the average lifetimes have a high temperature sensitivity ($Q_{10} \geq 3$).
4. The three conductance states display a similar ion selectivity for alkali cations.
5. The kinetics of complex events that display fluctuations between a main level and a sublevel are consistent with a single channel which can fluctuate between two open states and at least one closed state according to the kinetic scheme

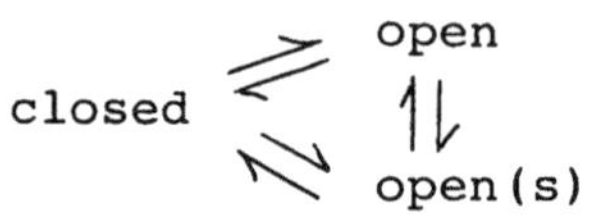

SCHEME V

with the condition that an opening to the substate directly from the closed state has a low probability.

C. Molecular Models of the AChR Channel

It is now generally accepted that the AChR channel is formed by an oligomeric protein that normally spans the postsynaptic membrane (30,31,32). The electrophysiological observations discussed above provide some clues to the molecular operation of this protein. It would appear that the AChR channel can exist in a number of distinctly different closed and open states. In the case of the open states their stability appears to be affected by (among other things) changes in temperature and the nature of permeating cations. A simple view is that in the presence of agonist the protein can fluctuate between a number of conformations. The temperature dependence would arise because the transitions from one conformation to another occurs by overcoming an energy barrier. Similarly, coulombic forces associated with ions binding to channel sites could alter the rates of conformational transitions. In this model it is assumed that the protein normally exists as a static structure and must be activated to undergo a conformational change. However, recent studies on the molecular dynamics of proteins (for review see 33, 34, 35) indicate a more complex picture. It has been demonstrated by a number of different techniques that proteins in equilibrium can exist in a large number of conformational substates, rapidly moving from one state to the next (35,36,37,38). The dwell times in each state may vary from nanoseconds to seconds (35). At high temperatures the substates are very short lived but at sufficiently low temperature the protein may remain in a particular substate for a longer duration (35). In these terms agonist binding to the AChR protein may act to stabilize specific substate conformations associated with either the conducting form of the channel or the desensitized form of the receptor. The channel while open may also fluctuate rapidly between substates and in the case of the AChR channels in embryonic muscle the substates are stable enough to be resolved at low temperatures (29). In such a model changes in the environment that alter external or internal interactions with or within the channel molecule could produce their effects on channel characteristics by shifting the spectrum of conformational fluctuations.

References

1. Katz, B., Miledi, R.: J. Physiol. 224, 665-699 (1972).
2. Anderson, C.R., Stevens, C.F.: J. Physiol. 235, 655-691 (1973).
3. Neher, E., Sakmann, B.: Nature 260, 779-802 (1976).
4. Neher, E., Sakmann, B., Steinbach, J.H.: Pflügers Arch. 375, 219-228 (1978).
5. Stevens, C.F.: Nature 270. 391-396 (1977).
6. Adams, P.R.: J. Physiol. 268, 291-318 (1977).
7. Ruff, R.L.: J. Physiol. 264, 89-124 (1977).
8. Marty, A.: J. Physiol. 278, 237-250 (1978).
9. Neher, E., Steinbach, J.H.: J. Physiol. 277, 153-176 (1978).
10. Van Helden, D.F., Hamill, O.P., Gage, P.W.: Nature 269, 111-113 (1977).
11. Ascher, P., Marty, A., Neild, T.O.: J. Physiol. 278, 177-206 (1978).
12. Gage, P.W., Van Helden, D.F.: J. Physiol. 289, 115-141 (1979).
13. Marchias, D., Marty, A.: J. Physiol. 297, 9-45 (1979).
14. Colquhoun, D., Hawkes, A.G.: Proc. R. Soc. B 199, 231-262 (1977); 221, 205-235 (1981).
15. Nelson, D.J., Sachs, F.: Nature 282, 861-863 (1979).

16. Colquhoun, D., Sakmann, B.: Nature (in press).
17. Katz, B., Thesleff, S.: J. Physiol. 138, 63-80 (1957).
18. Sakmann, B., Patlak, J., Neher, E.: Nature 286, 71-73 (1980).
19. Neher, E., Sakmann, B.: J. Physiol. 258, 705-729 (1976).
20. Dreyer, F., Walther, C., Peper, K.: Pflügers Arch. 366, 1-9 (1976).
21. Gage, P.W., Hamill, O.P.: J. Physiol. 298, 525-538 (1980).
22. Sakmann, B., Brenner, H.R.: Nature 276, 401-402 (1978).
23. Steinbach, J.H., Merlie, J., Heinemann, S., Bloch, R.: Proc. Nat. Acad. Sci. 76, 3547-3551 (1979).
24. Michler, A., Sakmann, B.: Develop. Biol. 80, 1-17 (1980).
25. Fischbach, G.D., Schuetze, S.M.: J. Physiol. 303, 125-137 (1980).
26. Neher, E.: In Techniques in Cellular Physiology (Baker, P.F., ed.) Elsevier, Amsterdam (1981).
27. Hamill, O.P., Sakmann, B.: J. Physiol. 312, 41-42P (1981).
28. Hamill, O.P., Marty, A., Neher, E., Sakmann, B., Sigworth, F.J.: Pflügers Arch. 391, 85-100 (1981).
29. Hamill, O.P., Sakmann, B.: Nature (in press).
30. Raftery, M.A., Hunkapiller, M.W., Strader, C.D., Hood, L.A.: Science 208, 1454-1457 (1980).
31. Schindler, H., Quast, U.: Proc. Nat. Acad. Sci. 77, 3052-3056 (1980).
32. Boheim, G., Hanke, W., Barrantes, F.J., Eibl, H., Sakmann, B., Fels, G., Maelicke, A.: Proc. Nat. Acad. Sci. 78. 3586-3590 (1981).
33. Williams, R.J.P.: Proc. R. Soc. B 200, 352-389 (1978).
34. Cooper, A.: Prog. Oxf. 66, 473-497 (1980).
35. Frauenfelder, H., Petsko, G.A., Tsernoglu, D.: Nature 280, 558-563 (1980).
36. Austin, R.H., Beeson, K.W., Eisenstein, L., Frauenfelder, H., Gunsalus, I.C.: Biochemistry 14, 5355-5373 (1975).
37. Munro, I.,Pecht, I., Stryer, L.: Proc. Nat. Acad. Sci. 76, 56-60 (1979).
38. Wagner, G., Wüthrich, K.: Nature 275, 247-249 (1978).

INVESTIGATION OF LIPOSOMES AND VESICLES RECONSTITUTED WITH ACETYLCHOLINE RECEPTOR EMPLOYING PERCOLL DENSITY GRADIENT CENTRIFUGATION

F. Spillecke and E. Neumann
Max-Planck-Institut für Biochemie, D-8033 Martinsried

Summary

In this report we present the study of uni- and multilamellar liposomes as well as vesicles reconstituted with acetylcholine receptor with the aid of Percoll, a recently introduced medium for density gradient centrifugation. We employ the Li^+ content as a sensitive marker for location and intactness of unilamellar vesicles. Furthermore, we show that the Li^+ content in combination with the lipid concentration allows to characterize the vesicles in terms of size. The use of Percoll proved to be useful in improving the purity of vesicles reconstituted with *Torpedo californica* acetylcholine receptor.

Introduction

Liposomes and vesicles resulting from reconstitution of membrane proteins have become an important subject of various investigations in membrane biology (1,2). It has been noted, that despite this wide attention only few methods for the purification or separation of vesicles are available (1). Usually, they belong to differential centrifugation or column chromatographic techniques (3,4). Both approaches are associated with some disadvantages. While differential centrifugation yields only a limited resolution gel filtration chromatography causes considerable dilution and matrix effects may alter the characteristics of the vesicle population. Therefore, we addressed the question of developing a different means of purifying or separating vesicles. We focused our interest on density gradient centrifugation employing Percoll. This material has been recently introduced and found application in work on subcellular fractionation (5,6) for instance. In this report, we demonstrate that density gradient centrifugation using Percoll adds to existing methods and might be useful in the study of reconstituted vesicles.

Experimental Section

Chemicals were usually of the highest grade available. Percoll was obtained from Pharmacia. Lipid analysis was performed by phosphate determination using Fiske and Subbarow (7). Ultracentrifugations were done either on a Spinco L50 (Beckman Instruments) or IEC B60 centrifuge. Densities were determined with a Zeiss refractometer in combination with a 10ml pycnometer. Li^+ concentrations were measured by flame emission spectroscopy (Pye Unicam SP1900).

Acetylcholine receptor was isolated from Torpedo californica electroplax tissue(Pacific Biomarine Laboratories) and purified by affinity chromatography (8). Radioactivity represents I^{125}-labeled α-bungarotoxin bound to acetylcholine receptor (AChR) as measured by a filter paper (DE 81) assay. Multilamellar vesicles were produced by slow rehydration of dried lipids or hydration accelerated by the addition of few small glass beads (9). Unilamellar liposomes and vesicles reconstituted with AChR were generated by cholate dialysis (10). For further details see figure legends and text.

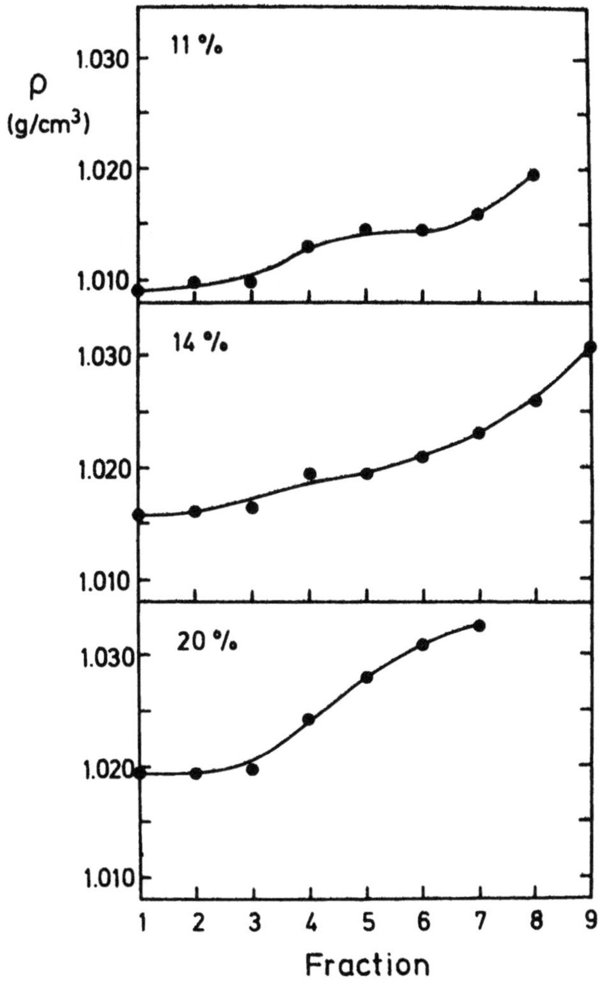

Fig. 1 Densities of gradient fractions at different Percoll concentrations in 100 mM NaCl, 5 mM Pipes, pH 7.4 at 4°C. The tubes are centrifuged for 45 min. at 9500 g.

Results and Discussion

Percoll gradients and phosphate determination

The utility of Percoll as a medium for density gradient centrifugation is exemplified in figure 1. It is shown how Percoll particles even at low concentrations are able to self-generate gradients of varying density during centrifugation. By varying the experimental conditions it is possible to investigate uni- and multilamellar liposomes as well as vesicles reconstituted with AChR. The lipid concentration in all our experiments is indicated by measuring the content of hydrolized phosphate and is compared with a standard curve of the same lipid source. The phosphate analysis is based on standard procedures but modified in order to simplify handling of large amounts of material and the testing of many samples. Additionally, Percoll was removed prior to phosphate analysis (unpublished results). A typical standard curve of such a lipid assay is presented in figure 2.

Unilamellar Vesicles

The unilamellar vesicles obtained by cholate dialysis were shown to be closed structures with diameters in the range of 100 nm by electron microscopy (data not shown) and flame emission spectroscopy of encapsulated Li^+ (figure 3). Vesicles filled with 1 mM Li^+ were put on a 3-step Percoll suspension containing layers of 5,10, and 15 % Percoll. As evident from the phosphate analysis most of the vesicles show up in the top part while vesicles of higher density occur in lower parts of the gradient. The corresponding amounts of Li^+ encapsulated in the vesicles are also shown in figure 3. The Li^+ content indicates the intactness of the vesicles since in preceding wash steps internal Li^+ would have been lost otherwise; it also constitutes a sensitive means of following them. The densities of the various fractions are given in figure 4.

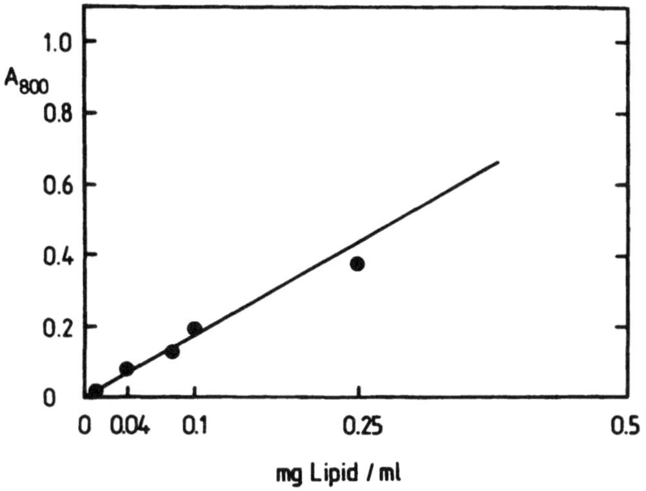

Fig. 2 Phosphate determination of phosphatidylcholine. The absorbance at 800 nm is a measure of the phosphate content of the sample.

The study of two independent informations such as density and lipid concentration or Li^+ content and lipid concentration allows to calculate important parameters of these vesicles with few simplifying assumptions. We concentrated on Li^+ content and lipid concentration because this approach appears to be more convenient and accurate. By considering the vesicles as spherical particles with a fairly homogeneous size distribution within the individual gradient fractions and neglecting small diffusional losses of Li^+ during handling, one obtains the following simple relationship,

$$r = \frac{[Li^+]}{[Lip]} \frac{v \alpha}{x} \qquad \text{and} \qquad \alpha = \frac{3 n_{Lip}}{c_{Li^+}}$$

where r represents the radius of the vesicles while v and x are correction factors for dilutions during the Li^+ and

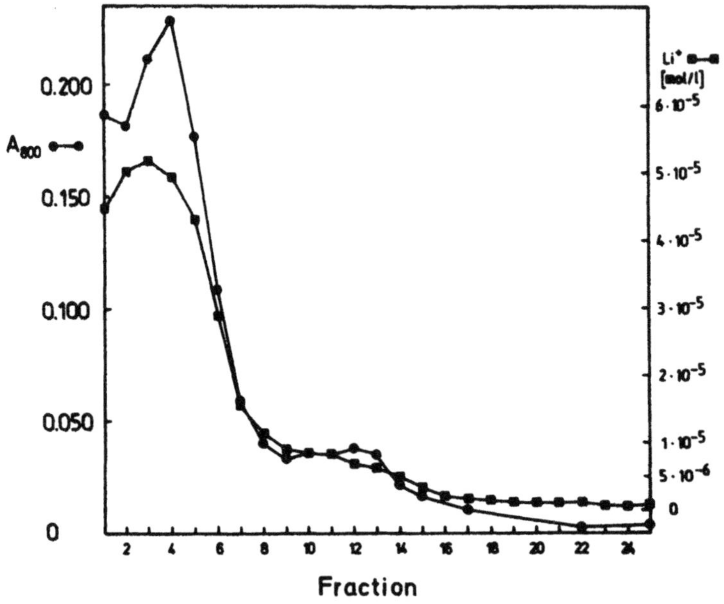

Fig. 3 Lipid and Li^+ content versus fraction number. The density gradient consisted of three layers with varying composition: 5 % Percoll, 50 mM NaCl, 5 mM Pipes, pH 7.4; 10 % Percoll, 100 mM NaCl, 5 mM Pipes, pH 7.4; 15 % Percoll, 100 mM NaCl, 5 mM Pipes, pH 7.4. Centrifugation for 45 min. at 9500 g and 4°C.

lipid assays; α is a constant for given experimental conditions. n_{Lip} is the number of lipid molecules per unit area and c_{Li^+} the Li^+ concentration inside the vesicles. $[Li^+]$ and $[Lip]$ are the experimental values as obtained from the respective assay. Using the numbers of figure 3 one calculates values around 90 nm for the radius of the vesicles. This slightly increased value is presumably due to a preceding centrifugation step which was applied in order to reduce the heterogeneity of the vesicle population and which leaves behind micelles and small vesicles.

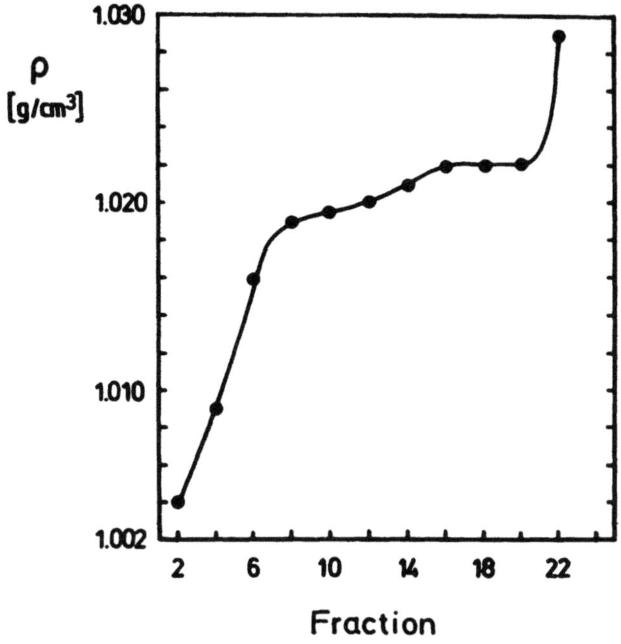

Fig. 4 Density versus fraction number of the Percoll gradient. For conditions of centrifugation see legend of figure 3.

Multilamellar Vesicles

Dispersions of multilamellar vesicles were formed by two different techniques as detailed in the experimental section. Interestingly, slow rehydration yields vesicles with a broad distribution in terms of size (figure 5). This probably reflects a great variation in the number of bilayer-sheaths per vesicle. On the other hand, most of the multilamellar vesicles obtained with the help of glass beads appear in a fairly narrow peak at lower density. It indicates that this preparation leads to fewer wrappings per vesicle and, also, results in less variation. At the bottom of the gradient a sharp band shows up which appears to be due to large lipid aggregates produced by the mechanical action of the glass beads.

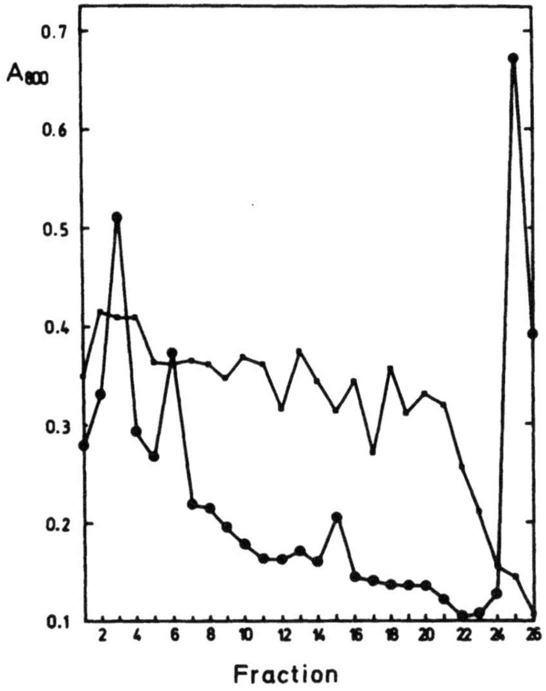

Fig. 5 Lipid content versus fraction number. The gradient was formed from 10 % Percoll, 100 mM NaCl, 5 mM Pipes, pH 7.4. Centrifugation for 45 min. at 9500 g and 4°C.

Vesicles Reconstituted with AChR

Fig. 6 shows the distribution of vesicles reconstituted with AChR if put on a Percoll suspension and centrifuged as given in the figure legend. The use of the Percoll method allowed protein aggregates or lipid vesicles associated with such aggregates to move further to higher densities. This was most obvious in a preparation were partial aggregation was induced by increasing the NaCl concentration. The radioactivity of the vesicle peak was reduced but increased in fractions of higher density (not shown). From the data in figure 6 one can calculate that approximately 300-400 receptor molecules (assuming four toxin sites per 500 000 d) occur on the average per vesicle. The significance of the shoulder observable in figure 6 is not clear as yet. Probably, it arises from vesicles with receptor aggregates.

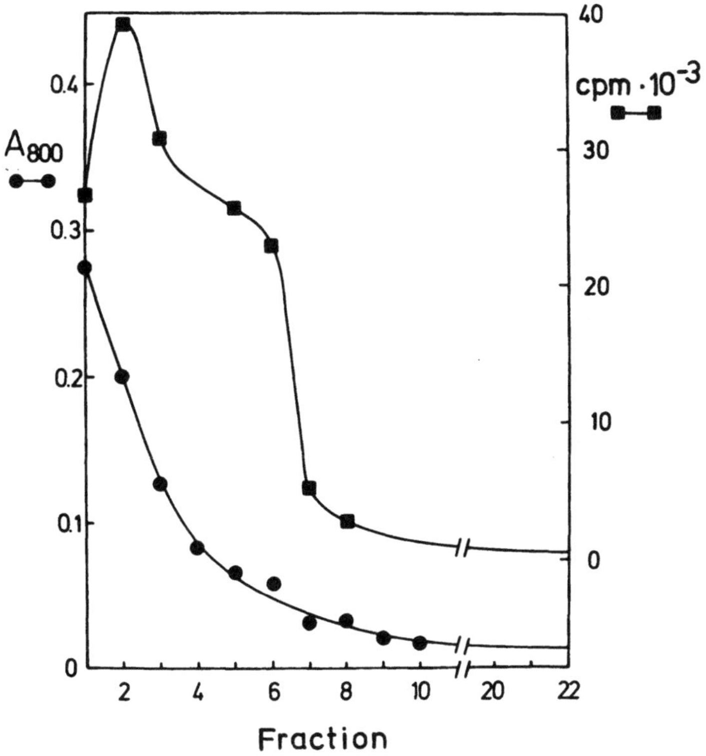

Fig. 6 Lipid content and toxin binding of AChR versus fraction number; 5 % Percoll, 50 mM NaCl, 5 mM Pipes, pH 7.4; for 45 min. 9500 g at 4°C applied.

The aim of this study is to show the utility of the Percoll technique applied to lipid vesicles, particularly, if reconstituted with membrane proteins such as AChR. The strength of this method is the adaptability to various experimental situations,however, it constitutes at the same time a certain drawback: the necessity for careful development of the experimental conditions to be used.

Acknowledgement. The technical assistance of F.Stocker and the financial support of the Stiftung Volkswagenwerk (grant I 34706) are greatfully acknowledged.

References

1. Szoka, F., Papahadjopoulos, D.: Ann. Rev. Biophys. Bioeng. 9, 467-5o8, (198o)
2. Changeux J.-P.: The Harvey Lectures, Series 75, Academic Press (198o)
3. Barenholz, Y., Gibbes, D., Litman, B. J., Goll, J., Thompson, T. E., Carlson F. D.: Biochemistry 16 28o6-281o (1977)
4. Huang, C.-H.: Biochemistry 8, 344-352 (1969)
5. Pertoft, H., Laurent, T. C.: Methods of Cell Separation Vol. 1, (Catsimpoolas, N.; Ed.), Plenum Press, New York, 25-65 (1977)
6. Grafenstein von, H., Neumann, E.: FEBS Letters 123 238-24o (1981)
7. Fiske, C. H., Subbarow, Y.: J Biol Chem 66 375-4oo (1925)
8. Chang, H. W., Bock, E.: Biochem 18, 172-179, 1979
9. Bangham, A. D., Hill, M. W., Miller, N. G. A.: Meth. Membr. Biol. 1, 1-68 (1974)
1o. Epstein, M., Racker, E.: J Biol Chem 253 666o-6662 (1978)

DOES ACETYLCHOLINE BIND COOPERATIVELY TO THE RECEPTOR?

E.K. Wolff, G. Fels and A. Maelicke
Max-Planck-Institut für Ernährungsphysiologie,
Rheinlanddamm 201, D-4600 Dortmund

Abstract

We have studied binding of acetylcholine (ACH) to membrane bound acetylcholine receptor (AChR) from Torpedo marmorata. Using tritiated ACH and an optimized assay protocol we were able to reduce the experimental error to less than 6% in the critical range of the binding curves. We found: (i) Acetylcholine binds to two distinct classes of saturable binding sites with weak positive cooperative interaction. (ii) Coupling of sites is very sensitive to the experimental conditions during the initial steps of the purification procedure. Positive cooperativity is best obtained when the tissue is homogenised in the presence of a protease inhibitor cocktail consisting of phenylmethylsulfonylfluoride (PMSF), EDTA and iodoacetamide. (iii) Aging of receptor preparations abolishes the positive cooperativity of ACH binding.

Introduction

Binding of ACH to postsynaptic acetylcholine receptors induces transient changes in ion permeability of this membrane. The ion flux through the receptor integrated ion-channel (1) relates to the doses of ACH by a sigmoidal function (2). Although central to the mechanism of cholinergic excitation it is still uncertain whether this sigmoidal shape of the dose-response curve

Neuroreceptors

is due to cooperative binding of the transmitter to its receptor or not. The answer to this question could indicate whether there is direct coupling, or additional intermediate steps are involved between transmitter binding and channel opening.

Previous binding studies employing membrane preparations from the electric organ of Torpedo were ambiguous in that some showed a single class of ACH binding sites (3,4,6), others indicated positive cooperativity of sites (5,6). Furthermore it has been shown that agonists bind via two classes of non-interacting or anti-cooperative sites to solubilized eel-receptor (7).

Because of its central role for any model of receptor function we have reinvestigated the binding of ACH to membrane preparations of Torpedo receptor. As with all previous studies the time resolution of our centrifugation assay is still too low to measure the active state of the receptor. Thus equilibrium binding studies rely on the assumption that long exposure of the receptor to ACH only changes the quantitative values but not the basic pattern of binding. Other limitations of previous studies we have tried to overcome: We have developed both a highly sensitive assay and suitable methods of data analysis and, most important, we have varied over a wide range the conditions of cell homogenization and membrane purification. We find that weak positive interactions between ACH sites remain even at equilibrium.

Materials and Methods

Membrane fragments enriched in acetylcholine receptor from Torpedo marmorata were prepared and characterized as described in reference (8). The buffer I contained 10 mM Tris-HCl, 100 mM NaCl, 1.6 mM KCl, 2 mM $CaCl_2$, 2 mM $MgCl_2$, pH 7.4, and varying protease inhibitors (1 μM Trasylol, 0.1 μg/ml Pepstatin A,

0.02% NaN_3, 0.1 mM PMSF, 50 mM benzamidine and/or 2 mM EDTA). The protease inhibitor buffer (buffer II) contained 10 mM NaPi, 10 mM NaN_3, 5 mM EDTA, 5 mM PMSF, 5 mM iodoacetamide, pH 7.5. The buffer used for the ultracentrifugation assay contained 20 mM Tris, 100 mM NaCl, pH 7.4; for experiments with bivalent ions the solutions were made 2 mM each in $CaCl_2$ and $MgCl_2$. An ultracentrifugation assay (9) employing the Beckman Airfuge was used to separate the receptor-ligand complex. The protocol has been described in detail in (8). [^{3}H]α-cobratoxin (4 Ci/mM) was prepared as described in (7). Acetylcholine esterase activity was measured by the method of Ellman et al. (10). Esterase concentrations (in moles of active sites per liters) were calculated using a turnover number of 8.5 x $10^5 min^{-1}$ (11). Protein concentrations were determined by the method of Lowry et al. (12) using an automatic technique developed by Dr. Ann Kipps of our laboratory. [^{3}H] ACH of 250 mCi/mM was bought from Amersham. All other chemicals and biochemicals were from BioRad, Calbiochem Behring, Merck, Pierce or Serva. Radioactive samples were counted in a Searle Mark III scintillation counter with a minimum of totally 400 counts per sample corresponding to a maximal statistical error of 5%.

Results

1. Preparation of ACHR-rich Membrane Fragments

The exact protocoll of the standard procedure to obtain highly enriched membrane fragments from Torpedo marmorata is described elsewhere (8). The results are outlined in Table 1. Preparations with either 1500-2000 or 3000-4000 nmol α-cobratoxin sites per g protein were used for further experiments. Various protease inhibitors were tested both in the homogenization and centrifugation buffers. Best results were obtained with an inhibitor cocktail consisting of EDTA, PMSF and iodoacetamide.

	purification step	protein mg	specific activity nmol toxinsites/g Protein	% esterase	toxinsite concentration
S_1	supernatant from low speed spin	400	50-150	10-20	$10^{-7}M$
P_2	pellet from high speed spin	30	800-1200	1-3	$10^{-7}M$
P_3	pellet from high salt/high speed spin	20	1200-1700	0.5-1.5	$10^{-7}M$
P_4	crude homogenate	15	1500-2000	0.5-1.5	$10^{-5}M$
	sonication	15	5-10% loss of toxinsites	5-10% loss of esteraseactivity	$10^{-5}M$
P_5	43.000 D depleted homogenate	13	2200-2500	0.1-0.3	$10^{-5}M$
	sepharose 6B chromatography				
	a) peak fraction		2800	0.4-0.7	$10^{-6}M$
	b) pool	7	2200	0.4-0.7	$10^{-7}M$
P_6	purified homogenate from sucrose gradient	7	3000-4000	0.2-0.4	$10^{-5}M$
	solubilized receptor		7000-8000		

Table 1: Purification of acetylcholine-receptor-rich-membrane fragments from the electric organ of Torpedo marmorata (values are given for a purification starting from 50 g electric organ)

This cocktail was also employed in large scale purifications and yields membrane fragments with sufficient concentration of binding sites (approximately 10^{-5}M α-cobratoxin binding sites).

2. Equilibrium Binding Assay

Since even the most purified membrane preparations still contain non-negligible amounts of acetylcholine esterase (see Tab. 1) acetylcholine binding must be measured in the presence of an esterase inhibitor, for which we used Tetram (O.O-diethyl-S-(ß-diethylamine)ethyl phosphothiolate). To obtain highly accurate binding data the experimental protocol was as follows: (a) For each assay point 4.00 ± 0.02 ml of membrane suspension in assay buffer containing 0.1 mg/ml BSA and 2 x 10^{-4}M Tetram were incubated for 15 min with 1.00 ± 0.03 ml of the appropriate amount of [^{3}H] ACH in assay buffer. (b) 3 aliquots of approximately 600 μl each of incubation mixture were weighted and counted for 10 min (density of the incubation mixture was 1.010 mg/ml at 20°C). (c) The membranes were pelleted by centrifugation for 15 min at 135.000 x g in 12 x 180 μl samples for each assay point. From the supernatants 3 aliquots of approximately 600 μl each are counted (exact amount determined by weight; density of the supernatant was 1.005 g/ml at 20°C). The concentration of the free [^{3}H] ACH (c_F) was determined from the supernatant while the concentration of bound ligand (c_B) is calculated from the total amount of ACH applied and c_F.

3. Binding Curves

Equilibrium binding of [^{3}H] ACH to Torpedo membrane fragments was determined at 20°C for ligand concentrations varying between 2 and 800 nM. Only specific but no non-specific binding of [^{3}H] ACH was detected. Displacement by 10^{-4}M decamethonium or cold ACH was complete over the whole applied concentration range. A representative binding curve is shown in Fig. 1.

At first view this curve seems to be fully hyperbolic in shape. In general, binding curves of this type indicate the presence of one single class of sites, while sigmoid curvature shows positive cooperativity (e.g. binding to the second site is with higher affinity than to the first). Differences in binding modes are better seen in the Scatchard representation (13).

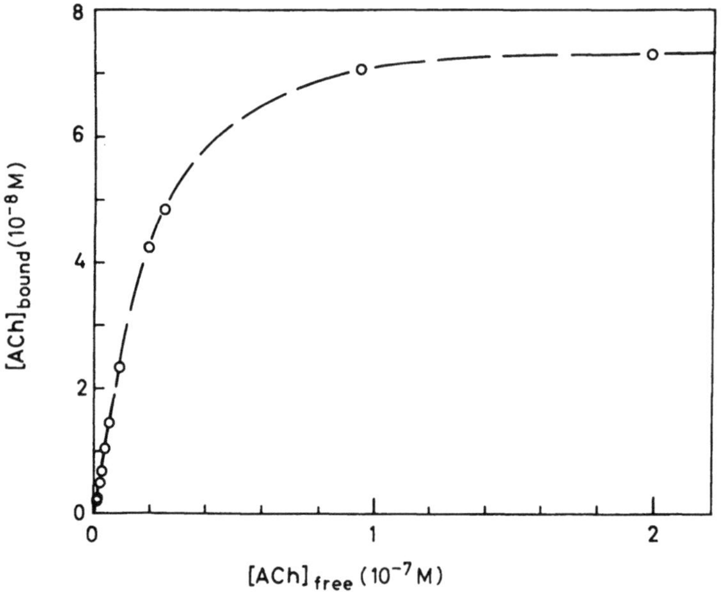

Fig. 1. Binding of [^{3}H] ACH to Torpedo marmorata membrane fragments as measured by ultracentrifugation assay. The assay buffer (pH 7.4) contained 2 mM $CaCl_2$ and 2 mM $MgCl_2$.

In this case a linear plot would be equivalent with a single class of binding sites and curved graphs would indicate the existence of two or more sites. In addition a concave curvature is evidence for positive cooperativity while negative cooperativity causes a convex curvature of the plot. Fig.2 represents the Scatchard presentation of the binding curve shown in Fig.1. Obviously, the experimental points are better fitted by a curved line then by a straight one. The same conclusion also holds when the error range of the experiments is considered. All points fall within the upper and lower error limits (dotted lines in Fig. 2) calculated from 55 pooled experiments (8). This error is less than 6% in the concentration range most sensitive for the determination of cooperativity and K_D-values

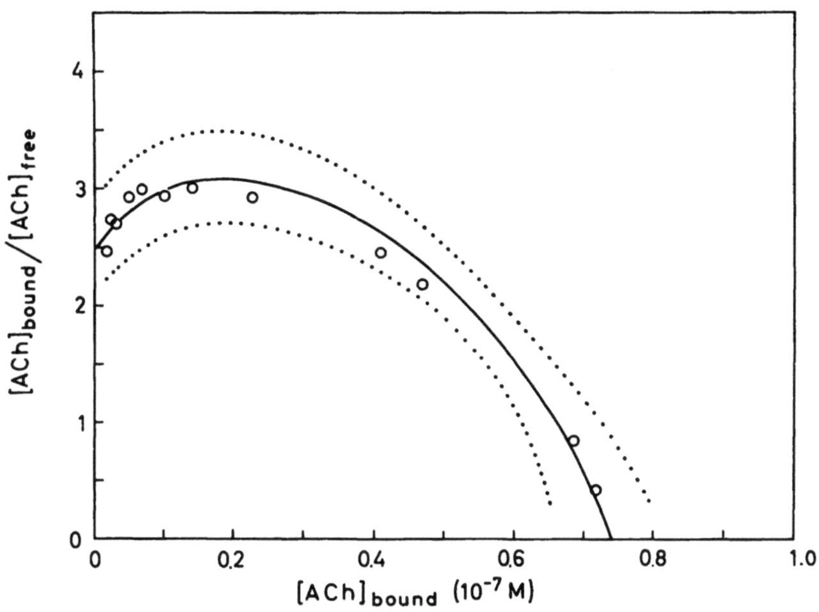

Fig. 2. Scatchard plot of [^{3}H] ACH binding to Torpedo marmorata membrane fragments freshly prepared in buffer I.

(up to about 90% saturation). The simplest model (14) to explain this ligand-receptor interaction assumes two independent ligand binding sites according to the following scheme.

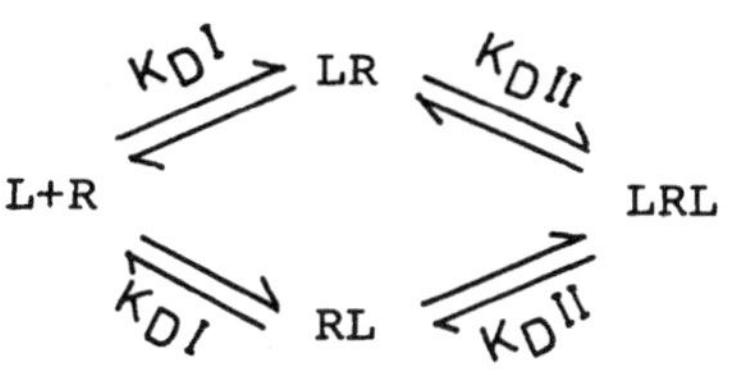

K_D-values for the two binding sites can be calculated (8) to $K_D I = 27 \pm 3$ nM and $K_D II = 8 \pm 2$ nM. It can be seen from these data as from the Fig.3 that the positive cooperativity is weak yielding a difference in K_D-values by a factor of only 2.5-5. Variation of the model would only influence the numerical values for the binding constants but not the shape of the curve (8).

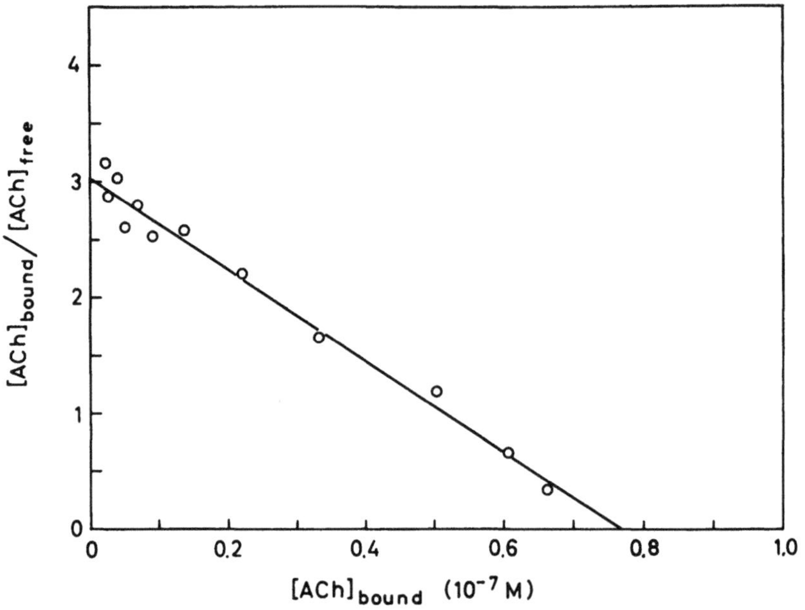

Fig. 3. Scatchard plot of an experiment as in Fig. 3 using the identical membrane preparation after five days.

In contrast to previously reported equilibrium binding studies with membrane bound AChR (3-6) we consistantly and reproducibly received concave Scatchard plots. To do so the Torpedo membrane fragments must be prepared under conditions that minimize proteolytic breakdown. Best results were obtained when PMSF, EDTA and iodoacetamide were used in the initial homogenization step.

Thus, if buffer systems without protease inhibitors are used, positive cooperativity of ACh-binding is only occasionally observed. Furthermore, even the best of our inhibitor cocktails do not suffice to conserve cooperativity of site interaction for longer periods of time. As shown representatively in Figs. 2 and 3, preparations tend to have curved Scatchard plots within the first few days changing to linear plots after 3 to 5 days of storage. At that stage the membrane preparations do not change this binding pattern any more except that the total number of sites slowly diminishes.

Discussion

In our study we report weak positive cooperative interactions of ACH-binding sites at the membrane bound acetylcholine receptor. This interaction may be weak because it is measured at equilibrium and not during the initial period of receptor exposure to ACH. We can show that cooperativity is ownly observed with preparations homogenized in the presence of suitable protease inhibitors and is only detectable during the first few days after preparation. This is evidence for considerable sensitivity of the receptor to knicking by a specific protease the nature of which is still unknown.

All these complications require more than the usual effort in conclusively proving or disproving cooperativity of transmitter binding. Only because the error of our assay is small enough to sensitively probe the whole range of the Scatchard plot (see Fig. 2), we can now confirm cooperativity at equilibrium. This makes it likely but does not prove cooperativity of ACH-binding to the actively ion-translocating receptor and, thus, can only provide circumstancial evidence for the sigmoid dose-response curve being caused by this mode of binding.

Acknowledgement

We are grateful to Dr. H. Prinz for valuable help and discussions. This investigation was supported by the Deutsche Forschungsgemeinschaft.

References

1. Boheim, G., Hanke, W., Barrantes, F.J., Eibl, H., Sakmann, B., Fels, G., Maelicke, A.: Proc. Natl. Acad. Sci. USA 78, 3586-3590 (1981).
2. Changeux, J.-P., Podleski, T.R.: Proc. Natl. Acad. Sci. USA 59, 944-950 (1968).
3. Raftery, M.A., Bode, J., Vandlen, R., Michaelson, D., Deutsch, J., Moody, T., Ross, M.J., Stroud, R.M. (1975) in: Protein-Ligand Interactions; eds. Sund, H. & Blauer, G. (Walter de Gruyter, Berlin), pp. 328-352.
4. Moore, H.-P.H., Raftery, M.A.: Biochemistry 18, 1862-1867 (1979).
5. Schiebler, W., Lauffer, L., Hucho, F.: FEBS Lett. 81, 39-42 (1977).
6. Heidmann, T., Changeux, J.-P.: Annu. Rev. Biochem. 47, 317-357 (1978).
7. Maelicke, A., Fulpius, B.W., Klett, R.P., Reich, E.: J. Biol. Chem. 252, 4811-4830 (1977).
8. Fels, G., Wolff, E.K., Maelicke, A., submitted for publication.
9. Neubig, R.R., Cohen, J.B.: Biochemistry 18, 5464-5475 (1979).
10. Ellman, G.L., Courtney, K.D., Andres, V.jr., Featherstone, R.M.: Biochem. Pharmacol. 7, 88-95 (1961).
11. Froede, H.C., Wilson, I.B.: Isr. J. Med. Sci. 6, 179 (1970).
12. Lowry, O.H., Rosebrough, N.J., Farr, A.L., Randall, R.J.: J. Biol. Chem. 193, 265-275 (1951).
13. Scatchard, G.: Ann. NY Acad. Sci. 51, 660-672 (1946).
14. Prinz, H., Maelicke, A., submitted for publication.

MOLECULAR FORMS OF THE ACETYLCHOLINE RECEPTOR PROTEIN FROM TORPEDO MARMORATA

R. Rüchel, D. Watters and A. Maelicke
Max-Planck-Institut für Ernährungsphysiologie,
Rheinlanddamm 201, D-4600 Dortmund, West-Germany

Abstract

The purified receptor from Torpedo marmorata electric organ exists in different interconvertible forms depending on both the type and concentration of detergent present, and the presence or absence of an intersubunit disulfide bridge. Receptor purified in the absence of sulfhydryl-blocking agents exists in two monomeric and two dimeric forms at very low detergent concentrations (0.01-0.05% Tween 80). At intermediate detergent concentrations (0.4% Triton X-100) one monomeric and one dimeric form are present. Only the monomeric form remains at high levels of detergent (2% Triton X-100). If receptor is purified in the presence of sulfhydryl-blocking agents, conversion of dimers into monomers by high concentrations of detergent does not occur. Disulfide-reducing agents convert dimers into monomers independent of whether the receptor's free sulfhydryl groups are blocked or not. These findings imply that dimer formation is primarily due to hydrophobic interactions between monomers. When these interactions are reduced by high levels of detergent the intersubunit disulfide bridge is dissociated at the expense of newly formed intra-subunit ones, as long as the sulfhydryl group(s) have remained unblocked.

Neuroreceptors

Introduction

The nicotinic acetylcholine receptor of electric fish is an integral membrane protein that remains tightly associated with its surrounding membrane during cell fractionation procedures. A variety of detergents can be employed to replace the surrounding lipids partially or completely and the resulting micellar preparations can be purified to apparent homogeneity of protein (1-3). Due to its absolute requirement for detergent to maintain solubility, purified receptor is micellar, and hence, microheterogeneous in nature. This has hampered quantitative studies of its basic molecular properties because conventional methods ordinarily depend in part on measurements related to either the density, the total charge or the numbers of particles of the solute being studied. Consequently, properties such as size and shape of the solubilized receptor have remained controversial.

This situation has prompted us to reinvestigate the molecular properties of the purified receptor from Torpedo marmorata by a combination of conventional together with relatively new techniques. As an alternative to the commonly employed sucrose gradient centrifugation technique we used polyacrylamide gradient gel electrophoresis (4) to study the properties of the receptor protein under non-denaturating conditions. In acrylamide gradient gels migrating species will slow down to zero mobility as they approach "pore limit". Consequently, the final separation pattern will not change by further electrophoresis and gel positions will reflect molecular weight and shape of the respective proteins. Applying this technique with a variety of buffer, detergent, salt and other conditions, we can show: (i) The solubilized receptor exists in two monomeric and two dimeric forms that are interconvertible. (ii) As the concentration of non-ionic detergent is increased, only one monomer and one dimer are apparent. (iii) The dimers can be dissociated into monomers by either disulfide reducing agents or detergents or both. (iv) Dissociation of disulfide linked monomers by detergents occurs by means of an internal sulfhydryl-disulfide exchange reaction and depends on the availability of suitably positioned sulfhydryl groups within the δ-subunits.

Materials and Methods

All materials employed, the purification procedure for acetylcholine receptor from Torpedo marmorata and the supporting biochemical procedures have been described elsewhere (5).

Gradient Electrophoresis and Isoelectric Focussing. - Electrophoresis in microgradient gels was performed as previously described (4,6). Continuous polyacrylamide gradient gels of 1-33% acrylamide and 2.5% crosslinkage were cast in glass capillaries of 32 mm length and 0.4 mm diameter (Brand, Wertheim), the gels averaging 20 mm in length. A discontinuous buffer system (0.2 M Tris-sulfate, pH 8.4 in the gel and 0.1 M Tris-glycine, pH 8.4 as running buffer) was employed. At 40 V per cm gel length, electrophoresis time is generally less than 1 h. Gels were pushed out of their glass capillaries by means of a steel wire and were stained with Coomassie blue R-250.

Except when noted otherwise, non-ionic detergents were incorporated into the gel at concentrations ranging from 0.01-2%. Ionic detergents were incorporated into the gels and added to the running buffer. For SDS-gel electrophoresis the sample contained 1%, and the running buffer 0.1%, of sodium dodecylsulfate. Samples were boiled under an atmosphere of nitrogen for 1 min. In some cases (see text) a disulfide reducing agent (dithiothreitol or ß-mercaptoethanol) was added to the sample prior to heat treatment. Approximately 30% lower field strength was applied to SDS gels as compared to gels run under non-denaturing conditions.

Results

Purified receptor from Torpedo was subjected to anodic discontinuous electrophoresis at pH 8.4 in parallel channels of gradient slab gels and in cylindrical microgradient gels. As examples we show in Fig. 1 the migration pattern of Torpedo receptor in a gradient slab gel.

Independent of the type of gel or the non-ionic detergent used Torpedo receptor contained one major component (monomer) migrating to a gel position in close proximity to horse ferritin. In addition various amounts of a larger (dimer) but no smaller components were observed. The receptor protein approached pore limit more slowly than ferritin, resulting in less defined bands and apparently larger molecular weight at shorter running times. The slow migration properties of the receptor complicated application of slab gels. We therefore used almost exclusively gradient microgels with their advantages of short running time (less than 60 min) and small sample requirements (5-10 ng of protein).

The observed receptor monomer and dimer were identical with those described by other groups (7-20) as shown by the following control experiments: (i) Receptor was incubated with various other detergents (Triton X-100, Tween 80, Emulphogene, Na-deoxycholate), at detergent concentrations of up to 10%; with up to 100 mM dithiothreitol; with chelating agents (EDTA, EGTA), and with combinations of these. Under no circumstances did we observed any smaller components than the one migrating close to ferritin. (ii) Receptor was prepared in the presence of either N-ethylmaleimide or iodoacetamide, or NaF or with higher concentrations of detergent throughout the preparation. With the exception of variations in the ratio of monomer and dimer, receptor protein obtained under these conditions had identical electrophoretic properties. (iii) Receptor was freed

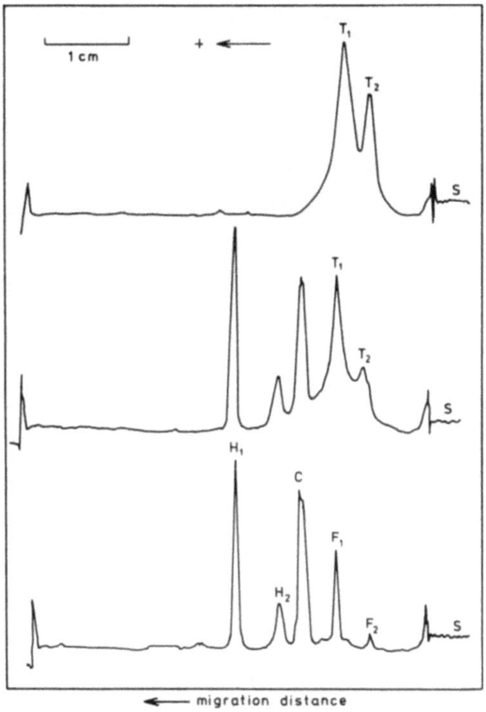

Fig. 1. Anodic electrophoresis of receptor from Torpedo marmorata and marker proteins in a 3-30% gradient polyacrylamide slab gel in the presence of 0.1% octyl glucoside.
(a) Optical density scan after staining with Coomassie blue of gel channel containing receptor from Torpedo marmorata. Peaks T_1 and T_2 both bound iodinated α-bungarotoxin; S designates the large pore spacer gel applied on top of the gradient gel.
(b) Optical density scan of adjacent gel channel containing a mixture of Torpedo receptor and marker proteins.
(c) Optical density scan of adjacent gel channel containing marker proteins only. H_1 and H_2 are human serum albumin monomer and dimer (MW = 69,000 and MW = 138,000), c is bovine catalase (MW = 232,000) and F_1 and F_2 are horse ferritin monomer and dimer (MW = 440,000 and MW = 880,000). In all cases samples were preincubated with 0.1% octyl glucoside and the gel contained the same detergent concentration throughout. A semilogarithmic plot of molecular weights versus migration distances in the gel yielded a molecular weight of the smaller receptor component (monomer) of MW = 440,000.

from attached detergent by washing hydroxylapatite-bound protein with 5.7 M urea in 0.005 M potassium phosphate buffer. This receptor while unable to bind toxin or other ligands still displayed in electrophoresis an apparent molecular weight larger than 350,000 for the smallest component. Furthermore, treatment of this receptor with DTT and/or EDTA did not cause any dissociation of the monomer. (iv) in both sucrose gradient centrifugation and equilibrium sedimentation studies we were able to reproduce the results previously obtained by others (6,19, 20). Hence, while electrophoretic techniques permit identification and characterization of the molecular forms of the receptor, they appear to yield erroneously high values for their molecular weight (10,11,17-19). The latter must be due to the method of standardizing the migration distances in gels. "Standard" proteins usually are neither integral membrane proteins nor glycoproteins. Furthermore, the receptor micelle may have considerable asymmetry.

The gel pattern of purified receptors depended on both type and concentration of detergent applied (Fig. 2). At very low detergent concentrations (0.01% Tween 80), not only the usual two but four bands were observed. They appeared to represent two pairs each of monomers and dimers. At intermediate detergent concentrations (0.4% Triton X-100) the pattern was reduced to one monomer and one dimer band, the latter one disappearing at high detergent concentrations (2% Triton X-100). Conversion between the various forms was reversible and all forms had toxin binding capacity. There existed significant variations in the effectiveness of detergents to convert dimers to monomers. While Emulphogene acted at the same concentration as Triton X-100, Tween 80 at 2-5% caused little or no conversion. The detergent effect depended also on ionic strength and temperature. Patterns were similar for fresh receptor preparations from the two <u>Torpedo</u> species while Electrophorus receptor consistently contained much less dimer.

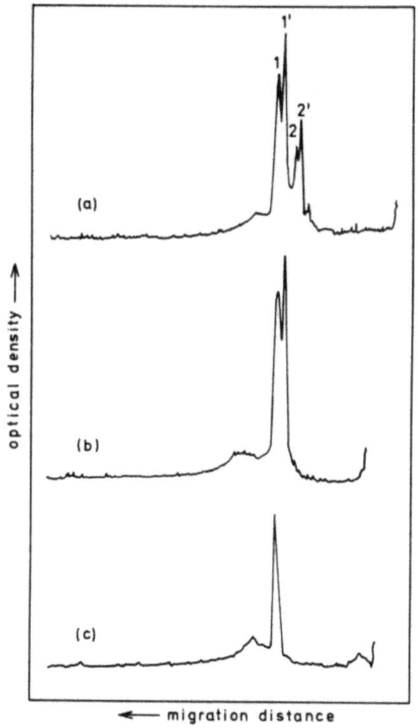

Fig. 2. Anodic electrophoresis of receptor from Torpedo marmorata in cylindrical gradient microgels in the presence of different detergent concentrations. (a) Receptor in 0.05% Tween 80, as desorbed from hydroxyapatite. (b) Aliquot of the same receptor preparation after incubation with 0.4% Triton X-100 for 30 min at 22°C. (c) Aliquot of the same receptor preparation after incubation with 2% Triton X-100 for 30 min at 22°C. Gels of samples a and b contained 0.1% octylglucoside, those of sample c contained 2% Triton X-100. Gel scans were aligned to indicate common gel positions although gradients may be slightly different in each gel. 1 and 1' denote gel positions of monomeric, 2 and 2' gel positions of dimeric receptor.

In view of earlier findings by others (16,19-21) the conversion of dimers into monomers by incubation with high concentrations of detergent was particularly surprising. The experiments were therefore repeated with receptor samples purified in the presence of the sulfhydryl blocking agents N-ethylmaleimide (NEM) and iodoacetamide. Such receptor samples commonly showed relatively higher amounts of dimers, and these dimers could not be converted into monomers by high concentrations of detergent. However, as was found previously (16,19) these as well as the unblocked dimers could be converted into monomers by the action of DTT. In addition, a combination of non-ionic detergent and DTT was more effective than either of these alone. Taken together, these experiments suggest that dissociation of dimers into monomers by non-ionic detergents crucially depends on the presence of certain unblocked and accessible intramolecular sulfhydryl groups.

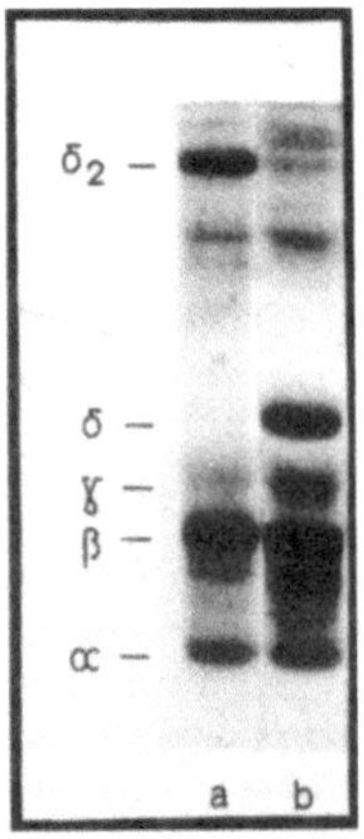

Fig. 3. SDS-gel electrophoresis of receptor from Torpedo marmorata. (left) receptor preparation rich in dimer, (right) same preparation after treatment with 100 mM dithiothreitol. Typically, receptor dimers displayed a pattern of bands corresponding to Mr of 40 x 10^3 (α), 50 x 10^3 (β) 57 x 10^3 (γ) and 130 x 10^3 (δ_2). In the presence of DTT the δ_2-band disappeared at the expense of another one corresponding to Mr of 65 x 10^3 (δ). The same effect is achieved by preincubation of intact receptor with 4% Triton X-100.

To test this hypothesis various mixtures of receptor monomers and dimers were subjected to SDS-gel electrophoresis. As shown in Fig. 3 the receptor dimers consisted of monomers linked by disulfide bridges between δ-subunits (16,19). The typical δ_2-band of such preparations disappeared when these were exposed to dithiothreitol or high concentrations of non-ionic detergents prior to SDS-gel electrophoresis. However, when receptor was first treated with iodoacetamide and then exposed to non-ionic detergent both the receptor dimer band(s) (Fig. 1,2) and the δ-dimer band (Fig. 3) remained unmodified. Thus, dissociations of receptor dimers by non-ionic detergents required the presence of a specific unblocked sulfhydryl group within each δ-subunit. If this group was blocked (by NEM or iodoacetamide) dimer dissociation by detergent did not occur. Consequently, non-ionic detergents do not directly reduce the disulfide bridges between δ-subunits but instead induce or promote a disulfide-sulfhydryl exchange reaction that leads to this dissociation.

Discussion

That receptor dimers can be dissociated into monomers by non-ionic detergents and, thus, not merely by disulfide reducing agents (16,19,21,22) is an interesting but not totally surprising result. A similar observation has previously been made by Aharonov et al. (23), who by ultracentrifugation studies showed the disappearance of the 13-S component in the presence of 1% Triton X-100. Since both their and our receptor preparations contained δ-subunit disulfide bridges, a governing role of hydrophobic forces in the formation of receptor dimers is suggested. This view is further supported by the fact that detergents such as Triton X-100 are more likely to contain oxidizing rather than reducing contaminants (24). The formation of a disulfide bond between δ-subunits is a specific rather than an accidental reaction because these bonds do not reappear with the solubilized receptor and only partially with the membrane-bound receptor (22) when these are incubated with oxidizing agents. Under the latter conditions abnormal disulfide bridge formation such as between ß-subunits has also been observed (22,25).

Although the formation of the δ-δ-disulfide bridge may require membrane components other than the receptor, their dissociation apparently does not. Thus, our findings argue against the postulate by Chang and Bock (16) of "a certain protein in the membrane that contains sulfhydryl groups both with unusual low redox potential and with close proximity to the receptor" which is responsible for the conversion of dimers into monomers during cell homogenisation procedures. Our studies show that dimers with the intersubunit disulfide bridge can be dissociated by the mere action of detergent as long as certain sulfhydryl groups remain free. Under these conditions the presence of high levels of non-ionic detergent forces a rearrangement of the intersubunit disulfide bridge into intramolecular ones thereby causing dissociation of the dimer. Probably, one particular sulfhydryl group is responsible for this effect. Not all receptor purification procedures may preserve the required steric arrangement between this sulfhydryl group and the disulfide bridge and, thus, only partial conversion of dimers into monomers by the action of detergents (12,13) or urea (26) may occur. In conclusion it appears that the "certain protein with sulfhydryl groups in close proximity to the receptor" is the receptor protein itself. Thus, given the appropriate conditions (high levels of detergent, particular states of the membrane environment) δ-δ-intersubunit disulfide bridges can dissociate spontaneously as a result of an internal sulfhydryl-disulfide exchange.

References

1. Maelicke, A., Fulpius, B.W., Reich, E.: Handbook of Physioly Section I, Part I, 493-519, American Physiological Society, Betheda, Md. (1977).

2. Heidmann, T., Changeux, J.-P.: Ann. Rev. Biochem. 47, 317-357 (1978).

3. Vandlen, R.L., Wu, C.S., Eisenach, J.C., Raftery, M.A.: Biochemistry 18, 1845-1854 (1979).

4. Ruechel, R.: Histochem. Cytochem. 24, 773-791 (1976).

5. Ruechel, R., Watters, D., Maelicke, A.: Eur. J. Biochem. 119, 215-223 (1981).

6. Ruechel, R., Mesecke, S., Wolfrum, D.I., Neuhoff, V.: Hoppe-Seyler's Z. Physiol. Chem. 354, 1351-1368 (1973).

7. Raftery, M.A., Schmidt, J., Clark, D.G., Wolcott, R.R.: Biochem. Biophys. Res. Comm. 45, 1622-1629 (1971).

8. Meunier, J.C., Olsen, R.W., Changeux, J.-P.: FEBS Letters 24, 63-68 (1972).

9. Bieseker, G.: Biochemistry 12, 4404-4409 (1973).

10. Hucho, F., Changeux, J.-P.: FEBS Letters 38, 11-15 (1973).

11. Martinez-Carrion, M., Sator, V., Raftery, M.A.: Biochem. Biophys. Res. Commun. 65, 129-137 (1975).

12. Edelstein, S.J., Beyer, W.B., Eldefrawi, A.T., Eldefrawi, M.E.: J. Biol. Chem. 250, 6101-6106 (1975).

13. Gibson, R.E., O'Brien, R.D., Edelstein, S.J., Thompson, W.R.: Biochemistry 15, 2377-2383 (1976).

14. Salvaterra, P.M., Mahler, H.R.: J. Biol. Chem. 251, 6327-6334 (1976).

15. Chang, R.S.L., Potter, L.T., Smith, D.S.: Tissue and Cell 9, 623-644 (1977).

16. Chang, H.W., Bock, E.: Biochemistry 16, 4513-4520 (1977).

17. Reynolds, J.A., Karlin, A.: Biochemistry 17, 2035-2038 (1978).

18. Hucho, F., Bandini, G., Suarez-Isla, B.A.: Eur. J. Biochem. 83, 335-340 (1978).

19. Hamilton, S.L., McLaughin, M., Karlin, A.: Biochem. Biophys. 79, 692-699 (1977).

20. Witzemann, K., Raftery, M.: Biochem. Biophys. Res. Comm. 81, 1025-1031 (1978).

21. Suarez-Isla, B., Hucho, F.: FEBS Letters 75, 65-69 (1977).

22. Hamilton, S.L., McLaughin, M., Karlin, A.: Biochemistry 18, 155-163 (1979).

23. Aharanov, A., Tarrab-Hazdai, R., Silman, I., Fuchs, S.: Immunochemistry 14, 129-137 (1977).

24. Ashami, Y., Catravas, G.N.: Anal.Biochem. 109, 55-62 (1980).

25. Weiland, G., Frisman, D., Taylor, P.: Mol. Pharmacol. 15, 213-226 (1979).

26. Sobel, A., Weber, M., Changeux, J.-P.: Eur. J. Biochem. 80, 215-224 (1977).

PROTEASE ACTIVITIES AND QUATERNARY STRUCTURE OF ACETYLCHOLINE RECEPTOR FROM TORPEDO CALIFORNICA. INHIBITION BY α' (43K) PEPTIDE

Giampiero Bandini, Jan Verdenhalven, and Ferdinand Hucho
Institut für Biochemie, Fachbereich Chemie der Freien
Universität Berlin, Arbeitsgruppe Neurochemie,
Fabeckstraße 34-36, 1000 Berlin 33, Germany

Introduction

The nicotinic acetylcholinereceptor protein (AChR) from the electric organs of electric fish has become the model system for neurotransmitter and hormone receptors, especially for the type of receptors which convert extracellular signals directly into permeability changes of the target cell membrane. AChR regulates directly an ion channel coupled to the transmitter binding protein. Alternatively, transmitter or hormone receptors are frequently coupled to an enzyme cascade converting signal- (transmitter or hormone) recognition into an intracellular effect. Prototype of the latter species is the ß-adrenergic receptor coupled to an adenylate cyclase also presented in this volume. AChR from electric fish is a favorite research object because it is readily available in large quantities and therefore an ideal object to study many of the basic questions of receptor biochemists (1). The vast literature about this protein has been comprehensively reviewed (2).

Results

1) Quaternary structure. The quaternary structure of AChR was under dispute until recently especially because conflicting subunit patterns have been published probably due to pro-

tease contaminations in the preparations of many laboratories. Based on endgroup determinations and initial sequencing work (3) it is now widely accepted, that the AChR from Torpedo californica is a pentamer of MW 27o,ooo (± 10%) (4) consisting of four different polypeptide chains and having an overall polypeptide composition $\alpha_2\beta\gamma\delta$. Recent computer analysis of high resolution electron microscopic pictures of receptor-rich membranes isolated from Torpedo electric organs (5) has shown that the AChR protein is an asymmetric molecule with a horseshoe appearance rather than a doughnut shape as assumed earlier. We investigated the quaternary structure in more detail by a nearest neighbour analysis of the various polypeptide chains using cleavable bifunctional cross-linkers and SDS polyacrylamide gel electrophoresis in two dimensions. The results of this analysis is summarized in the structural model (1) presented in fig. 1. This model contains the following features:

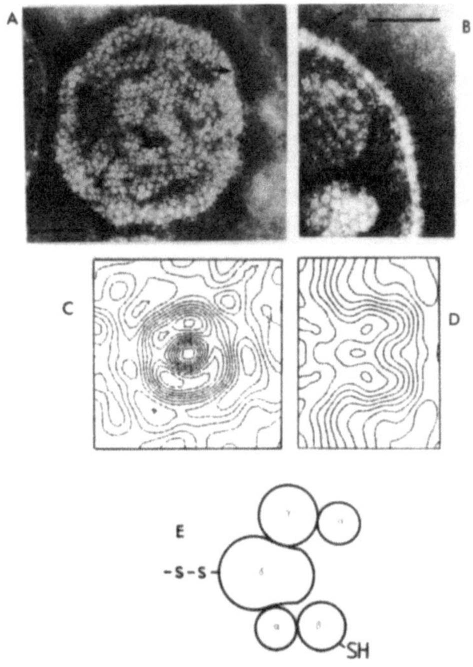

Fig 1: Ultrastructure of nAChR.
(A,B) Electron micrographs of negatively stained receptor rich membranes (19). Calibration bars represent 50 nm.
(C,D) The results of computer image-averaging (5) applied to electron micrographs of negatively stained, membrane-bound nicotinic acetylcholine receptor from T. marmorata. The height of the contour plots corresponds to 128 Å; the contours represent lines of equal density. Resolution as presented: 20 Å.
(C) A projection along an axis perpendicular to the membrane plane.
(D) A cylindrical average of several of the side views, which are visualized along the edges of microsacs (see also B). This corresponds essentially to a projection along an axis parallel to the membrane plane. Both projections represent receptor monomers. It becomes

clear that about half of the receptor molecule extends from the membrane into the outer medium. This hydrated portion of the molecule has a cavity, 40 - 50 Å deep and about 25 Å wide, around which the mass is distributed in an approximately three-fold manner, but without strict axial symmetry. This gives rise to the overall horseshoe appearance in E. (Reproduced with kind permission of H.P. Zingsheim).
(E) Structural model of nAChR based on nearest neighbour analysis with bifunctional cross-linkers.

a) The AChR is an asymmetric pentameric protein.
b) The AChR molecule is linked via a disulfide bridge to a second AChR molecule, forming a dimer the functional significance of which is not yet clear. The dimerisation is mediated by the δ-polypeptide chain.
c) The two α-polypeptide chains which have been shown to contain the binding sites for cholinergic ligands (6, 7) are not neighbours and are placed in different chemical environments. This is relevant for the interpretation of binding studies and kinetic experiments.
d) One α-chain is in contact with each of the other three polypeptide chains.
e) Several SH- (and further S-S) groups are present on the various polypeptides.

All the contacts included in the model have been proven by the cross-linking method mentioned above and by the application of photoaffinity derivatives of α-bungarotoxin known to be bound by the α-chains of the receptor but after photoactivation also reacting covalently with the δ-chain (8, 9). This reaction could be modulated by cholinergic effectors indicating not only a structural but also a functional relationship between α- and δ-polypeptide chains in the receptor complex.
The model of course gives no hint as to the location of the ion channel regulated by agonist binding to the α-chains. Recent photoaffinity labeling experiments with derivatives of ion channel ligands (local anaesthetics) have presented evidence that the δ-chain may be involved in the ion translo-

cation process (10).

2) Protease activities in AChR-rich membranes.
Considerable confusion existed until recently concerning the true quaternary structure of the AChR and many alternative subunit compositions have been published (2). This confusion apparently was caused by proteolytic activities in the receptor preparations. Proteolysis could be largely eliminated during AChR preparation by protease inhibitors and EDTA (11).

One central theme in receptor research is the regulation of receptor concentration in postsynaptic membranes (12). Regulation of AChR synthesis is under thorough control but there is also evidence that regulation of AChR degradation plays a considerable role in this respect. Half live of AChR in the subsynaptic membrane of the neuromuscular endplate is in the order of 14 days, in the extrasynaptic membrane only 7 hours (12). In pathological states as in Myasthenia gravis AChR degradation appears to be enhanced by an autoimmune response. Bifunctional AChR antibodies have been shown to stimulate AChR degradation (13).

Because of the possibility that the observed proteolytic activities are not only a nuisance for the preparative biochemists but are of significant and possibly specific physiological importance we describe in this paper some of its properties. In a preliminary study we have shown that especially in crude AChR preparations most of the proteolytic activity is of lysosomal origin, can be released by sonication and detergents and has pH optima at acidic pH values (14). Now we describe a proteolytic activity which is still present in the purest AChR membrane preparations and which shows considerable differences as compared to the aforementioned lysosomal proteases. This proteolysis may be regulated by the α' peptide, a peripheral protein, which can be extracted from AChR-rich membranes by treatment at alkaline pH (15). This polypeptide which has a MW of 43.000 was at times considered to be the only other AChR component besides the ligand-binding α-chain (16) and thought to be the ion channel of the AChR (10, 17, 18).

Proteolysis in crude homogenates of Torpedo electric tissue was assayed with typical exogenous protease substrates (casein, hemoglobin) (14). The first routine purification steps, especially the "high-salt-wash" (19) removes this activity from AChR-rich membranes. In addition to the properties mentioned above this lysosomal protease activity was found to be partly inhibited by phenylmethanesulfonyl-fluoride (PMSF) or EDTA. With our purest membranes obtained by sucrose density gradient centrifugation (19) virtually no proteolysis of exogenous substrates was observed. For an assay of this proteolytic activity which is obviously endogenous to the AChR membranes only endogenous membrane proteins were used as substrates, and proteolysis was qualitatively monitored by changes in the band pattern of AChR-rich membranes on SDS-polyacrylamide gel electrophoresis.
Fig. 2 (top) shows that all AChR bands (α, α', β, γ, δ) are degraded by this protease after prolonged (three day) incubation. It is important to point out that also the uppermost band in the gel (arrow) which most likely represents an ATPase located on an impurity in most AChR-membrane preparations (4) ist digested. Fig. 2 (bottom) whows several other important features of the endogenous protease: The protease is present in all membrane containing fractions of the density gradient. Furthermore, the partially degraded AChR protein shown on this gel indicates that degradation starts with the α polypeptide chain the other chains being well preserved at this stage. This is a characteristic

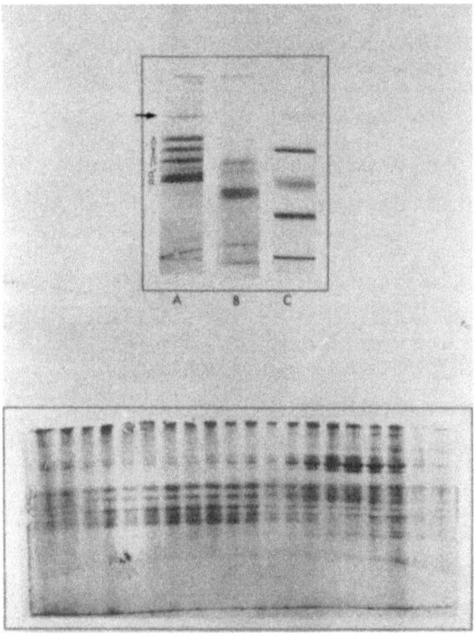

Fig. 2: Endogenous protease activity in AChR-rich membranes:

Top: A, control, SDS polyacrylamide gel of AChR-rich membranes showing the characteristic integral membrane proteins α, β, γ, δ, and the peripheral protein α'. B, the same preparation after three days incubation at pH 8.4 and room temperature. C, calibration standards.
Bottom: SDS polyacrylamide gel electrophoresis of various fractions of a sucrose density gradient, the final purification step of the AChR-rich membranes (19); top of the gradient to the right. These fractions also were incubated at room temperature and the gels show that proteolysis began with the α-protein in all receptor containing fractions. Arrow: see text.

difference as compared to the lysosomal proteases mentioned above and even to exogenous proteases as trypsin or chymotrypsin which digest the γ and δ chains first a fact which led to the interpretation that these and the β chain are not even part of the receptor complex (2). Finally in contrast to the degradation by exogenous trypsin (20) the degradation product of MW 27.000 characteristically obtained by this method is not observed (but see below!). The degradation products are apparently small enough to escape during electrophoresis.

While the exogenous (lysosomal) proteases have pH optima below pH 7 the endogenous protease shows little activity at neutral or acidic pH values. We assay it routinely at pH 8.4 but because of the lack of a truely quantitative assay we do not yet know if this is really the optimal pH.

Effect of EDTA and PMSF on the endogenous protease: Proteolysis was strongly inhibited by EDTA and EGTA, suggesting that it requires divalent ions, especially Ca^{2+} for activity. PMSF, the irreversible inhibitor of serin proteases, had little if any inhibitory effect (fig. 3). For further investigations we therefore omitted EDTA from the membrane preparation to preserve maximal protease activity. In these preparations α was slightly degraded.

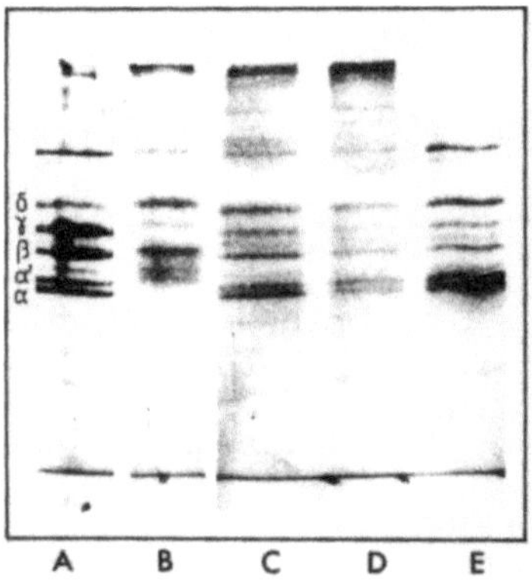

Fig. 3: Effect of EDTA and PMSF on the endogenous protease:

A and E, control, AChR-rich membranes stored at 4° C. B, the same membranes stored for three days at room temperature (pH 8.4, 0.02 % NaN_3), C, as B, but with 0.1 mM EDTA, EGTA gives identical results.
D, as B but with 0.1 mM PMSF.

Proteolysis of the AChR complex appears
›eptide chain. Therefore it is not sur-
›inding with high affinity to this poly-
thereby the whole complex against pro-
:ig. 4). α-bungarotoxin preserves the

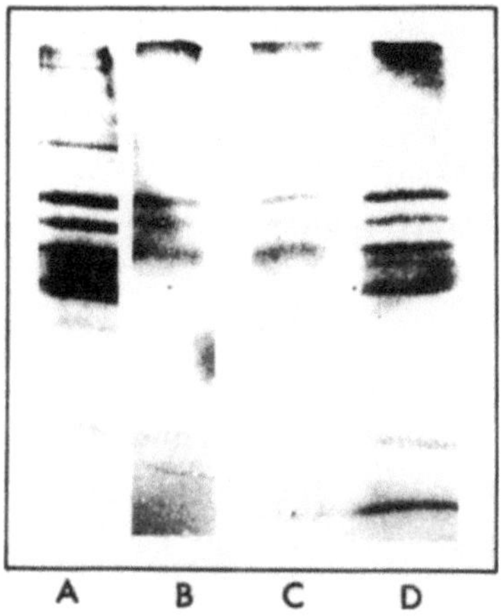

Fig. 4: Effect of cholinergic effectors on the endogenous protease:

A, control, AChR-rich membranes stored at 4°C. B, incubated for three days at room temperature in the presence of 1 mM carbamoylcholine, pH 8.4, 0.02% NaN_3. C, as B but instead of carbamoylcholine incubation was in the presence of 0.1 mM of the antagonist flaxedil. D, incubation in the presence of 0.0015 mM bungarotoxin.

original band pattern of AChR on SDS polyacrylamide gel. Neither the antagonist flaxedil (10^{-4} M) nor the agonist carbamoylcholine (10^{-3} M) have a comparable effect. Carbamoylcholine (10^{-3} M) also does not stimulate proteolytic degradation (not shown in the figure).

Reducing agents. A considerable stimulation of AChR proteolysis is observed in the presence of dithioerythritol (DTE) (fig. 5A). Instead of the three day incubation neccessary to

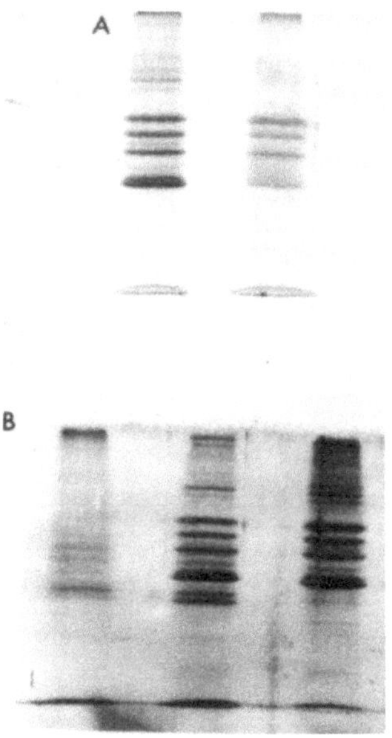

Fig. 5: Stimulation of degradation by DTE:

A, left: SDS polyacrylamide gel of AChR-rich membranes after 6 hrs incubation at 36°C; right: the same as left but incubation was in the presence of 1 mM DTE.
B, left track: AChR-rich membranes incubated with o.1 µg/ml trypsin O.1 mM DTE, 6 hrs at 36°C and pH 8.O; middle: the same as left track: but incubation was in the absence of DTE; right track: control, incubation without trypsin or DTE. No degradation was observed, not even by the endogenous protease, because its activity is low at pH 8.O.

visualize AChR degradation in the absence of DTE in the presence of DTE a significant effect was apparent already after 5-6 hours. Here again it was the α-polypeptide which was degraded first.

This effect is probably not due to thiol activation of the protease but to activation of the substrate AChR by reduction. This is evident from the observation (fig. 5B) that degradation of AChR by trypsin is also strongly stimulated by DTE.

Protease activity is membrane dependend: The proteolytic activity under investigation is membrane bound. Not even on a continuous sucrose density gradient the enzyme is removed. Obviously, also the substrate has to be membrane bound (fig.6).

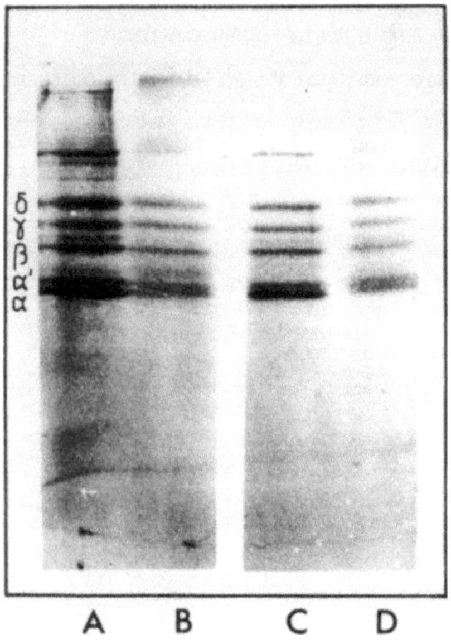

Fig. 6: Inhibition of endogenous protease by detergents:

A, control, AChR-rich membranes stored at 4° C. B, C, and D, incubation in the presence of 1 % cholate, SDS, and desoxylysolecithin, respectively. The band pattern is basically preserved.

Disolved in 1 % SDS no degradation was observed, but even in 1 % cholate or 1 % desoxylysolecithin degradation was much less than in the absence of these detergents (for comparison see fig. 2, top, middle track).

Virtually no degradation was observed after prolonged incubation of the receptor-rich membranes with soluble enzymes as albumin or β-galactosidase (not shown). On the other hand the amount of proteolytic activity appears to be variable. Different preparations are degraded to various extent under comparable experimental conditions. Because of the lack of a quantitative assay this conclusion is based as in all the experiments described here only on qualitative comparison of electrophoresis gel band patterns.

Effects of pH 11-treatment on endogenous protease activities:

It has been shown that losely adsorbed peripheral proteins especially the α' polypeptide chain can be removed from the receptor membrane by treatment at alkaline pH (pH 11) (15). Under these conditions the proteolytic activity is not removed indicating that it is an *integral* membrane component (fig.7). On the contrary after alkaline extraction degradation is significantly enhanced (fig.7) This finding hints at a stabilizing (protective) function of the α' peptide.

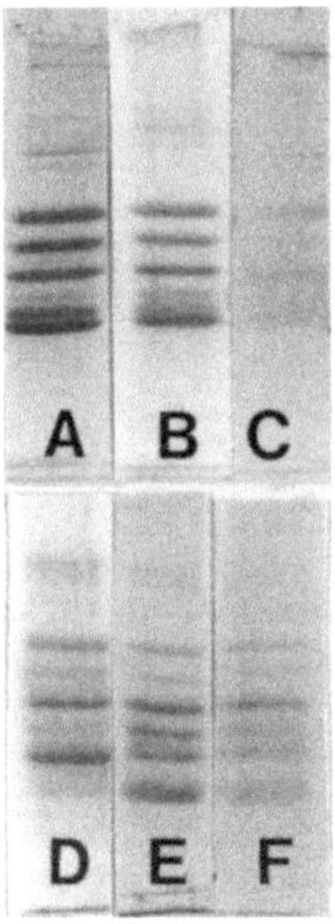

Fig.7: Endogenous protease activity in AChR-rich membranes extracted at alkaline pH (pH 11 treatment according to (15)):

(A) SDS polyacrylamide gel electrophoresis of AChR-rich membranes stored at 4°C. The same membranes stored 48 hrs at 36°C, in absence (B), in presence (C) of 1mM DTE. pH 11-treated membranes (α' is absent) incubated at 4°C, (D), at 36°C in absence (E) and presence (F) of 1 mM DTE. Comparison of (B) and (E) shows that degradation is more pronounced in the pH 11-treated membranes.

Discussion:

It has been claimed (16) that the cholinergic receptor from Torpedo electric tissue consists of only two different polypeptide chains, α(M_r 4o.ooo) and α'(M_r 43.ooo), β,γ and δ being probably impurities. It is now widely accepted that this claim was based on proteolysis of the receptor protein.
From the experiments presented here and elsewhere (14) it is obvious that the method of preparation leading to the α,α' -

AChR (16) contained several elements stimulating proteolysis: reducing agents, rendering AChR more susceptible to proteolysis and sonication releasing proteases most probably from lysosomes (14). The protease inhibitor applied, PMSF, on the other hand has very little effect because neither the proteases with acidic pH optima nor the basic protease described here are inhibited by this reagent to a great extent.

Is the protease detected in highly purified AChR membranes specific for the nicotinic acetylcholine receptor? This is a central question relevant for the problem of regulation of AChR degradation. We believe that the answer is no: this conclusion is mainly based on the observation that in addition to proven AChR components other polypeptides previously shown to be impurities in receptor rich membrane preparations are also degraded. Reversible AChR ligands neither inhibit nor stimulate proteolysis significantly. On the other hand it is obvious that proteolytic degradation of the receptor complex can be *regulated* specifically by several exogenous and endogenous factors, by the redox state of the cystein side chains, the Ca^{2+} concentration and the practically irreversible AChR ligand α-bungarotoxin. The latter observation is in agreement with cell biological studies which have indicated that the average lifetime of receptors complexed with α-bungarotoxin was selectively lengthened to 22 hours (12).

Most interesting is the considerable stimulation of proteolytic degradation by alkaline extraction. Of course it is premature to conclude from this observation that α' stabilizes and protects the AChR membrane against degradation, because in addition to this abundant protein several minor components are extracted as well which could be responsible for this effect. But several authors have supplied evidence that the peripheral protein α', which is most likely located on the internal side of the postsynaptic membrane, plays a stabilizing role. Although its removal does not change the binding and ion translocating capabilities of the AChR, it renders the

AChR more susceptible to heat inactivation (21), and the receptors in the membrane become more mobile (22).

Conclusion

There is a protease activity endogenous to the AChR-rich membrane which is not necessarily specific for the AChR but may be regulated by specific endogenous factors relevant for the regulation of receptor density in the postsynaptic membrane.

The quaternary structure of AChR from vertebrate endplates is unknown but immunological investigations have shown that this protein is not grossly different from electric fish AChR. In a recent publication (23) it has been proven that even the α'(43 K)-protein can be found in mammals. There it is localised in the endplate region supporting our hypothesis that the difference in the turnover of subsynaptic and extrasynaptic AChR is due to the regulatory function of the (43 K)-protein which may be absent from extrasynaptic receptors.
It will be interesting now to investigate further the properties of the endogenous protease and to find out whether it is regulated by the phosphorylation state of the AChR and by antibodies directed against the receptor.

Acknowledgements

This work was supported by the Land Berlin, the Deutsche Forschungsgemeinschaft and the Fonds der Chemischen Industrie.

References

1. Hucho,F.: TIBS 6, 242-245 (1981)
2. Heidmann,T., Changeux,J.-P.: Ann.Rev.Biochem. 47, 317-357 (1978)
3. Raftery,M.A., Hunkapiller,M.W., Strader,C.D., and Hood,L.E.: Science 208, 1454-1457 (1980)
4. Hucho,F., Bandini,G., Suárez-Isla,B.A.: Eur.J.Biochem. 83, 335-340 (1978)
5. Zingsheim,H.P., Neugebauer,D.-Ch., Barrantes,F.J., Frank,J.: Proc.Natl.Acad.Sci. USA 77, 952-956 (1980)
6. Reiter,M.J., Cowburn,D.A., Prives,J.M., Karlin,A.: Proc. Natl.Acad.Sci. USA 69, 1168-1172 (1972)
7. Hucho,F., Layer,P., Kiefer,H.R., Bandini,G.: Proc.Natl. Acad.Sci. USA 73, 2624-2628 (1976)
8. Witzemann,V., Muchmore,D., Raftery,M.A.: Biochemistry 18, 5511-5517 (1979)
9. Hucho,F.: FEBS Letters 103, 27-32 (1979)
10. Sobel,A., Heidmann,Th., Hofler,J., Changeux,J.-P.: Proc. Natl.Acad.Sci. USA 75, 510-514 (1978)
11. Raftery,M.A., Vandelen,R.L., Reed,K.L., Lee,T.: Cold Spring Harbor Symp. Quant.Biol. 40, 193-202 (1976)
12. Fambrough,D.M.: Physiol.Reviews 59, 165-227 (1979)
13. Appel,S.H., Anwyl,R., McAdams,M.W., Elias,S.: Proc.Natl. Acad.Sci. USA 74, 2130-2134 (1977)
14. Baumann,H., Bayer,H., Hucho,F.: Hoppe Seyler's Z.Physiol. Chem. 362, 190 (1981)
15. Neubig,R.R., Krodel,E.K., Boyd,N.D., Cohen,J.B.: Proc.Natl. Acad.Sci. USA 76, 690-694 (1979)
16. Sobel,A., Weber,M., Changeux,J.-P.: Eur.J.Biochem. 80, 215-224 (1977)
17. Blanchard,S.G., Raftery,M.A.: Proc.Natl.Acad.Sci. USA 76, 81-85 (1979)
18. Eldefrawi,A.T., Eldefrawi,M.E., Albuquerque,E.X., Oliveira, A.C., Mansour,N., Adler,M., Daly,J.W., Brown,G.B., Burgermeister,W.B., Witkop,B.: Proc.Natl.Acad.Sci. USA 74, 2172-2176 (1977)
19. Schiebler,W., Hucho,F.: Eur.J.Biochem. 85, 55-63 (1978)
2o. Bartfeld,D., Fuchs,S.: Biochem.Biophys.Res.Commun. 89, 512-519 (1979)
21. Saitoh,T., Wennogle,L.P., Changeux,J.P.: FEBS Letters 108, 489-484 (1979)

22. Barrantes,F.J., Neugebauer,D.-Ch., Zingsheim,H.P.: FEBS Letters 112, 73-78 (1980)

23. Froehner,S.C. Gulbrandsen,V., Hyman,C., Jeng.A.Y., Neubig, R.R., Cohen,J.B.: Proc.Natl.Acad.Sci., USA 78, 5230-5234 (1981)

TRIPHENYLMETHYLPHOSPHONIUM: A NEW ION CHANNEL LIGAND OF THE NICOTINIC ACETYLCHOLINERECEPTOR

Leander Lauffer
Freie Universität Berlin, Fachbereich Chemie,
Institut für Biochemie, Arbeitsgruppe Neurochemie,
Fabeckstraße 34-36, 1000 Berlin 33

Introduction

The lipophilic cation triphenylmethylphosphonium and the related compound tetraphenylphosphonium are widely used as membrane potential sensors on whole cells (1,2), subcellular fractions like synaptosomes (3) and membrane vesicles (4). These cations accumulate into the membrane-enclosed compartment, when a potential (interior negative) is generated across the membrane. Using radioactively labeled ions, it is possible to determine the amount of ions accumulated by simple filtration assays (5). The concentration difference of cations between inside and outside can be used to calculate the membrane potential with the NERNST-equation.

We intended to apply this method for the investigation of the potentials across membranes of vesicles prepared from the electric organ of *Torpedo marmorata*.

Surprisingly, we found that with these vesicles accumulation of triphenylmethylphosphonium is not only voltage-dependent but is also stimulated in a voltage independent manner by a variety of cholinergic effectors.

Neuroreceptors

Abbreviations:

HEPES: N-2-Hydroxyethylpiperazine-N'-2-ethanesulfonic acid
(H_{12}-)HTX: (perhydro-) histrionicotoxin
PCP: 1-(1-Phencyclohexyl)piperidine (phencyclidine)
$TPMP^+$: Triphenylmethylphosphoniumbromide

Materials and methods:

(^3H)-TPMP: 36 Ci/mMol, NEN, (^3H)-PCP: 48 Ci/mMol, NEN, (^3H)-acetylcholine: 50-100 mCi/mMol, NEN, ^{22}NaCl: 200 μCi/ml, NEN. All other reagents were of the highest commercially available purity.

Preparation of acetylcholinereceptor-rich membrane fragments: As described in (6): 90 g of electric tissue from Torpedo marmorata (stored frozen at -60°C) are cut into small pieces and homogenized with a Waring blendor for 3 min. at maximum speed in 180 ml 0,02 M sodium phosphate buffer, pH 7,4, containing 2 mM ethylenediaminetetraacetate, 0,1 mM phenylmethylsulfonylfluoride and 0,4 M NaCl. This and all subsequent steps are performed at 2° C. The homogenate is centrifuged 90 min at 27 000 x g, and the supernatant is discarded. The pellet is suspended in 90 ml of 0,02 M sodium phosphate buffer, pH 7,4, containing 2 mM ethylenediaminetetraacetate and 0,1 mM phenylmethylsulfonylfluoride with a Waring blendor at low speed (3 min). The suspension is centrifuged 90 min at 39 000 x g. The pellet is suspended and centrifuged again, and after this second wash the pellet is suspended in 35 ml of the same buffer. After 10 min centrifugation at 1 000 x g each 7 ml of the supernatant are layered on top of 55 ml of a continuous sucrose gradient (25-50 % w/v sucrose in distilled water containing 0,02 % NaN_3). Centrifugation is performed for 6 h at 59 000 x g in a Beckman SW 25 rotor. The gradient is fractionated in 2-ml portions. The purest fractions (usually 4 to 5

2-ml fractions containing about 0,3 mg of protein/ml) yielding membranes with predominantly the four receptor polypeptide chains (more than 85 %) are suspended in 60 ml distilled water, centrifuged 30 min at 20 000 x g and the pellet from these gradients is resuspended in 2,5 - 3 ml of the desired medium.

(^{3}H)-TPMP$^+$- and (^{3}H)-PCP-binding to acetylcholinereceptor-rich membrane fragments:
The membrane suspension obtained by the preparation described above is incubated overnight at 4° C in either Na-rich medium, containing 160 mM NaCl, 5 mM KCl, 2 mM $CaCl_2$, 0,1 mM phenylmethylsulfonylfluoride, 10 mM HEPES pH 7,4 or K-rich medium, containing 165 mM KCl, 2 mM $CaCl_2$, 0,1 mM phenylmethylsulfonylfluoride, 10 mM HEPES pH 7,4. Binding is measured at 20° C-22° C. The filters used (EHWP 02500 Celotate filters, pore width 0,45 µm, Millipore, Neu-Isenburg) are soaked in Na-rich medium containing 10 mg/ml bovine serum albumine at least 2 hrs prior to use. Binding reaction is started by tenfold dilution of the membrane suspension in either Na- or K-rich medium containing 1 mg/ml bovine serum albumine and additional reagents and ligands as described in the results section. At the indicated time intervals, the binding reaction is stopped by diluting 100 µl of reaction mixture with 3 ml icecold Na-rich medium containing 1 mg/ml bovine serum albumine followed by rapid filtration. The filters are washed twice with 3 ml icecold Na-rich medium containing 1 mg/ml bovine serum albumine and counted with 0,2 ml H_2O and 5 ml Supertron (Kontron, München) in a liquid scintillation counter.

(^{3}H)-acetylcholine-binding to acetylcholinereceptor-rich membrane fragments:
Binding is measured at 20° C by an equilibrium centrifugation assay. The membrane suspension (protein concentration: 0,5 mg/ml - 0,15 mg/ml) is incubated 30 min at room temperature with 10^{-4} M eserine to block acetylcholineesterase-function. After

5 min incubation with the desired (^{3}H)-acetylcholine-concentration, 165 µl aliquots are centrifuged for 30 min in a Beckman airfuge. Before and after centrifugation aliquots are counted in 5 ml Supertron (Kontron, München) in a liquid scintillation counter to give total and free concentration of (^{3}H)-acetylcholine, respectively.

^{22}Na-efflux:

As described in (7). Receptor-rich microsacs from the combined peak fractions of the sucrose gradient are collected by 30 min centrifugation at 20 000 x g and suspended in Na-rich medium (see above) to a final protein concentration of 5 - 10 mg/ml. The suspension is incubated overnight with 20 µCi/ml ^{22}Na at 4° C. The incubation mixture is diluted 140-fold in icecold Na-rich medium. Aliquots of 1 ml are filtered through Millipore filters (0,45 µm pore width) at the time intervals indicated in the figures.

Results:

Voltage-dependent and carbamoylcholine-stimulated (^{3}H)-TPMP^{+}-accumulation:

Receptor-rich membrane fragments were incubated over night in K-rich medium (for composition of K-rich and Na-rich medium: see "methods"). By dilution into Na-rich medium the "physiological" situation should be simulated and a K-diffusion potential be generated. In fact, accumulation was stimulated following dilution into Na-rich medium compared to the one observed in K-rich medium (fig. 1A). We did not try to evaluate the values obtained in terms of membrane potentials for two reasons: (i) we have not yet determined the internal volume of the vesicles obtained with our preparation and (ii) we found that accumulation of (^{3}H)-TPMP is not only voltage-dependent, as is shown in the following paragraphs.

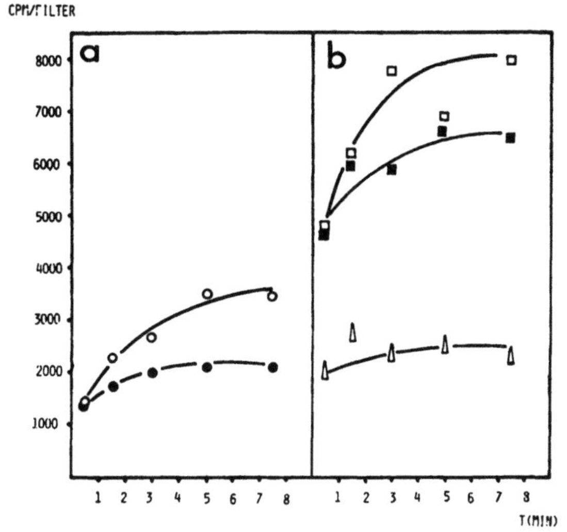

Fig. 1: (^{3}H)-TPMP$^+$-binding to acetylcholinereceptor-rich membrane fragments

Protein concentration was 0,26 mg/ml, membranes equilibrated in K-rich medium. Concentration of (^{3}H)-TPMP$^+$ was 130 nM. A) Membrane suspension was diluted into either K-rich (-●-) or Na-rich (-○-) medium. B) Dilution medium contained 10^{-5} M carbamoylcholine. Membrane suspension was diluted either into K-rich (-■-) or Na-rich (-□-) medium. (-△-): Membrane suspension was incubated 10 min at roomtemperature with 10^{-5} M α-bungarotoxin prior to dilution into Na-rich medium.

In fact, we feel that the results presented in this paper justify the use of the term "(^{3}H)-TPMP$^+$-binding" rather than "(^{3}H)-TPMP$^+$-accumulation".

Dilution in the presence of the cholinergic agonist carbamoylcholine (10^{-5}M) resulted in even larger amounts of (^{3}H)-TPMP$^+$ bound to or in the vesicles (fig. 1B). This is in contrast to theoretical predictions, as one would expect the acetylcholinereceptor ion channel to be opened by the agonist, the membrane to be depolarized and accumulation inhibited.

The stimulating effect of carbamoylcholine could be antagonized by preincubating the acetylcholinereceptor-rich membranes with α-bungarotoxin.

We conclude from this fact that carbamoylcholine-action on (^{3}H)-TPMP$^+$-accumulation is mediated by its binding to the cholinergic site of the acetylcholinereceptor-complex rather than an unspecific effect on e.g. the vesicle membrane. This assumption is further justified by control experiments which show that carb does not stimulate (^3H)-TPMP-accumulation into membrane vesicles prepared from crayfish axons, which posess no acetylcholinereceptor (data not shown).

Bound (^3H)-$TPMP^+$ can be displaced by unlabeled $TPMP^+$:

Binding of (^3H)-$TPMP^+$ in the presence of carbamoylcholine seems to be specific as indicated by (^3H)-$TPMP^+$-displacement by unlabeled $TPMP^+$(fig.2).

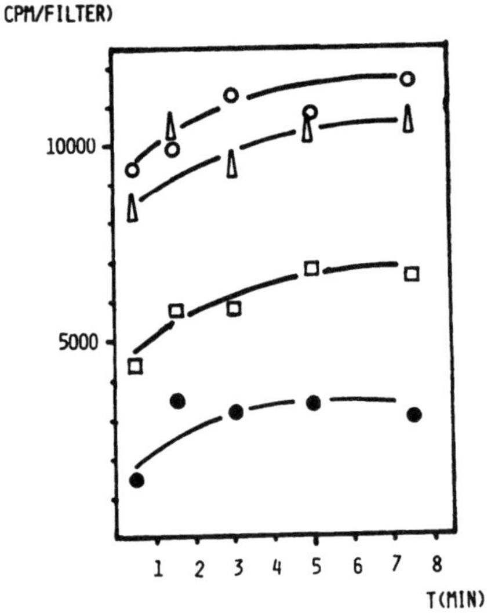

Fig.2: Displacement of (^3H)-$TPMP^+$ by unlabeled $TPMP^+$
Protein concentration was o,84 mg/ml, membranes equilibrated in K-rich medium. Concentration of (^3H)-$TPMP^+$ was 7o nM.
(-●-): Binding following dilution into Na-rich medium.
Open symbols: Binding in the presence of $1o^{-5}$ M carbamoylcholine.
(-o-): Without further additions
(-△-) binding in the presence of a tenfold, (-□-) binding in the presence of a hundredfold excess of unlabeled $TPMP^+$.

In the experiment (fig.2) highest concentration of unlabeled $TPMP^+$ was 7 μM, in the presence of 5 mM $TPMP^+$ (a condition where we define binding of (^3H)-$TPMP^+$ to be "unspecific"), binding would have been further reduced to about 2% of the maximal value (data not shown, compare fig.6).

This observation demonstrates that voltage-dependent (^{3}H)-TPMP^{+}-accumulation into receptor-rich membrane vesicles contributes only a small part of total (^{3}H)-TPMP^{+} binding: voltage-dependent accumulation is expected to be virtually independent of (^{3}H)-TPMP^{+}-concentration in the range used in this experiment. Raising the TPMP^{+}-concentration should have a diminishing effect on the membrane potential dependent (^{3}H)-TPMP^{+}-accumulation only in the millimolar range, because the potential is generated by a concentration gradient of K-ions as high as 165 mM : 16,5 mM.

Dose-response curve for carbamoylcholine:

Half-maximal stimulation of (^{3}H)-TPMP^{+}-binding occurs with 10^{-6} M carbamoylcholine (fig. 3). This value is close to the K_D of the non-desensitized acetylcholinereceptor for agonist binding (8). However, we do not think this correlation to be signicant, because carbamoylcholine stimulated (^{3}H)-TPMP^{+}-binding as well with desensitized acetylcholinereceptor-complex: Desensitization of receptor by 10 min preincubation with 10^{-4} carbamoylcholine did not alter the affinity for (^{3}H)-TPMP^{+}.

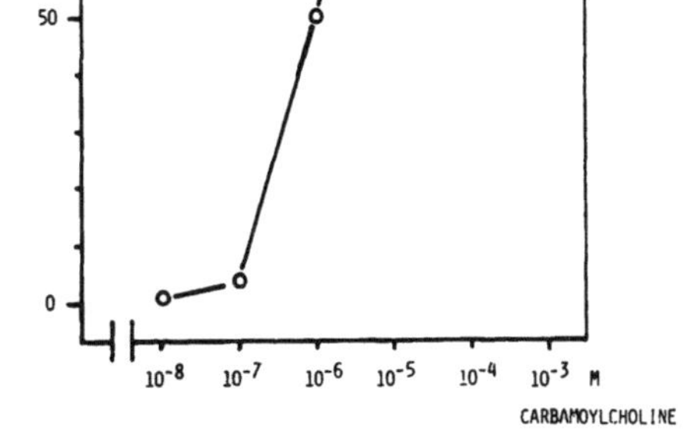

Fig. 3: Dose-response curve for the action of carbamoylcholine

Protein concentration was 0,84 mg/ml, membranes equilibrated in K-rich medium. Concentration of (^{3}H)-TPMP^{+} was 100 nM. Points represent the plateau values of the time-dependent (^{3}H)-TPMP^{+}-binding after dilution into Na-rich medium (the plateau is reached in 5-10 min, compare figs. 1,2) in the presence of the indicated concentrations of carbamoylcholine. 0%: Binding in the absence, 100 %: Binding in the presence of 10^{-5} M carbamoylcholine.

Various cholinergic ligands affect (^{3}H)-TPMP$^{\pm}$-binding:

It is clear from the data shown in fig.4, that both agonists and antagonists stimulate (^{3}H)-TPMP$^{\pm}$-binding: only α-bungarotoxin and the local anesthetic tetracaine (fig.4A) inhibit, acetylcholine, decamethonium and d-tubocurarine (fig.4B) stimulate (^{3}H)-TPMP-binding.

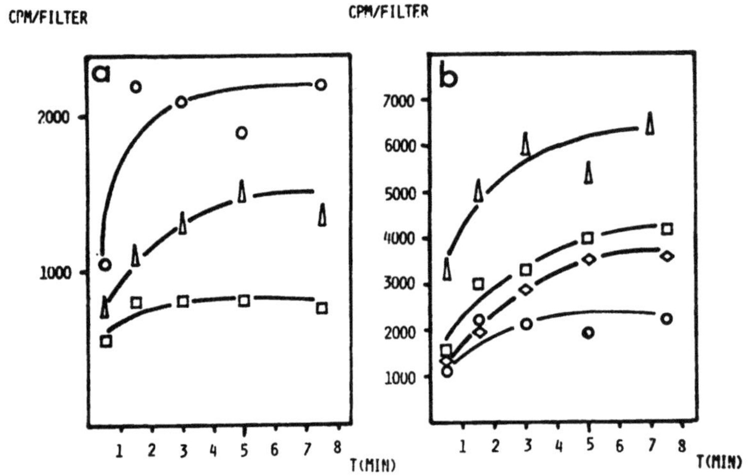

Fig. 4: Effect of cholinergic ligands on (^{3}H)-TPMP$^+$-binding

Protein concentration was 0,26 mg/ml, membranes equilibrated in K-rich medium. Concentration of (^{3}H)-TPMP$^+$ was 90 nM. A) Inhibiting effectors. (-o-): Binding following dilution into Na-rich medium; in the presence of 10^{-4} M α-bungarotoxin (-▵-) or 10^{-4} M tetracaine (-□-). B) Stimulating effectors. (-o-): Binding following dilution into Na-rich medium; in the presence of 10^{-4} M decamethonium (-◇-), 10^{-4} M d-tubocurarine (-□-), or 10^{-4} M acetylcholine (-▵-).

Effect of TPMP$^+$ on (^{3}H)-acetylcholine-binding:

(^{3}H)-acetylcholine-binding was determined by equilibrium centrifugation in the presence of various concentrations of TPMP$^+$ (fig.5). Up to 10^{-5} M TPMP$^+$, (^{3}H)-acetylcholine-binding appears virtually not to be influenced (K_D = 3 x 10^{-8}M);

in the presence of 10^{-3} M $TPMP^+$ affinity for acetylcholine seems slightly reduced; drastic effects can only be observed with 10^{-2} M $TPMP^+$, here, K_D appears to be increased tenfold and the number of binding sites is reduced to 50 %.

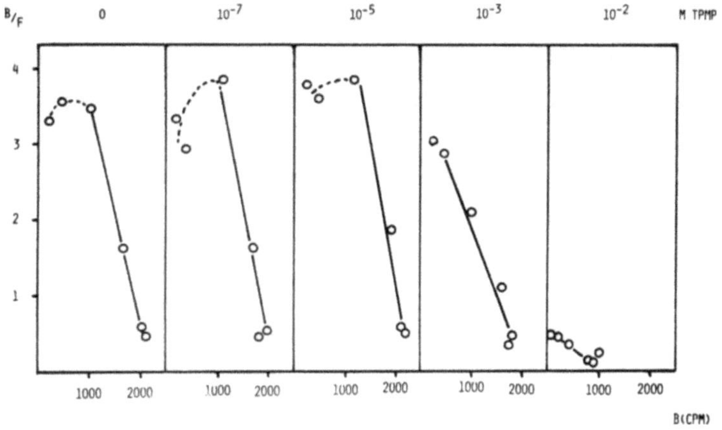

Fig. 5: Scatchard-analysis of binding of (^3H)-acetylcholine to acetylcholinereceptor-rich membrane fragments in the presence of various concentrations of $TPMP^+$

Protein concentration was 0,14 mg/ml, binding was measured in Na-rich medium. A) (^3H)-acetylcholine-binding without further additions, B-E) binding in the presence of $TPMP^+$ as indicated.

The possibility exists that $TPMP^+$ in high concentrations exerts detergent-like effects; this hypothesis will be tested in the future as well as will be investigated the significance of the probable disappearance of positive cooperativity of acetylcholine-binding (broken lines in fig. 5A-C) with increasing concentrations of $TPMP^+$.

Binding of (^3H)-$TPMP^+$ to acetylcholinereceptor-rich membrane fragments:

Whereas (^3H)-acetylcholine-binding is inhibited only by high

$TPMP^+$-concentrations, saturable binding of $TPMP^+$ can be shown in comparably low concentration (fig.6). Analysis of the binding data shows that carbamoylcholine provokes an about tenfold decrease in K_D (K = 13 μM in the absence, K_D = 1,5 μM in the presence of $1o^{-5}$ M carbamoylcholine without altering the maximal number of binding sites. The further increase of specific (^3H)-$TPMP^+$-binding in the presence of (^3H)-$TPMP^+$-concentrations higher than about 15 μM was observed in two independent experiments and probably reflects the existence of a low affinity binding site, the nature of which has not yet been investigated.

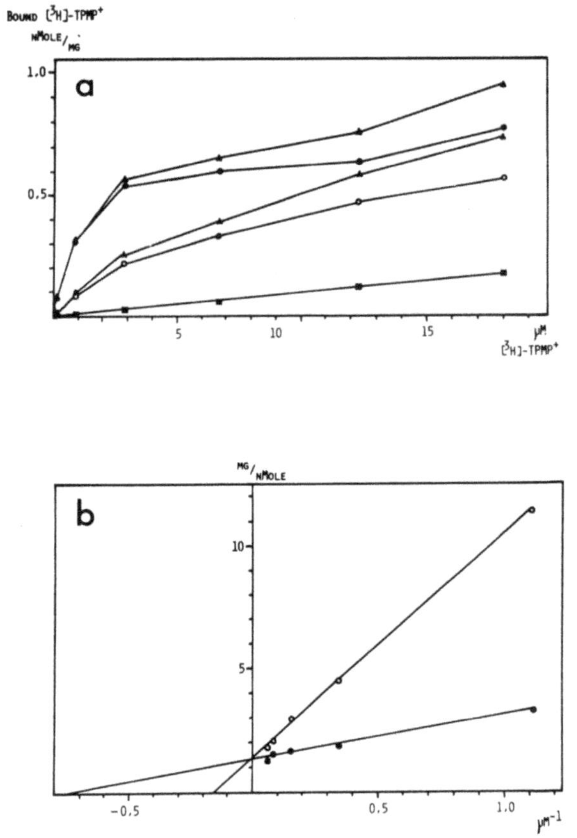

Fig.6: Binding of (^3H)-$TPMP^+$ to acetylcholine-receptor-rich membrane fragments

Protein concentration was o,23 mg/ml, membranes equilibrated in Na-rich medium. A) Direct representation of binding data. Each point is the mean value of two determinations 5 min and 5,5 min after dilution into Na-rich medium. Closed symbols: Binding in the presence of $1o^{-5}$ M carbamoylcholine. Open symbols: Unstimulated binding, no further additions. (-■-): Unspecific binding in the presence of 5 mM $TPMP^+$, amounts to the same value with and without carbamoyl choline. (-△-,-▲-): Total binding and (-○-,-●-): Specific binding; unspecific binding subtracted from total binding. B) Double reciprocal plot of the data for specific binding. (-○-): Binding in the absence and (-●-): Binding in the presence of $1o^{-5}$ M carbamoylcholine

TPMP$^+$ blocks ^{22}Na-efflux from acetylcholinereceptor-rich membrane vesicles

A convenient method of measuring acetylcholinereceptor-function *in vitro* is monitoring the ^{22}Na-efflux after dilution of preloaded acetylcholinereceptor-rich membrane vesicles (7). Efflux can be stimulated by cholinergic agonists, e.g. carbamoylcholine. In the experiment shown in fig.7 efflux stimulated by 10^{-5} M carbamoylcholine was slightly reduced by 10^{-4} M TPMP$^+$ and completely blocked by 10^{-3} M TPMP$^+$ in the dilution medium.

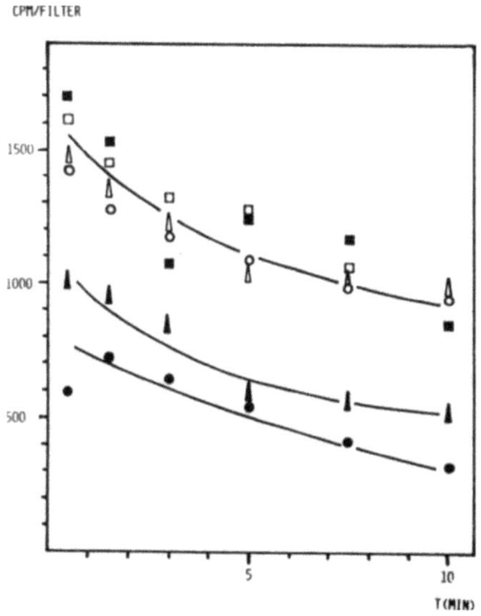

Fig. 7: Effect of TPMP$^+$ on ^{22}Na efflux from acetylcholine-receptor-rich membrane fragments

Protein concentration was 6 mg/ml. Efflux was measured in Na-rich medium. Open symbols: Leakage; closed symbols: Efflux in the presence of 10^{-5} M carbamoylcholine. (-o-,-●-): Control without TPMP$^+$; (-△-, -▲-): Efflux in the presence of 10^{-4} M TPMP$^+$ in the dilution medium and (-□-,-■-): Efflux in the presence of 10^{-3}M TPMP$^+$ in the dilution medium.

The blocking effect of TPMP$^+$ on the ion channel could be potentiated by preincubating the receptor-rich vesicles with the agent, in this case, efflux stimulation was fully inhibited by 10^{-5} M TPMP$^+$ (fig.8), a concentration where (^{3}H)-acetylcholine-binding is not yet blocked.

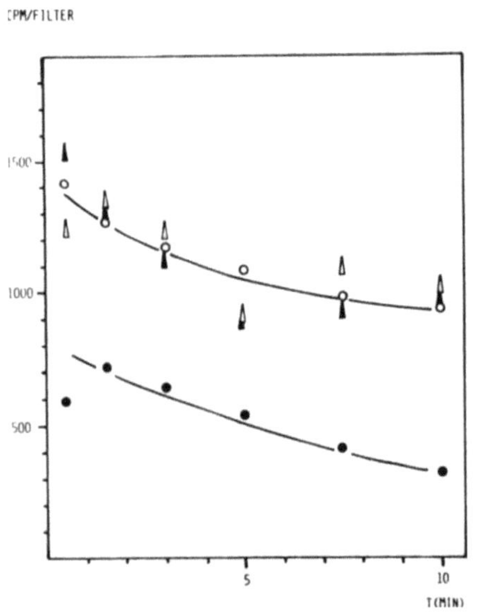

Fig. 8: Effect of preincubation with TPMP$^+$ on ^{22}Na efflux from acetylcholinereceptor-rich membrane fragments

Protein concentration was 6 mg/ml, efflux was measured in Na-rich medium. Open symbols: Leakage, closed symbols: Efflux in the presence of 1o^{-5} M carbamoylcholine.
(-o-,-●-): Control without TPMP$^+$, same as in fig.7, (-△-,-▲-):Prior to dilution the membrane suspension was incubated 1o min at room temperature with 1o^{-5} M TPMP$^+$, the dilution medium equally contained 1o^{-5} M TPMP$^+$.

TPMP$^+$ is a competitive inhibitor of (^{3}H)-PCP-binding

To test the possibility that TPMP$^+$ is an ion channel ligand we investigated the effect of TPMP$^+$ on (^{3}H)-PCP-binding. PCP is a general anesthetic and hallucinogen and was shown to bind to the ion channel of the acetylcholinereceptor complex thereby blocking ion translocation (9,1o). Binding of PCP is also stimulated by cholinergic agonists (1o); we could confirm this observation (fig.9). Specific binding of (^{3}H)-PCP either in the absence or presence of carbamoylcholine is completely blocked by TPMP$^+$ (fig.1o). Unspecific binding in this experiment was determined in the presence of 5 mM amantadine, which was previously shown to be a channel ligand (11,12). All three compounds are competitive with respect to binding to the acetylcholinereceptor-complex; amantadine not only blocks (^{3}H)-PCP-binding, but (^{3}H)-TPMP$^+$-binding as well (data not shown).

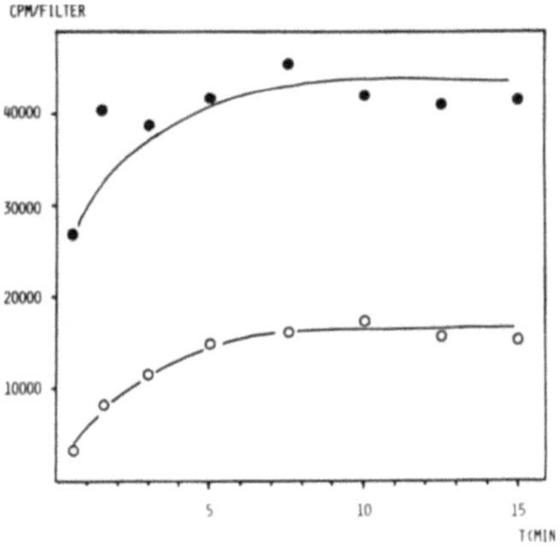

Fig. 9: (^{3}H)-PCP-binding to acetylcholinereceptor-rich membrane fragments

Protein concentration was 0,8 mg/ml, membranes equilibrated in Na-rich medium. Concentration of (^{3}H)-PCP was 23 nM. (-o-): Binding in the absence and (-●-): Binding in the presence of 10^{-5} M carbamoylcholine.

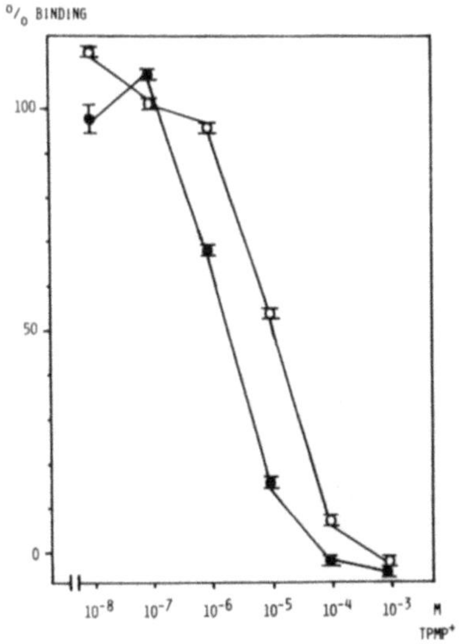

Fig. 10: Displacement of (^{3}H)-PCP by TPMP$^+$

Protein concentration was 0,65 mg/ml, membranes equilibrated in Na-rich medium. Concentration of (^{3}H)-PCP was 8,75 nM. Aliquots were filtered 5 min and 5,5 min after dilution into Na-rich medium. Bars represent upper and lower values, symbols are mean values. (-o-): Binding in the absence and (-●-): Binding in the presence of 10^{-5} M carbamoylcholine. 100 %: Binding in the absence of TPMP$^+$; (-o-): 0,34 pMole/mg protein, (-●-): 1,36 pMole/mg protein. 0 %: Binding in the presence of 2 mM amantadine; (-o-): 0,06 pMole/mg protein, (-●-): 0,13 pMole/mg protein.

The values for half-maximal displacement of (^{3}H)-PCP-binding by TPMP$^+$ (2 x 10^{-6} M in the presence, 10^{-5} M in the absence of carbamoylcholine) are in good agreement with the K_D-values found in the direct binding experiment (compare fig.6); however, substantiation of this correlation must wait till the K_D for (^{3}H)-PCP-binding is determined with Torpedo marmorata vesicles which has not yet been accomplished.

Discussion of results:

The ion-translocating part of the receptor-complex ("ion-channel" or "ionophore") so far has been investigated predominantly using radioactively labeled perhydrohistrionicotoxin (H_{12}-HTX), a derivative of an alkaloid isolated from the skin of the colombian frog Dendrobates histrionicus (13-18). Only recently, PCP was introduced for the same purpose (9, 10, 19). There are striking similarities in the binding characteristica of these "channel ligands" with those of $TPMP^+$. Binding of all three compounds is stimulated by cholinergic agonists. This effect is inhibited by antagonists (α-bungarotoxin); antagonists alone (d-tubocurarine) however stimulate binding also but to a lesser degree.
By increasing agonist concentration beyond a certain value, stimulation of at least $TPMP^+$- and H_{12}-HTX-binding is decreased. Local anestetics inhibit binding of channel ligands. H_{12}-HTX, PCP and $TPMP^+$ block the ion channel at concentrations where there is no effect on binding of cholinergic agonists. However, there is one important difference between $TPMP^+$ on the one hand and H_{12}-HTX and PCP on the other: stimulation of binding of the last two drugs is inhibited by desensitization; in fact, for this reason H_{12}-HTX has been proposed as a tool for monitoring different functional states of the receptor-complex; in contrast, desensitization has no effect on $TPMP^+$-binding.

One must bear in mind however, that even with PCP and H_{12}-HTX desensitization does not reduce binding completely to the unstimulated level.

In addition, there are strong indications suggesting differences in the binding sites of the ion channel for H_{12}-HTX and PCP: affinities obtained for various channel drugs (adiphenine, dibucaine, dimethisoquine, piperocaine, procaine, quinacrine, tetracaine, amantadine) determined by inhibition of either PCP-

or H_{12}-HTX-binding are different (10). Furthermore, affinity of piperocaine for PCP-binding sites is enhanced tenfold following receptor stimulation, whereas it is reduced by 90 % for H_{12}-HTX-binding sites (10, 20).
We conclude from this evidence, that channel ligands do not necessarily bind to identical sites, although they appear to bind competitively. Thus we would like to introduce $TPMP^+$ as a new channel ligand, the properties of which can be summarized as follows:
$TPMP^+$ is a lipophilic cation exhibiting affinity for the ion channel of the acetylcholinreceptor complex and blocking it upon binding. Its binding site is coupled with the binding site for the usual cholinergic effectors; binding is stimulated by both receptor activation and binding of antagonists and is not inhibited by desensitization.
Recently a report on the effects of lipophilic cations (tetraphenylarsonium, tetraphenylphosphonium and $TPMP^+$) on motility and other physiological properties of the bacterium Bacillus subtilis has been published (21). The authors found major changes in various parameters, including swimming speed and frequency of tumbling. They concluded from their evidence that lipophilic cations perturb the process of conversion of the protonmotive force into work. Whether this fact can be related with a similar channel blocking activity as described here should well be worth further investigation.

References

1. Vacata,V., Kotyk,A., Sigler,K.: Biochim.Biophys.Acta 643, 265-268 (1981)
2. Komor,E., Tanner,W.: Eur.J.Biochem. 70, 197-204 (1976)
3. Ramos,S., Grollman,E.F., Lazo,P.S., Dyer,S.A., Habig,W.H., Hardegree,M.C., Kaback,H.R., Kohn,L.D.: Proc.Natl.Acad. Sci. USA 76, 4783-4787 (1979)
4. Schuldiner,S., Kaback,H.R.: Biochemistry 14, 5451-5460 (1975)
5. Kaback,H.R.: Methods Enzymol. 31, 698-709 (1974)
6. Schiebler,W., Hucho,F.: Eur.J.Biochem. 85, 55-63 (1978)
7. Kasai,M., Changeux,J.-P.: J.Membr.Biol. 6, 1-80 (1971)
8. Sugiyama,H., Changeux,J.-P.: Eur.J.Biochem. 55, 505-515 (1975)
9. Albuquerque,E.X., Tsai,M.-C., Aronstam,R.S., Witkop,B., Eldefrawi,A.T., Eldefrawi,M.E.: Proc.Natl.Acad.Sci. USA 77, 1224-1228 (1980)
10. Eldefrawi,M.E., Eldefrawi,A.T., Aronstam,R.S., Maleque,M.A., Warnick,J.E., Albuquerque,E.X.: Proc.Natl.Acad.Sci. USA 77, 7458-7462 (1980)
11. Albuquerque,E.X., Eldefrawi,A.T., Eldefrawi,M.E., Mansour,N.A., Tsai,M.-C.: Science 199, 788-790 (1978)
12. Tsai,M.-C., Mansour,N.A., Eldefrawi,A.T., Eldefrawi,M.E., Albuquerque,E.X.: Mol.Pharmacol. 14, 787-803 (1978)
13. Elliot,J., Raftery,M.A.: Biochem.Biophys.Res.Commun. 77, 1347-1353 (1977)
14. Sobel,A., Heidmann,T., Hofler,J., Changeux,J.-P.: Proc. Natl.Acad.Sci. USA 75, 510-514 (1978)
15. Eldefrawi,M.E., Eldefrawi,A.T., Mansour,N.A., Daly,J.W., Witkop,B., Albuquerque,E.X.: Biochemistry 17, 5474-5484 (1978)
16. Elliot,J., Raftery,M.A.: Biochemistry 18, 1868-1874 (1979)
17. Eldefrawi,M.E., Aronstam,R.S., Bakry,N.M., Eldefrawi,A.T., Albuquerque,E.X.: Proc.Natl.Acad.Sci. USA 77, 2309-2313 (1980)
18. Aronstam,R.S., Eldefrawi,A.T., Pessah,I.N., Daly,J.W., Albuquerque,E.X., Eldefrawi,M.E.: J.Biol.Chem. 256, 2843-2850 (1981)
19. Oswald,R., Changeux,J.-P.: Proc.Natl.Acad.Sci. USA 78, 3925-3929 (1981)
20. Aronstam,R.S., Eldefrawi,A.T., Eldefrawi,M.E.: Biochem. Pharmacol. 29, 1311-1314 (1980)
21. Zaritsky,A., Macnab,R.M.: J.Bacteriol. 147, 1054-1062 (1981)

SYNTHESIS OF A CONJUGATE OF LACTOPEROXIDASE AND α-BUNGAROTOXIN. LABELING OF ACETYLCHOLINE RECEPTOR COMPONENTS WITH THE CONJUGATE.

Jan Verdenhalven and Leander Lauffer
Institut für Biochemie, Fachbereich Chemie der Freien Universität Berlin, Arbeitsgruppe Neurochemie, Fabeckstraße 34-36, 1000 Berlin 33, Germany

Summary

Lactoperoxidase iodinates protein tyrosin residues in presence of iodide and H_2O_2. Under certain conditions the iodination occurs specifically and not via free I_2. α-bungarotoxin is a snake venom toxin which binds nearly irreversibly to acetylcholine receptors. For coupling α-bungarotoxin (M_r = 8000) to lactoperoxidase (M_r = 80 000) covalently we used the periodate method (1) and separated the coupling products by a prepacked column (LKB TSK-G-4000, SW 600 mm). The column fractions were assayed for peroxidase activity and acetylcholine receptor binding. A fraction containing both properties showed a M_r of 88 000 - 104 000 as shown by sodium dodecyl sulfate electrophoresis. We concluded that one to three molecules of α-bungarotoxin were coupled to one molecule of lactoperoxidase. The conjugate might be a useful tool for topographic studies of the postsynaptic membrane and the synaptic cleft. After binding the conjugate to membrane-bound acetylcholinereceptor and removing the unbound conjugate by washing, centrifugation etc. only protein components of the closer environment of the receptor should become radioactively labeled by addition of ^{125}iodide and H_2O_2, These components could be easily analysed by dodecyl sulfate electrophoresis and autoradiography.

Abbreviations

AChR: acetylcholinereceptor, α-BTX: α-bungarotoxin,
LPO: Lactoperoxidase

Introduction

α-bungarotoxin (M_r 8000) belongs to a group of basic peptides from the venom of the snake <u>Bungarus multicinctus</u> (2). It is composed of 74 amino acid residues in known sequence, 6 of which are lysine residues. Four of these can be modified without loss of toxicity (3), in addition to other residues which are not essential for biological activity of the peptide (4, 5). α-bungarotoxin (α-BTX) is neurotoxic because it binds nearly irreversibly to the acetylcholinereceptor (AChR) thereby blocking synaptic transmission (6).

Lactoperoxidase (LPO) is a hemoprotein with a M_r of 80 000. It contains several sugar- and lysineresidues (7). Unlike horseradishperoxidase, which is very unspecific, LPO catalyses the iodination of tyrosine with iodide and H_2O_2 (8). Using this activity LPO became a tool for the examination of the orientation of membrane proteins (9). Our idea was to combine the specific iodination of LPO with the specific binding of α-BTX in a protein-protein-conjugate. In contrast to the conventional LPO-technique, the conjugate should be selective for only a few components of the membrane: the acetylcholinereceptor and its surrounding.We call the conjugate mediated iodination "affinity-iodination".

Materials

All chemicals were of the highest commercially available purity and purchased from Merck (Darmstadt, Germany), α-bungarotoxin was purchased from Boehringer (Mannheim, Germany) and

Sigma (München, Germany); lactoperoxidase was from Sigma also. Torpedo californica was obtained alive from Biomarine Supply Inc. (Venice, California).

Methods

Synthesis of the conjugate

1 mg of LPO and 2 mg of α-BTX with tracer quantities of ^{125}I-α-BTX (prepared according to 10) are incubated in 50 µl of 0,1 M Na/PO_4 pH 4,5 with 5 µl of 0,1 M $NaIO_4$ at room temperature for one hour. The mixture is cooled in an ice bath and 5 µl of a freshly prepared solution of $NaBH_4$ (20 mg/ml) is added. After three hours incubation at 0° C the mixture is centrifuged for 5 min in an Eppendorf centrifuge 5412 to remove insoluble reaction products. The supernatant is neutralized with 150 µl of 0,1 M NH_4CH_3COO and chromatographed on an LKB TSK-G-4000, SW 600 mm column using the same buffer for elution. 0,5 ml-fractions were collected and assayed for molecular weight of the components by SDS-electrophoresis (11), for protein concentration (12), for peroxidase activity (13), for AChR-binding (14), and for radioactivity (in dioxane/omnifluor 8 g/l as scintillation coctail).

Affinity-iodination of purified AChR-vesicles

Affinity-iodination is carried out in a two-step-procedure. In the first step the conjugate is bound to AChR-vesicles and the unbound conjugate is removed by centrifugation in a Beckman airfuge for 15 min at full speed. In the second step the resuspended pellet is incubated with H_2O_2 and ^{125}iodide and the vesicles are separated from the excess of ^{125}iodide by centrifugation. First step: 50 µg of AChR (prepared according to (15)) in 100 µl of 0,1 M Na/PO_4 pH 7,4 containing 1 ng of the conjugate are incubated for 30 min at 25° C. To remove the unbound conjugate the vesicles are spun down at full speed for 15 min in a Beckman airfuge. The excess conjugate remains in

the supernatant.
Second step: The pellet of the first step is resuspended in 150 µl 0,1 M Na/PO_4 pH 7,4 with 1 µCi carrier-free ^{125}iodide (Amersham) and 0,1 mM H_2O_2. After 5 minutes of incubation at 25° C the membranes are centrifuged. The pellet is prepared for SDS-electrophoresis according to Laemmli (11). Electrophoresis is performed in 10 % polyacrylamide tube gels. The gels are stained, destained, scanned at 550 nm with a Zeiss PMQ 3 photometer, and than sliced in 1 mm slices with a Joyce/Loebl gel slicer. The radioactivity of each slice is counted in a Kontron Gamma counter.
To account for unspecific binding of the conjugate, the same procedure as above is performed with AChR-vesicles in the presence of 20 µM cold α-BTX.

Results

Synthesis of the conjugate

For cytochemical localization of acetylcholinreceptors the use of a horseradish peroxidase-α-bungarotoxin conjugate has been reported (16, 17). The published two step synthesis is not suitable for lactoperoxidase, because LPO is even more basic than α-bungarotoxin (with 33 lysine residues) and therefore the coupling procedure will predominantly result in LPO-LPO self conjugation. We developed a one step procedure with a twentyfold excess of α-BTX at low pH, which is a modification of the periodate method (1). The sugar residues of the LPO were oxidized to aldehydes with sodium periodate in the presence of α-bungarotoxin. During the incubation Schiff-bases between the amino groups of the toxin and the nascent aldehyde functions of the LPO were formed. LPO-LPO self conjugation was diminished by the excess of α-bungarotoxin. For stabilization of the conjugate the Schiff-bases were reduced with sodiumborohydride. The reaction mixture was chromatographed on an LKB TSK-G-4000 column (fig. 1).

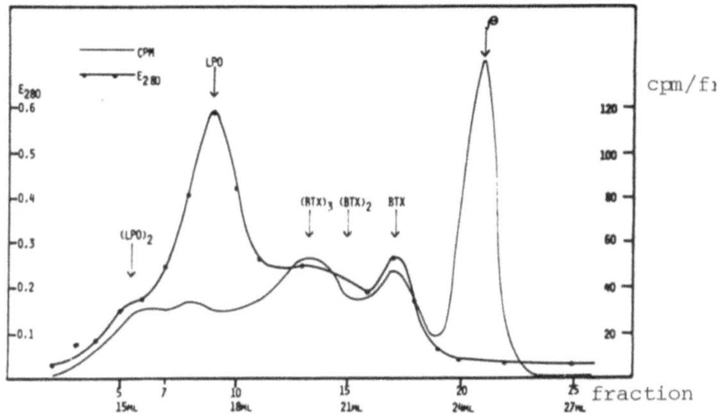

Fig. 1: Chromatography of a conjugation-reaction mixture:

1 mg lactoperoxidase were conjugated with 2 mg α-BTX after oxidation with 0,1 M $NaIO_4$ as described in the text. Chromatography was carried out on an LKB TSK-G-4000 column eluted with 0,1 M NH_4CH_3COO at 4 ml/h; 0,5 ml fractions were collected. Optical density was monitored by a Gilson flow-photometer, radioactivity was measured by counting 50 μl aliquots of each fraction in 5 ml dioxane (omnifluor 8 g/l) in a Kontron MR 300 liquid scintillation counter.

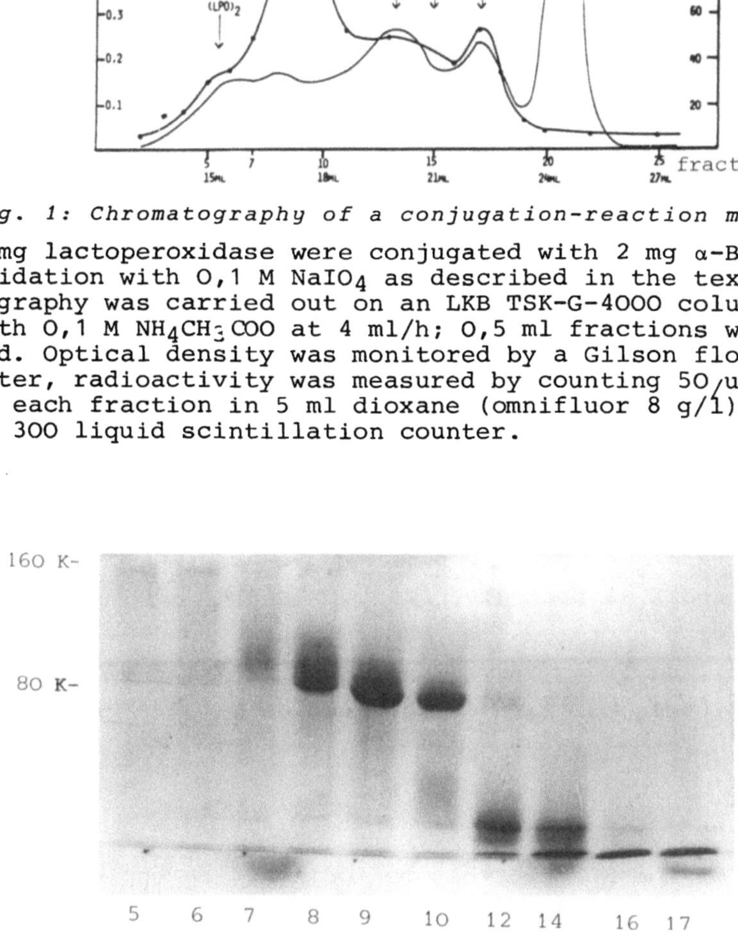

Fig. 2: SDS-electrophoresis of column fractions

Coomasie-stain of an SDS-electrophoresis of 50 μl of column fractions (fig.1) as indicated. Slot 5 and 6: high-molecular weight-conjugates; Slot 7: conjugates with M_r of 88 000 - 104 000; Slot 8: conjugates with small contributions of unlabeled LPO; Slot 9+10: monomeric LPO; Slot 12-17: low-molecular weight components, predominantly α-BTX.

Despite the excess of toxin only one to three molecules of toxin were coupled to one molecule of LPO.
The SDS-electrophoresis of fraction 7 in figure 2 shows a conjugate with Mr of 88 000 - 104 000 corresponding to a 1 : 1 to 1 : 3 ratio of LPO to α-BTX.
This fraction is nearly free of monomeric LPO and high-molecular-weight conjugates and essentially free of unconjugated α-bungarotoxin. It represents 0,1 mg protein. Therefore the yield is about 10 % with respect to LPO. In a hundredfold excess it completely blocks the binding of ^{125}I-bungarotoxin to AChR (data nor shown). The peroxidase activity of the conjugate is 50 U/mg, which is 60 % of that of the purest commercially available LPO which we used for conjugation.
The radioactivity pattern in figure 1 is not a good quantitative indication for α-BTX labeling because the ^{125}I -α-BTX tracer becomes partially deiodinated by $NaBH_4$-reduction and the free ^{125}iodide gives a separated peak. In addition, self iodination of the LPO occurs.
α-BTX elutes in broad peaks containing mono-, di- and trimers of the toxin. Dimerisation occurs spontaneously and commercially obtained α-BTX always contains mono- and dimer molecules. In addition, α-BTX as purchased from Boehringer (Mannheim) is contaminated with proteases (G. Bandini and F. Hucho, personal communication), so it is very likely that proteolysis contributes to the inhomogeneities in the elution pattern of the column.

Affinity iodination

All subunits of the receptor become iodinated by the conjugate (fig. 3). The non receptor peptide of Mr 100 000, which is thought to be the major subunit of the Na/K-ATPase is labeled as well. So far, the radioactivity pattern of the gel as determined in the gel slices is identical to the coomasie stain (not shown). However, a peptide of a Mr of 35 000 becomes labeled as well; this peptide is not detectable in the coomasie stain and was not identified as an AChR component so far. In the controlexperiment with AChR vesicles preincubated with α-BTX the amount of radioactivity incorporated in all peptides is markedly reduced.

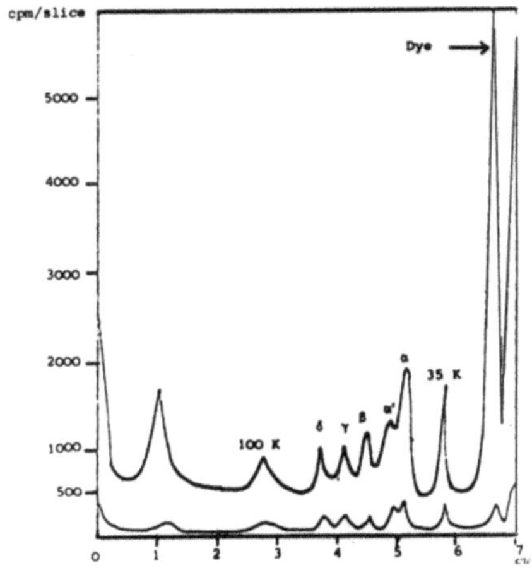

Fig. 3: Affinity-iodination of purified acetylcholinereceptor-rich membrane fragments

Procedure is described in the text. Upper trace: labeling was carried out with native AChR-vesicles; lower trace: membrane vesicles were blocked with α-BTX and than used for affinity-labeling.

Discussion of results

A conjugate of α-BTX and LPO could be synthesized. This conjugate still binds to the AChR and still retains peroxidase-activity. Whether the conjugate is suitable for affinity-iodination, has been investigated with purified AChR-rich membranes. These membranes not only contain AChR receptors, but in addition a peptide of M_r 100 000, probably on distinct membrane fragments (18). This peptide is thought to be the major subunit of the Na/K-ATPase and as such does not form an integral part of the receptor complex (18). However, it has been iodinated to the same extent as the receptor subunits. Of course this fact makes specifity of affinity-iodination questionable. Two possible explanations may account for unspecific labeling:

(i) We do not know the orientation of the conjugate's LPO-residue. It might well be that the active site is oriented towards the external medium and not to the vesicle surface, therefore not finding tyrosine residues as appropriate substrates. With a substrate lacking the LPO produces free $^{125}I_2$ (9). This molecule could freely diffuse and label peptides which are not in close vicinity of the binding site.

(ii) Membranes containing the M_r 100 000 peptide can associate with receptor containing vesicles, thus coming within reach of the conjugate. This is the more likely explanation for the apparent unspecificity of the affinity iodination: We do not assume that unspecific binding of the conjugate to the M_r 100 000 peptide containing membrane fragments leads to their iodination, because by blocking AChR-rich membrane fragments with α-BTX labeling of all peptides including the one of M_r of 100 000 could be prevented.

Despite possible artifacts caused by unspecific labelling, affinity-iodination might prove to be a valuable tool for elucidation of receptor and synaptic cleft structure. With this technique we found a M_r 35 000 peptide which is iodinated with high efficiency. Though it is not visible in the coomasie stained gel, radioactivity is incorporated to an amount comparable to the receptor subunits. This peptide is not known to be part of the receptor complex. We do not believe that unspeific labeling may account for the comparatively high degree of iodination of this peptide. Instead we conclude from our experiments that this peptide is present in small amounts, but in an orientation which makes it easily accessible for the conjugate. Presumably its location is at the periphery of the receptor complex. Since its occurence in purified membranes is quite substoichiometric with respect to the AChR the possibility exists that it is only loosely associated with the complex and that the main amount is lost during the preparation.

References

1. Nakane,P.K., Kawoi,A.: J.Hist.Cyt. 22, 1084 (1976)
2. Tu,A.T.: Ann.Rev.Biochem. 42, 235 (1973)
3. Karlson,E., Eaker,D., Ponterius,G.: Biochim.Biophys.Acta 257, 235 (1972)
4. Hucho,F.: FEBS Lett. 103, 27 (1979)
5. Mebs,D.: Proceedings of the Third Symposium on Plant, Animal & Microbial Toxins, eds. G.Habermehl, D.Mebs, 9, (1978)
6. Raftery,M.A., Vandlen,R.L., Reed,K.C., Lee,T.: Cold Spring Harbour Symposia on Quantitative Biology, Vol. XL, 193 (1976)
7. Rombauts,W.A., Schroeder,W.A., Morrison,M.: Biochemistry 6, 2965 (1976)
8. Morrison,M.: Ann.Rev.Biochem. 45, 861 (1976)
9. Hubbard,A.L., Cohn,Z.A.: J.Cell.Biol. 55, 390 (1972)
10. David,G.S.: Biochem.Biophys.Res.Comm. 48, 464 (1972)
11. Laemmli,U.K.: Nature 227, 680 (1970)
12. Lowry,O.H., Rosebrough,N.J., Farr,A.L., Randall,R.J.: J.Biol.Chem. 193, 265 (1951)
13. Boehringer GmbH: Biochemica Information, 2, 104 (1975)
14. Hartig,P.R., Raftery,M.A.: Biochemistry 18, 1146 (1976)
15. Schiebler,W., Hucho,F.: Eur.J.Biochem. 85, 55 (1978)
16. Vogel,Z., Maloney,G.J., Ling,A., Daniels,M.P.: Proc.Natl. Acad.Sci. USA 74, 3268 (1977)
17. Lentz,T.L., Mazurkiewic,J.E., Rosenthal,J.: Brain Res. 132, 423 (1977)
18. Hucho,F., Bandini,G., Suarez-Isla,B.: Eur.J.Biochem. 83, 335 (1978)

INTERACTIONS OF THE MEMBRANE-BOUND ACETYLCHOLINE RECEPTOR WITH THE NON-RECEPTOR PERIPHERAL ν-PEPTIDE.

F. J. Barrantes
Max-Planck-Institut f. biophysikalische Chemie, Göttingen, FRG.

Introduction

Knowledge of the native molecular organization of the acetylcholine receptor (AChR) _in situ_ and the molecular mechanisms involved in the formation and maintenance of this structure have up to now remained inaccessible to direct experimental demonstration. The significance of this knowledge becomes apparent when looking at various biologically relevant phenomena. For example, the ontogenetic changes in AChR-controlled channel properties, i.e. changes from the embryonic type of gating into the adult (junctional) type operating in the normal synapse, seem to be associated with (though not strictly temporally coincident with) corresponding changes in the structural organization of AChR molecules (see review in ref. 10). Aggregational phenomena, whose mechanisms are still unknown, result in the formation of AChR patches by recruitment of a population of diffusely distributed, relatively mobile molecules having short half-lives. Localization and stabilization characterize the mature assembly of receptors in the adult synapse. A severely hindered translational and rotational mobility, and about 8-fold longer half-lives further characterize the densely packed junctional AChR (10,2).

In this chapter I shall review recent work and present new experimental data from my own laboratory to illustrate the relationship between the _various_ oligomeric states of the AChR and a non-receptor protein, the ν-peptide (M_r 43 000), which we have specifically postulated to be involved in AChR organization (5). The frequent inference that the dimeric,

Neuroreceptors

13S form of the AChR is the "native" one (8,11) does not inevitably follow from the present findings. A spectrum of discrete AChR oligo-meric forms associated with an unperturbed redox equilibrium appears to be a more realistic, albeit less elegant (or simpler) working hypothesis for understanding receptor organization *in situ*. A concrete role for the ν-peptide is postulated in this context. *In vitro* the ν-peptide appears to exert influence on (and/or participate in) an equilibrium between receptor monomers+dimers on the one hand, and higher oligomeric forms on the other. Predominantly dimeric AChR preparations are associated with the presence of the ν-peptide, which cannot be extracted by usual procedures. Depletion of the peptide from standard membranes alters the proportion of monomers and dimers with respect to the multimeric species, as if certain constraints were normally exerted by the ν-peptide on high-order associations of AChR molecules. These changes are paralleled by an increase in the translational and rotational freedom of the AChR, enabling the observation of rotational mobility of individual, 9S AChR monomers among the otherwise densely-packed and comparatively immobile receptor oligomers.

Materials and Methods.

Torpedo marmorata young specimens of less than 40 cm in length were obtained from the Marine Biological Station at Arcachon, France, and kept in an aquarium for at least for two days before killing by pithing. The preparation of the AChR-rich membrane fractions was carried out in medium I (0.1 mM phenylmethane- sulphonylfluoride, 1 mM ethylenediamino tetraacetic acid (EDTA) and 0.02% NaN_3 in double distilled water), medium II (the isotonic buffered solution of ref. 12). Media III and IV were as I and II but with the addition of 10 mM *N*-ethylmaleimide. Fish were layed on ice for 5 min before pithing. The electric tissue, free of peripheral connective tissue envelope, was chopped into small pieces and washed with ice-cold, argon-bubbled and extensively degassed medium. All these operations took less than 5 min. The chopped tissue was made 1:1 (w/v) with medium and homogenized for 30 s in a Virtis 60 homogenizer at 10 000±500 r.p.m. A series of tests were conducted to determine the optimal time/speed combination, which resulted in less damage being sustained by the membranes (see criteria under Results) and an admissible proportion of non-disrupted tissue. Calibration of the homogenizer speed was accomplished by measuring the frequency of the shaft spinning in actual operation with the aid of a He-Ne laser focused on the shaft, and photodiode recording of a mark on the metal cylinder. Adjustments had to be made to obtain less than 5% departures from nominal speed in actual performance. Homogenates were centrifuged 10 min (4,300 x*g*) in a Sorvall SS34 rotor. Pellets were resuspended, re-homogenized as above in the corresponding medium and the combined supernatants were filtered through two layers of 0.2 mm nylon mesh. The filtrate was centrifuged for 2 h in a Sorvall GSA rotor (19,750 x*g*). Supernatants were discarded. Only the whitish pellet was resuspended by gentle swirling, made to 70 mM sucrose, and homogenized in a Teflon-glass vessel at 800 r.p.m. for 30 s. Samples of 20 ml were applied atop discontinuous sucrose gradients (12 ml 1.44 *M*, 20 ml 1.28 *M*, and 8 ml 1.14 *M* sucrose in one of the above media and centrifuged in a Beckman SW 25.2 rotor for 6 h (71,000 x*g*).About 5 ml each of 0.6 *M* and 1.22 *M* sucrose were injected as in Fig. 1 before extraction of the samples, which were subsequently stored in sealed tubes at -196°C. Protein determinations and toxin binding assays were carried out as in (1 and 3) using $[^3H]$-α-bungarotoxin and the DEAE-cellulose filter assay . The sidedness of the membrane vesicles was determined as described by Hartig and Raftery (12). Extraction of peripheral proteins from receptor membranes was done at 2°C, with one or two cycles (1h, pH 10.8) as in ref. (4), i.e. slightly modifying the original description given in ref. 15. Thiol group modification of the purified membranes, gradient centrifugation experiments, polyacrylamide gel electrophoresis and electron microscopy were done as in ref. (3,4). *Torpedo* actin was a gift from Dr. K. Zechel. Preparation of monospecific antibodies against the ν-peptide followed the protocol described in ref. (4). Affinity chromatography-purified immunoglobulins G against the ν-peptide were tested for specificity by the immune blotting technique using a slight modification to the technique reported in ref. (18). Localization of the antigenic determinants of the ν-peptide by fluorescence techniques was carried out on normal membranes, those depleted of the ν-peptide as above, and normal membranes treated with 0.1% saponin (9) for 30 min. Upon labelling with anti-ν-peptide IgG, membranes were incubated with rhodamine-labelled anti rabbit IgG and fluorescence measurements carried out as in ref. (4).

Results

Standardized purification of AChR membranes. The fractionation scheme outlined under Material and Methods departs little from currently used preparative techniques. The few modifications introduced, however, sufficed to optimize and standardize the measurable variables for the simultaneous preservation of a) structural integrity of the membranes; b) original polypeptide composition (i.e. in the absence of proteolytic degradation), and c) the redox state of the thiol groups therein. An additional requisite was the obtainment of homogeneous vesicles of relatively large size for reasons illustrated below. The minimization of those fractionation steps involving mechanical disruption of the tissue was found to be crucial to meet the above criteria. Thus, sonication was omitted, homogenization strength was reduced and its optimal time/speed combinations were found and standardized. The distribution of toxin binding activity and polypeptide composition of membranes varied as a function of medium tonicity, presence or absence of protease inhibitors or alkylation of the membranes ab initio or not, among several parameters explored. Fig. 1 illustrates two such distributions, i) using a hypotonic Ca-depleted medium containing mainly EDTA as protease inhibitor (Fig. 1) and ii) the isotonic medium of ref. (12). The vesicle distribution in such media follows Donnan equilibria, which determine the isopycnic position of the vesicles.* Though typical preparative methods were used, the purity of the fractions and the fulfillment of the above criteria ("minimal disruption conditions") become apparent. Refractionation of the membranes through a continuous gradient in detergent, after alkaline treatment for 1 h, is also illustrated in Fig. 1.

---

* Note: Differences between the results of ref. 12 and those recently reported by Jeng et al. (Biochim. Biophys. Acta 646:411-421) are most likely due to the same phenomenon.

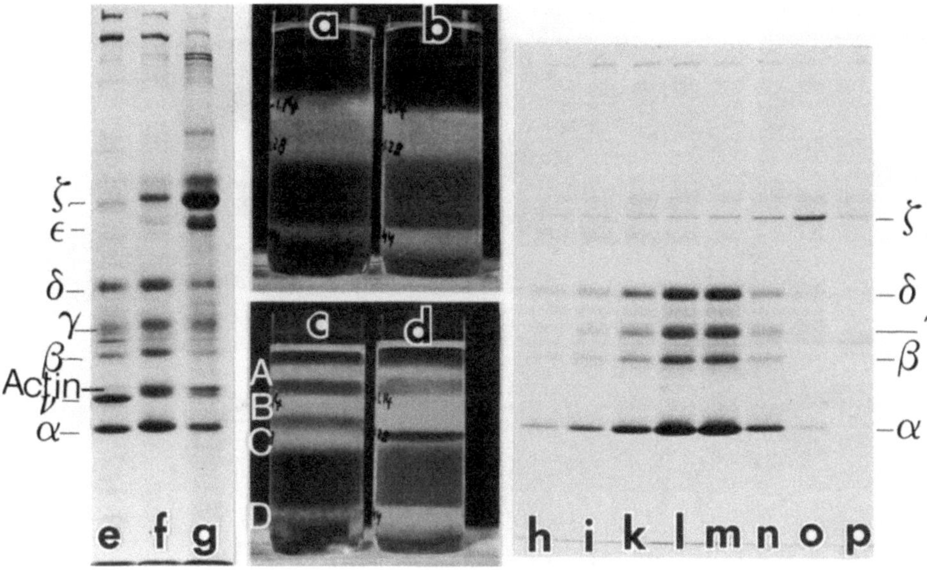

Fig. 1. a and b are preparative discontinuous gradient centrifugations in medium I or II respectively, and c and d the same after injection of the sucrose cushions. Traces e,f,g are SDS-gel profiles of fractions D,C and B respectively. Alkaline-extracted, detergent-solubilized D fraction submitted to DTT reduction and centrifugation in a linear 5-20% sucrose gradient is shown in h-p.

Fig. 2 illustrates the morphology of the "D" fraction obtained as in Fig. 1. The "structural integrity" criterion (see above) appears to be met. The vesicles, having mean diameters of 1.1±0.4 µm, are densely covered with the 7-8 nm receptor particles, as seen in end-on and lateral views. The high particle density (10 000±1000/μm^2) hinders the observation of the oligomeric organization. Up to recently, descriptions of this feature have relied on the solubilization of the receptor protein in detergents, and subsequent gradient or analytical centrifugation. (An alternative approach has been the reconstitution of solubilized AChR in lipid vesicles for morphological characterization, ref. 7). It is however possible to directly observe the receptor arrangement within and outside the membrane without resorting to solubilization by detergents (4). This is due to the fragility of alkaline-extracted vesicles, which disrupt upon drying onto

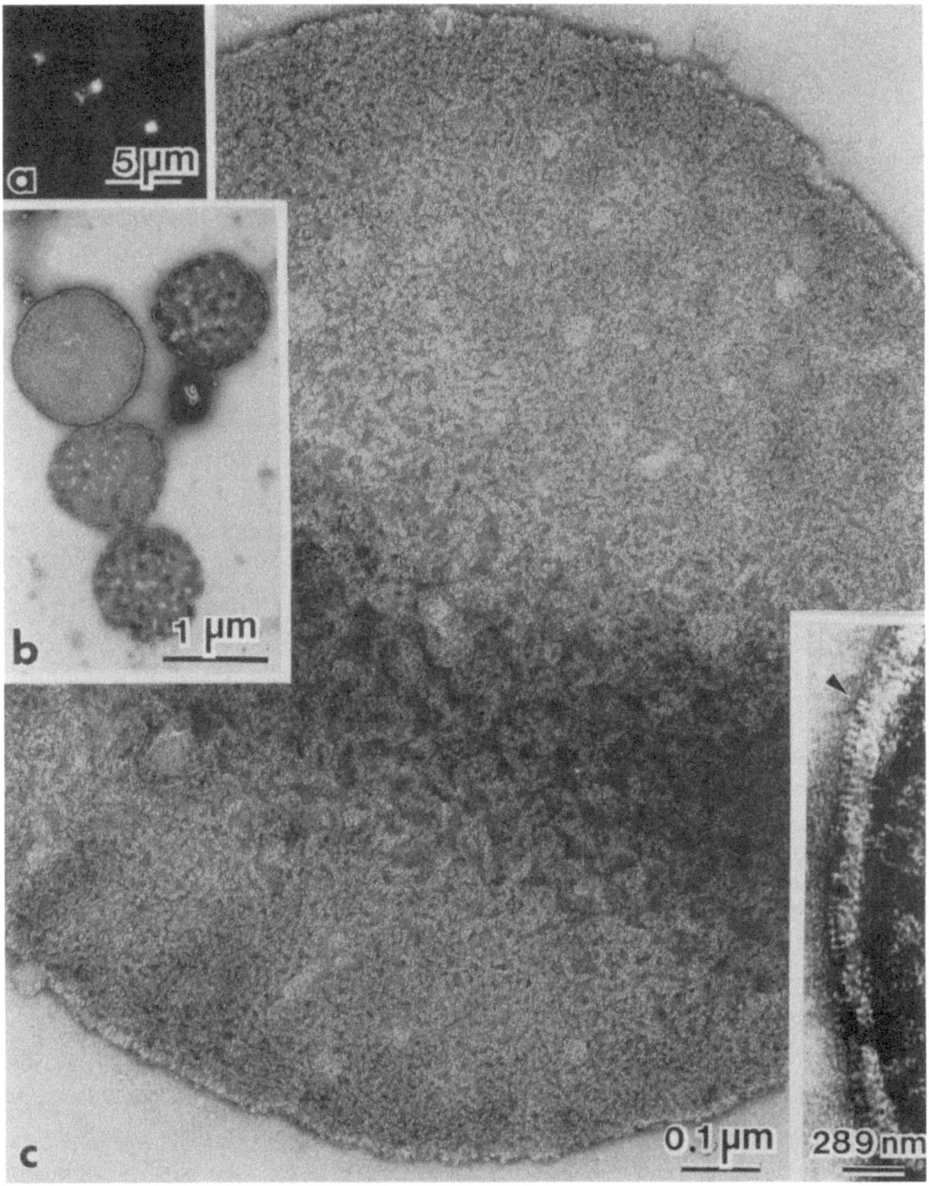

Fig. 2. a) Rhodamine-α-bungarotoxin labelled fraction "D" as observed in the light microscope. b) Panoramic electron micrograph illustrating size distribution of membranes. c) Dense AChR particle coverage of the membranes. Notice size of vesicle. Inset: Edge view of microsac, showing AChR protrusions towards the external face of the vesicle. All preparations were obtained from the experiment illustrated in Fig. 1. b, c and inset are micrographs of specimens contrasted with 1% uranyl acetate (ref. 4).

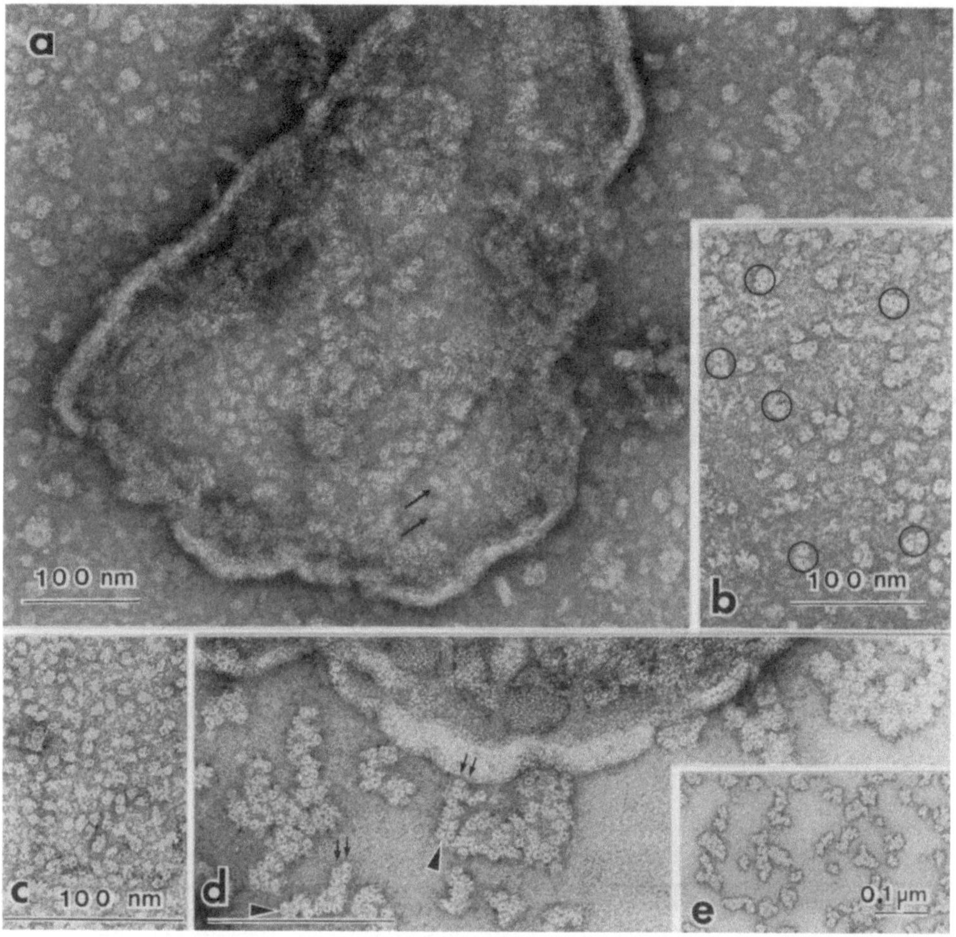

Fig. 3. Direct visualization of acetylcholine receptor oligomeric forms in alkaline-stripped membranes sheared on hydrophilic carbon supports (5). a) Standard membranes after 2 x 1h alkaline extraction (ref. 4). Arrows indicate membrane-associated doublets. Such particles predominate in both standard (alkaline-extracted) or b)NEM-membranes. c) Single particles, more abundant in dithiothreitol-reduced membranes. d) DTNB-reoxidized membranes. Arrows and arrowheads point to particle double rows sheared from the membrane remnants, similar to the receptor aggregational forms described by Heuser and Salpeter (13) in intact electrocytes. e) discrete distribution (n finite, see Fig. 4) of DTNB-treated particle aggregates, at even 10 x higher protein concentration as that used in d. This suggests a limited extension of long-range forces keeping receptor-receptor associations even after separation from the membrane environment and extraction of the ν-peptide. See Fig. 4 for statistics of particle size distribution.

hydrophilic carbon supports (5) and exhibit increased particle dispersion, facilitating the statistical processing of receptor arrangement (4). As seen in Fig. 3, receptor particles within the remnants of alkaline-extracted membranes (but not subjected to thiol modification) an in their immediate vicinity occur as single units, and aggregates of two, four or more particles. Doublets of the single particle predominate, but are not the only component, in normal or N-ethylmaleimide (NEM)-treated membranes (Fig. 3b). Single particles predominate in DTT-reduced samples (Fig. 3c). Treatment with 5,5'-dithio-bis-(nitrobenzoic acid) results in higher oligomeric species (Fig. 3d). The distribution of particle diameters shows concurrence with sedimentation profiles obtained in gradient centrifugation experiments (Fig. 4).

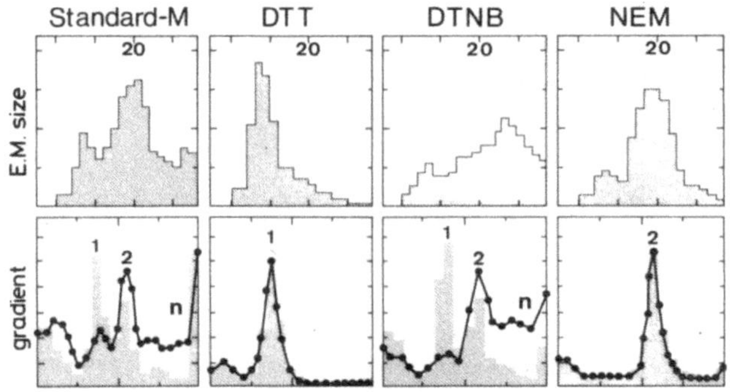

Fig. 4

Fig. 4. Correlation between particle sizes in alkaline-extracted membranes (upper panels) and AChR molecular species in gradient centrifugation (lower panel). Thiol treatments as indicated. NEM corresponds to the "NEM-membranes". In upper panel 20 nm is indicated for reference. In lower panel 1 = 9S monomer; 2 = 13S dimer; n = oligomers; filled circles = alkaline extracted membranes; dashed areas = control, non-extracted membranes in Triton. Notice absence of oligomers in DTT-reduced and NEM-membranes and relative changes in species distribution after alkaline extraction.

The involvement of the ν-peptide in the thiol-dependent AChR interconversions is apparent from the previous experiments: Extraction of the peptide shifts species distribution to higher oligomeric forms. Further, DTNB re-oxidation of NEM-membranes prevents the penetration of the AChR peptides into acrylamide gels in the absence of reducing agents, but not that of the ν-peptide (ref. 4). In <u>standard</u> membranes, DTNB reoxidation results in <u>segregation</u> of the ν-peptide from the AChR (Fig. 5). Upon Triton X-100 solubilization, the peptide appears in the insoluble residue (Fig. 5<u>b</u>), together with other non-receptor peptides, being absent from the Triton extract which solubilizes the AChR (Fig. 5<u>a</u>). The ν-peptide does not penetrate the gel even in the absence of DTNB reoxidation (Fig. 5<u>c</u>).

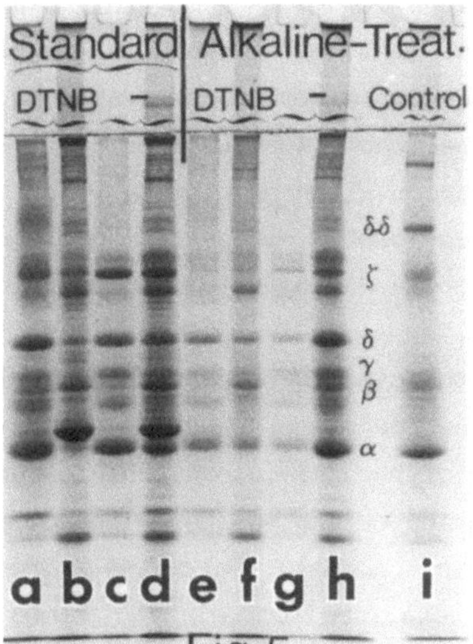

Fig 5

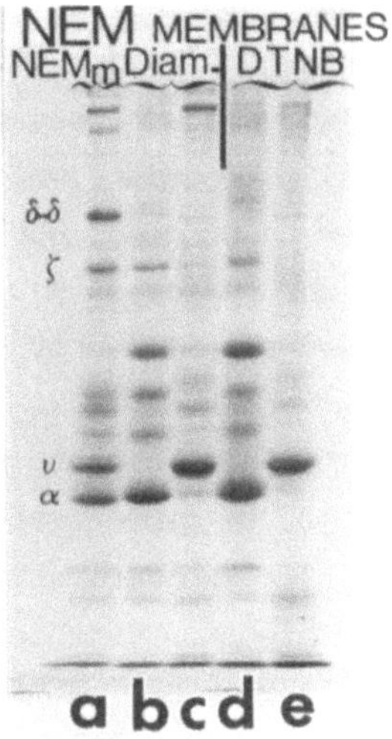

Fig 6

In alkaline-extracted membranes, depleted of the ν-peptide, the same thiol treatments do not hinder penetration of AChR peptides (Fig. 5<u>e</u>-<u>h</u>). Notice that the δ-subunit is essentially dimeric (Fig. 5<u>i</u>). Diamide reoxidation yields the same results (Fig. 6, but see ref. 11). All these experiments are suggestive of extensive cross-linking, via mixed disulphide formation (without involvement of the δ-subunit) between receptor and ν-peptide.

A further association between the two proteins was shown previously (ref. 4): Although alkaline stripping readily solubilizes the ν-peptide, actin and other non-receptor peptides from native and reduced membranes, alkaline treatment was <u>ineffective</u> in extracting the peptide from

NEM-membranes. The higher proportion of 13S, dimeric species, is found to be correlated with the lack of extraction of the ν-peptide.

Immune sera raised against the ν-peptide and subsequently purified by affinity chromatography to yield monospecific IgG's can be shown to react specifically with the ν-peptide by the very sensitive immune blotting technique (18). The monospecific anti-ν-peptide IgG could be used in an indirect immunofluorescence assay to demonstrate that the antigenic determinants of the peptide in the AChR membranes are mainly exposed to the inner, "cytoplasmic" side of the membrane: Rhodamine-labelled goat anti-rabitt IgG is bound predominantly to membranes treated with 0.1% saponin (ref. 4) a procedure which permeabilizes the AChR vesicles to molecules larger than Mr 450 000 without altering binding properties or the morphology of the vesicles (9). As expected, membranes depleted of the ν-peptide showed significantly lower labelling with monospecific IgG.

The influence of the ν-peptide on the dynamic properties of the AChR receptor could also be demonstrated by the use of phosphorescence anisotropy measurements (6). Two derivatives of the quasi-irreversible curaremimetic α-bungarotoxin (eosin-5'-isothiocyanate and eosin-5'-iodoacetamide) were employed to label the AChR in normal, alkaline-extracted, and thiol-modified membranes. Finite rotational correlation times (10-26 μs) were observed under two conditions: a)after DTT-reduction (20°C) or b) after depletion of the ν-peptide (39°C). Under the assumption that the AChR behaves as a rigid cylindrical body embedded in the membrane, its rotation about its symmetry axis (perpendicular to the plane of the membrane) is described by an anisotropy function of the type:

$$r(t) = \alpha_1 e^{-t/\phi} + \alpha_2 e^{-4t/\phi} + \alpha_3 \qquad (1)$$

where ϕ, the rotational correlation time, is given by:

$$\phi = 4 V \eta / k \quad T \qquad (2)$$

Only the volume of the AChR embedded in the membrane needs be considered. Quantitative sructural data from our previous electron microscope observations (20) and more recent freeze-etching, rotary shadowing experiments (H.P. Zingsheim and F.J. Barrantes, submitted) yielded information on the average diameter of the AChR in end-on views (i.e. perpendicular to the membrane) and the receptor moiety protruding from the membrane surface, roughly 100 nm^3 in volume (about 5.5 nm thick). This corresponds to a mass of about 100 000 dalton (Fig. 7).

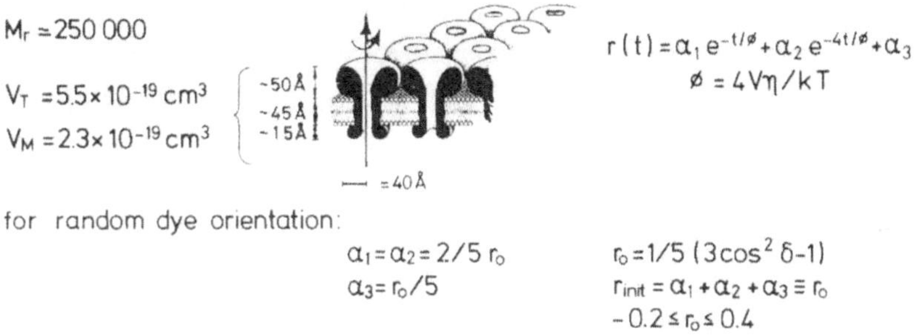

Fig. 7. Diagramatic representation of receptors embedded in the membrane, rotating about main molecular axis. Total and intramembranous volumes (V_T, V_M) of AChR, principal dimensions, and anisotropy function r(t) are given. Ideal random dye orientation conditions yield the above α coefficients.

Since the cytoplasmic-protruding moiety is about 1.5 nm thick (ref. 16,14 and Zingsheim and Barrantes, unpublished), the membrane domain can be calculated. Of a total volume of $5.5x10^{-19}$ cm^3 (the $\underline{M}_r$ 250 000 monomer) a 4.5 nm lipid bilayer would accomodate $2.3x10^{-19}$ cm^3. The other parameter needed in eq. (2) above is the membrane viscosity, η . Values of about 4 Poises were experimentally obtained (B. Rivnay, M. Shinitzky, F.J. Barrantes, unpublished). The calculated ϕ is 90 μs. Alternatively, the rotational correlation time expected for a $\underline{M}_r$ 250 000 AChR monomer with the dimensions given above and a partial specific volume of 0.73 cm^3 g^{-1} and an intramembranous moiety of $\underline{M}_r$ 100 000 yields ϕ(calc) = 49 μs. The observed correlation times, 13-26 μs is in acceptable agreement with the maximal range $\phi_{cal}/4$-ϕ_{cal} =12-90 μs, compatible with the motion of individual, 9S monomeric AChR. Since this motion could be observed only after reduction of the receptor or in ν-peptide-depleted membranes, and NEM-membranes did not yield observable anisotropy decays even after alkaline extraction, these experiments reinforce the hypothesis presented in the Introduction concerning the participation of the ν-peptide in AChR molecular states. Specifically, it follows that the 13S dimer, or higher oligomeric forms, lack the rotational mobility characteristic of the monomer.

Discussion

Biochemical, structural, immunological and spectroscopic studies have been used to investigate some of the possible relationships between the AChR oligomeric organization and the non-receptor ν-peptide. Depletion of this peptide does not hinder the thiol-dependent AChR interconversions. The presence or absence of the ν-peptide does influence, however, the original redox equilibrium (4). Thus, ν-peptide-depleted membranes show a slight shift to higher oligomeric states upon reoxidation as compared to "complete" membranes. Conversely, membranes from which the ν-peptide cannot be extracted (the "NEM-membranes") are made predominantly of 13S, dimeric species. The diagram below (Fig. 8) summarizes the present working hypothesis:

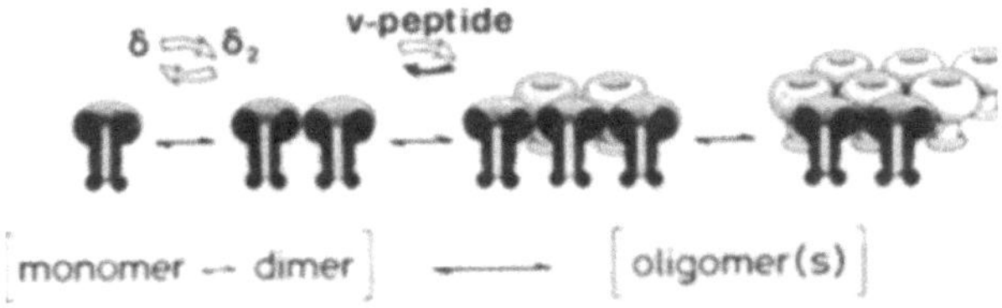

Fig. 8

Two equilibria would be operative in AChR membranes, one between monomer and dimers, controlled basically through δ-δ bonding /cleavage, and a second one between the two latter species and higher oligomeric forms. In the native excitable membranes this redox balance has been proposed to depend not only on the redox state of the receptor itself but on the multiple contributions from other constituents (3). It was further proposed that a protein having "unusually low redox potential and a close proximity to the receptor" as suggested by Chang & Bock (8) could materialize in the ν-peptide, envisaged as a "redox buffering system" normally impairing the high-order associations of the AChR which occur in its absence (see 4). Given the predominant cytoplasmic exposure of the antigenic determinants of the ν-peptide (4), in agreement with recent studies from other laboratories showing disappearance of electron dense material from alkaline-extracted membranes (17) or resistance of the peptide to proteolytic attack form the outer membrane face (19), it is likely that the effects of the ν-peptide are mediated from the inside of the electrocyte.

Partly supported by grant Ba 671/3-2 (Deutsche Forschungsgemeinschaft).

References

1. BARRANTES, F. J. 1978. J. Mol. Biol. 124:1-26.
2. BARRANTES, F. J. 1979. Ann. Rev. Biophys. Bioeng. 8:287-321.
3. BARRANTES, F. J. 1980. Biochemistry 19:2957-2965.
4. BARRANTES, F. J. 1981. J. Cell Biol. in press.
5. BARRANTES, F. J., D.-Ch. NEUGEBAUER, and H. P. ZINGSHEIM. 1980. FEBS Lett. 112:73-78.
6. BARTHOLDI, M., F. J. BARRANTES and T. M. JOVIN. 1981. Eur. J. Biochem. in press.
7. CARTAUD, J., J.L. POPOT, and J.P. CHANGEUX. 1980. FEBS Lett. 121:327-332.
8. CHANG, H.W. and E. BOCK. 1977. Biochemistry 16:4513-4520.
9. COHEN, J. B., N. D. BOYD, A. Y. JENG, D. C. MEDYNSKI, R. S. NEUBIG, P. ST JOHN and N. S. SHERA 1980. in Psychopharmacology of Neurotransmitter Receptors (Yamamura, Olsen, Usdin, eds.). Elsevier North Holland, pp. 47-62.
10. FAMBROUGH, D. E. 1979. Physiol. Rev. 59:165-227.
11. HAMILTON, S.L., M. McLAUGHLIN, and A. KARLIN. 1979. Biochemistry 18:155-163.
12. HARTIG, P.R., and M. A. RAFTERY. 1979. Biochemistry 18:1146-1150.

13.HEUSER, J. E. and SALPETER, S. R. 1979. _J. Cell. Biol. 82:_15-173.

14.KLYMKOWSKY, M.W., and R. M. STROUD. 1979. _J. Mol. Biol. 128:_319-334.

15.NEUBIG, R. R., E. K. KRODEL, N. D. BOYD, and J. B. COHEN. 1979. _Proc. Natl. Acad. Sci. U. S. A. 76:_690-694.

16.ROSS, J., M. W. KLYMKOWSKY, D. A. AGARD, and R. M. STROUD. 1977. _J. Mol. Biol. 116_:635-659.

17.SEALOCK, R., and KAVOOKJIAN, A. 1980. _Brain Res. 190:_81-93.

18.TOWLIN, H., T. STAEHELIN and J. GORDON. 1979. _Proc. Natl. Acad. Sci. U. S. A. 76:_4350-4354.

19.WENNOGLE, L. P. and J. P. CHANGEUX. 1980. _Eur. J. Biochem. 106:_381-393.

20.ZINGSHEIM, H. P., D.-Ch.NEUGEBAUER, F. J. BARRANTES, and J. FRANK. 1980. _Proc. Natl. Acad. Sci. U. S. A_. 77:952-956.

DETECTION AND CHARACTERISATION OF MONOCLONAL ANTIBODIES TO THE ACETYLCHOLINE RECEPTOR BY SOLID-PHASE IMMUNOASSAY

D. Watters* and A. Maelicke

Max-Planck-Institut für Ernährungsphysiologie,
Rheinlanddamm 201, D-4600 Dortmund

Abstract

Monoclonal antibodies have been produced against the acetylcholine receptor from Torpedo marmorata. These were detected and characterised using the rapid and sensitive technique of enzyme-linked immunosorbent assay (ELISA). Of the twenty anti-Torpedo acetylcholine receptor AChR antibodies studied, three cross-react with AChR from Electrophorus electricus, three cross-react with rat myotubes in culture and one with cultured sympathetic ganglion cells (chick embryo). The ELISA assay was also used to differentiate between antibodies binding at or distant to the acetylcholine binding site. Six of the antibodies bind at or near the ligand-binding site. By a solid-phase immunoassay using tritium labelled antibodies it was shown that these six antibodies bind to two distinct areas at the receptor.

Introduction

An animal immunised with acetylcholine receptor produces a range of antibodies, each the exclusive product of a single clone of

*Present address:

Dept. of Pharmacology, John Curtin School of Medical Research, Australian National University, P.O. Box 334, Canberra, 2601 Australia lymphocytes. Hybridoma technology allows the isolation of these individual clones providing a number of antigenic-site specific antibodies, each directed to different parts of the receptor. With these as tools we hope to gain further insight into the structure of the acetylcholine receptor and how it functions in neurotransmission. In this communication we describe a number of monoclonal antibodies including six which bind to the acetylcholine-binding site. They identify distinct antigenic sites at the receptor.

Materials and Methods

Solubilised acetylcholine receptors were purified from the electric organs of *Torpedo marmorata* and *Electrophorus electricus* as described previously (1): Receptor preparations in phosphate buffer (0.1 M pH 7.4) containing 0.05% Tween 80 were stored as sterile solutions at $4^{o}C$. Crude membrane fragments from *Torpedo marmorata* were prepared as described in an accompanying article (2).

Balb/c or Balb/c x C57BL/6 (F1) mice were immunised with purified *Torpedo* receptor and the spleen cells fused with NS-1 (K chain secreting) or X63.Ag8.653 (non-secreting) myeloma cell lines, according to published procedures (3,4). Positive hybrids were identified using an enzyme-linked immunosorbent assay (5). Either peroxidase-labelled anti-mouse IgG (Nordic) or alkaline phosphatase-labelled anti-mouse IgG (Miles) were used. The peroxidase reaction was carried out using 2,2'-azino-di-(3-ethylbenzthiazoline sulfonic acid) (ABTS, 0.25 mM) and H_2O_2 (0.18 mM) in 0.1 M phosphate buffer pH 6.8. p-Nitrophenylphosphate (1.7 mM in 0.1 M glycine-NaOH pH 9.8, containing 1 mM $MgCl_2$) was the substrate for alkaline phosphatase. The extent of reaction was determined in both cases by absorbance measurement at 405 nm in a Gilford EIA Manual Reader. Instead of using purified receptor as antigen in the ELISA test, it was also possible to use crude membrane fragments or cultured cells fixed with glutaraldehyde (6). Rat myotubes and chick embryo sympathetic ganglion cells were used in this way.

Antibodies were labelled biosynthetically with $[^3H]$ leucine (7). For competitive binding assays, polyvinylchloride microtiter plates were coated with receptor and incubated with labelled culture supernatant in the presence of unlabelled supernatants from other clones. Counts bound per well were usually of the order of 3000 to 20.000 being reduced to between 800 and 3000 when competiton between two antibodies occurred. If no competition occurs it can be assumed that two antibodies bind to mutually exclusive antigenic sites.

Results and Discussion

The concentration of AChR required to saturate the Gilford Cuvettes was determined as shown in Fig. 1. A dilution of 1:300 of our standard preparation (corresponding to 5 x 10^{-9}M toxin binding sites) resulted in maximum amount of receptor attached as determined by using excess developing antibody. The amount of receptor bound per well of a polyvinyl microtiter plate was shown by binding of $[^{125}I]$α-bungarotoxin to be of the order of 10^{-13} moles. A similar amount is expected to bind to the Gilford Cuvettes.

Figure 2 shows a serial dilution curve of rabbit anti-Torpedo AChR antiserum. Background absorbance values, as measured by controls with normal rabbit serum and uncoated cuvettes, are very low.

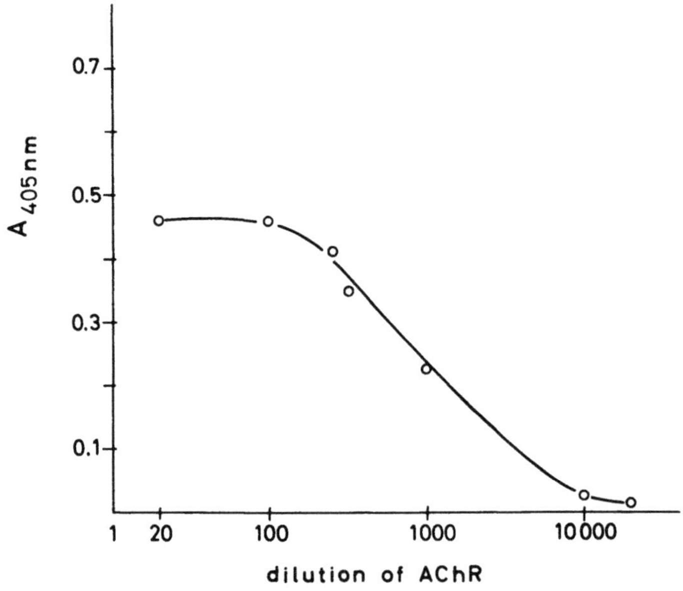

Fig. 1. Determination of the concentration of AChR required to coat the ELISA Cuvettes. 200µl of solutions of AChR (in 0.1 M $NaHCO_3$ pH 9) at different concentrations were allowed to bind overnight at 4°C. Excess antigen was removed by washing with phosphate-buffered saline containing 0.05% Tween 20 (PBS-Tween). Rabbit anti-*Torpedo* AChR antiserum was added in excess, followed after washing, by peroxidase-labelled goat anti-rabbit IgG. Reaction volumes were always 200µl and reaction times with substrate varied from 30 to 120 minutes, but were kept constant within each experiment.

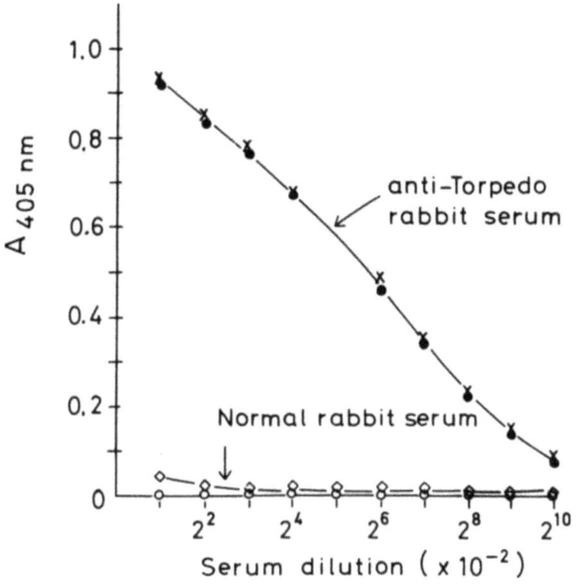

Fig. 2. Serial dilution (1 in 2) of rabbit anti-Torpedo AChR antiserum (● and x), duplicate measurements); (◇), normal rabbit serum; and (o), cuvettes not coated with receptor.

The ELISA is sensitive to between 10^{-13} and 10^{-14} moles per 0.2 ml sample in agreement with Norcross et al. (5). This sensitivity is more than adequate for detection of monoclonal antibodies in cell culture supernatants (~10μg/ml or 6 x 10^{-11} moles/ml). A serial dilution curve of one monoclonal antibody (mAb) to Torpedo AChR is shown in Fig. 3. This medium had a titre of about 1 in 2^{11} (approximately 1 in 2000). No attempt was made in this study to quantitate the ELISA, as the amount of antibodies in the culture supernatant varies with the time in culture and is of little consequence for the purpose of this work. The reaction time with substrate was not always kept constant from one experiment to the next, since comparisons were always made with appropriate controls within each experiment.

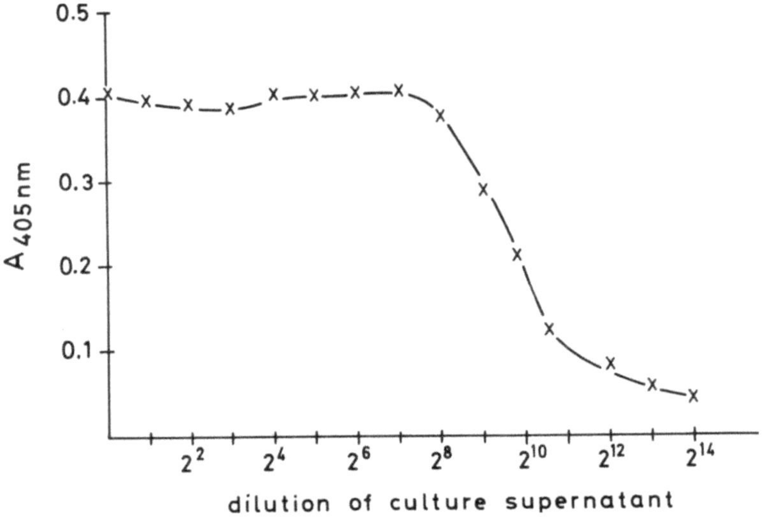

Fig. 3. Serial dilution (1 in 2) of culture supernatant from one clone producing anti-<u>Torpedo</u> AChR antibodies (clone 8, see Table 1).

The ELISA not only offers a very simple, rapid and sensitive method of screening large numbers of hybrids for positive clones, with the added advantages of requiring non-radioactive reagents of long shelf-life, but also can be used to further characterise the various types of anti-AChR antibodies. Fig.4 shows that two different classes of antibody can be distinguished - those binding at the ligand binding site (e.g. mAb 5) and those binding distant to this site (e.g. mAb 16). Table 1 summarises the properties of twenty monoclonal antibodies as determined by ELISA. The first six in the table are directed against a region at or near the acetylcholine binding site, since antibody binding is decreased in the presence of cholinergic ligands.

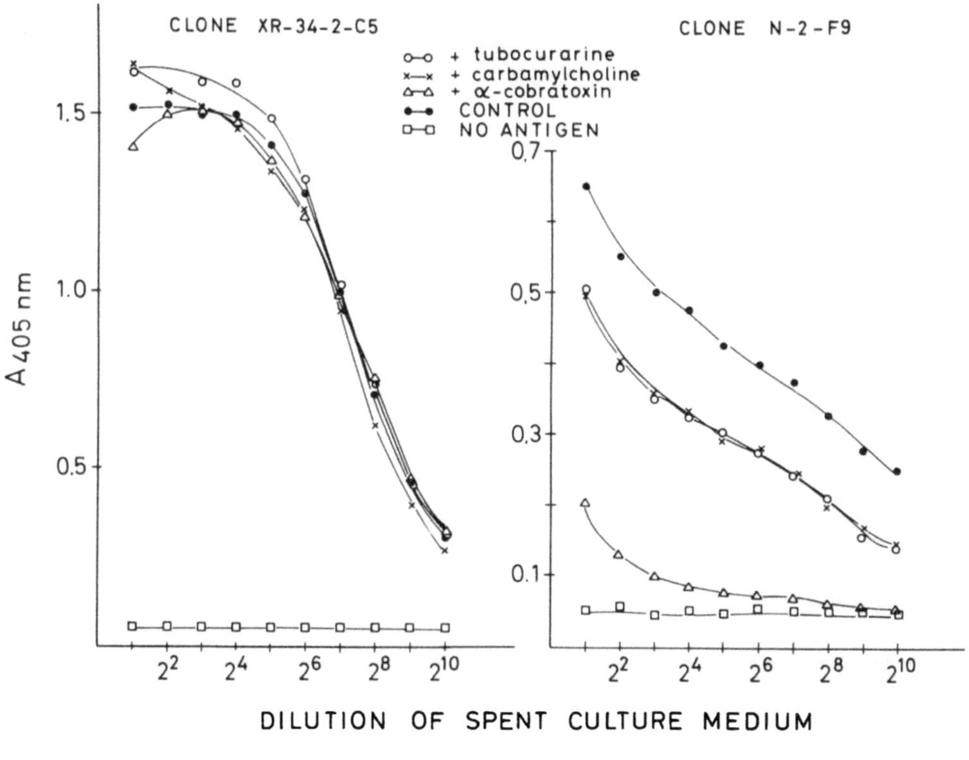

Fig. 4. Serial dilution (1 in 2) curves of culture supernatants in the presence and absence of cholinergic ligands, present at high concentration. Each curve was obtained by adding 200μl of ligand in PBS-Tween to each well of a strip of 10 cuvettes. To cuvette 1, 200μl of medium was added, mixed and 200μl transferred to the next cuvette, and so on. Cholinergic ligands were added at the following concentrations: carbamylcholine (2 mM), d-tubocurarine (1 mM) and α-cobratoxin (1μM).

TABLE 1

mAb	Hybridoma Clone	IgG subclass	Cross-reactivity with receptor from Electrophorus	Rat Myotubes	Sympathetic Ganglia	Inhibition by α-cobratoxin
1	1-A4-C8	2a				+
2	2-B4-12	2a				+
3	5-6-1-D6	1				+
4	1-C3-C9	3				+
5	N-2-F9	2b		+	+	+
6	XR-6-G10	2a	+	+		+
7	A-1-G11		+			
8	NA-19-E11	1				
9	1-B6-B10	2a				
10	XR-33-E7	1				
11	XR-16-B3	2a		+		
12	XR-64-F11	1				
13	XR-41-G6	1				
14	NB-20-C6	1				
15	NA-23-E4	2a				
16	XR-34-2-C5	1				
17	XR-26-D2	1				
18	XR-46-H8		+			
19	1-D2-F10	1				
20	H-5-E9	1				

Table 1: Characteristics of the monoclonal antibodies (mAb) as studied by ELISA.
IgG subclass was determined by Ouchterlony double immunodiffusion of ammonium sulphate concentrated medium against anti-mouse IgG subclass specific antisera (Nordic).
Cross-reactivity with cultured rat myotubes and chick embryo sympathetic ganglion cells was determined by ELISA on glutaraldehyde fixed cultures (6).

As can be seen from Table 1, one of the six antibodies directed at the ligand binding site (mAb 6) cross-reacts with muscle and Electrophorus AChR. mAb 5 cross-reacts with muscle and sympathetic ganglion AChR.

Competition between mAbs for Antigenic Sites.

Most of the twenty antibodies listed in Table 1 were labelled internally with [^{3}H] leucine. Labelled culture supernatant from one clone was allowed to bind to receptor coated microtiter plates in the presence of unlabelled culture supernatants from other clones in turn. The experiment was repeated for each labelled antibody. Two antibodies can be assumed to bind to non-overlapping sites if the binding of one is not inhibited by the other. Partial or complete inhibition of one antibody by another implies that both antibodies bind to overlapping or identical antigenic determinants, but the extent of overlap cannot be determined in these experiments. About ten overlapping immunogenic region have been distinguished so far using these antibodies. mAbs 17 and 19; 9 and 10; 12 and 14; and 7 and 8, form pairs of antibodies which compete strongly with one another and define four separate antigenic sites.

When the binding of antibodies 1 to 6 (anti-ligand binding site) was studied in this way some interesting observations emerged. The binding of mAb6 was inhibited by all of mAbs 1 to 5 as might be expected. The binding of mAbs 1 to 4 was inhibited by mAbs 1 to 4 and mAb 6 but only very slightly if at all by mAb 5. The binding of mAb 5 was inhibited only appreciably by mAb 6. The data for these experiments is shown in Table 2.

TABLE 2

cpm bound per microtiter well [a]

unlabelled mAbs	[^{3}H] mAb 5	[^{3}H] mAb 1	[^{3}H] mAb 6
-	11.000	6.000	20.000
1	10.700 [b]	1.300	15.700
2	9.500	2.500	13.500
3	10.000	2.500	16.000
4	10.000	2.100	14.500
5	3.500	4.700	13.000
6	5.000	1.500	4.000

a) The amount of counts bound per well depends on the incorporation of [^{3}H] leucine into antibody, which is never the same from one clone to the other or in different labelling experiments.

b) The affinity of mAb 1 is three times lower than that of mAb 5 and fifteen times lower than that of mAb 6. The same unlabelled culture supernatant 1 was used to inhibit labelled mAbs 5 and 6, therefore the lack of effect of antibody 1 cannot be due to differences in affinity.

The affinities of binding for these two antibodies to receptor immobilised on microtiter plates have been measured and differ only by a factor of 3 (mAb 5 having the higher affinity). Because mAb 5 does not displace mAb 1 from the receptor (Table 2), this lack of inhibition cannot be explained by differences in affinities of the antibodies for the receptor. Antibodies 1 and 5 are thus directed at different antigenic determinants.

Conclusion

We have made a small library of monoclonal antibodies to the acetylcholine receptor from Torpedo marmorata using solid-phase immunoassays for detection and characterisation. Apart from the obvious advantages of the ELISA, it has the added advantage in the case of the acetylcholine receptor, that it allows detection of antibodies directed against the ligand binding site. This site is covered by labelled α-toxin in the standard radioimmunoassay for anti-AChR antibodies (8). Antibodies to the ligand binding site should prove to be most useful in the study of receptor function in neurotransmission. As shown in Table 2, the anti-ligand binding site antibodies bind to various regions of the receptor. The antibodies also compete in different fashions with small cholinergic ligands (9).

Using tritium labelled antibodies and a solid-phase assay similar to ELISA, one can directly determine the binding affinity, therefore the conclusions drawn from ELISA can be supplemented by quantitative assays. Using this set of assays we can develop powerful tools to study the topography and function of this neurotransmitter receptor.

Acknowledgements

We thank Dr. Georges Köhler (Basel Institute for Immunology) for helpful discussions and Helga Burghardt for excellent technical assistance.

References

1. Rüchel, R., Watters, D., Maelicke, A.: Eur. J. Biochem. 119, 215-223 (1981).
2. Wolff, E., Fels, G., Maelicke, A.: submitted for publication.
3. Köhler, G., Milstein, C.: Nature 265, 495-497 (1975).
4. Fazekas de St. Groth S., Scheiddegger, D.: J. Immunol. Methods 35, 1-21 (1980).
5. Norcross, N.L., Griffith, I.J., Lettieri, B.A.: Muscle and Nerve 3, 345-349 (1980).
6. Stocker, J.W., Malavasi, F., Trucco, M.: Immunological Methods, Vol. 2 (Lefkovitz, I. and Pernis, B., eds.) pp. 299-308 (1981) Academic Press, New York
7. Pink, J.R.L., Ziegler, A.: Immunological Methods, Vol. 1 (Lefkovitz, I. and Pernis, B., eds.) pp. 169-179 (1979) Academic Press, New York
8. Tzartos, S.J., Rand, D.E., Einarson, B.L., Lindstrom, T.M.: J. Biol. Chem. 256, 8635-8645 (1981).
9. Watters, D., Maelicke, A.: in preparation.

THE STRUCTURALLY ORGANIZED REACTIONS OF ACETYLCHOLINE IN THE BIOELECTRIC SIGNAL TRANSMISSION

Eberhard Neumann
Biophysical Chemistry, Max-Planck-Institut für Biochemie
D-8033 Martinsried/München, Germany

Introduction

Nerve impulses and other membrane potential changes in excitable cells result from transient permeability changes of the excitable membranes to ions, in many cases channel-selectively to Na^+, K^+, Ca^{2+} or Cl^- ions. The changes in the ion flows are transient; they are conformationally controlled by membrane-bound channel gating proteins. The gating reactions responsible for opening and closing steps of the ion pathways in excitable membranes appear to involve, in general, <u>bimolecular reactions</u> coupled to intramolecular <u>conformational changes</u> and short-lived <u>metastability</u> of the iontransporting configuration of the gating system (1).

The molecularly most thoroughly studied ion-flow gating phenomena are those which are associated with the acetylcholine (AcCh) system. According to the original concept of Nachmansohn (1953) a proper stimulus releases AcCh from a storage site; the chemical activator then binds to the (at that time hypothetical) acetylcholine receptor protein (AcChR) and induces a conformational change to an open, ion-conducting structure. The enzyme acetylcholinesterase (AcChE) rapidly hydrolyzes the AcCh and thereby terminates the receptor-mediated permeability increase (2,3).

After a first chemical formulation (4) of the reaction of AcCh(A) with the receptor (R) by del Castillo and Katz (1957), a more modern version of formulating the AcCh gating concept is pictured in figure 1, where the flow nature of the AcCh mediated gating is indicated (5).

Indeed, meanwhile evidence has accumulated that AcCh regulates transmembrane ion flows by direct interactions with the two membrane associated proteins AcChR and AcChE. The intrinsic function of the nicotinic AcChR is the gating of Na^{+}-K^{+} flows via AcCh-induced structural changes leading to open and closed channel states; the esterase limits the availability of AcCh.

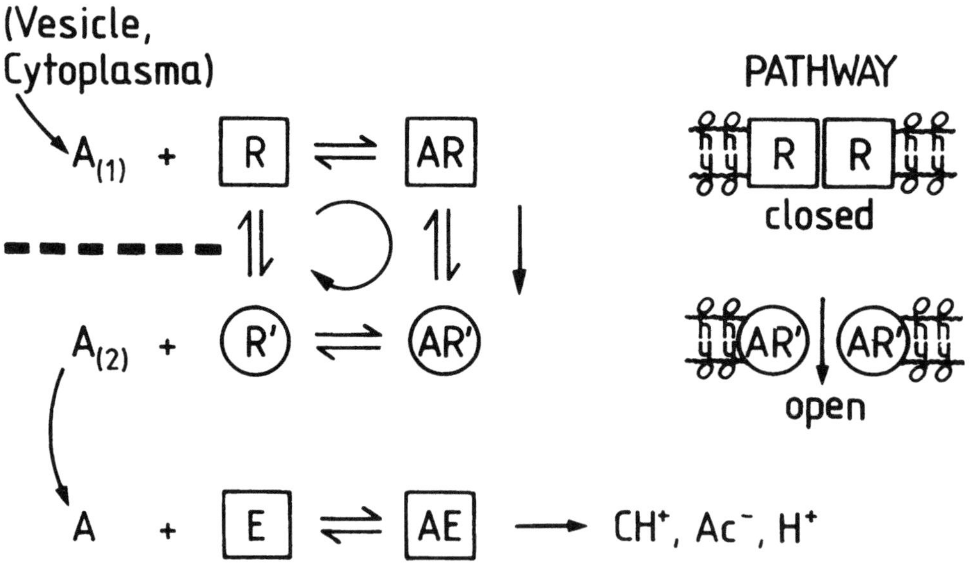

Figure 1: Conformational concept of acetylcholine (A) mediated ion flow gating by acetylcholine receptor converting, upon AcCh binding from a closed (R) to an open structure R', and esterase(E)hydrolysing the AcCh ion to choline (Ch^{+}), acetate (Ac^{-}) and H^{+} ions.

The reactions of AcCh with AcChR and AcChE occur in micro-reaction spaces near the excitable membranes. In figure 2 the so far most extensively studied reaction space of AcCh is enlarged, showing that the receptors are accumulated in post-synaptic parts, but are also present in presynaptic parts of excitable membranes (6) as far as can be judged from the α-bungarotoxin binding believed to be specific for (nicotinic) AcChR. Reaction products of esterase activity are found along all excitable biomembranes and in particular in the synaptic gap. Because the enzyme is in part intrinsically membrane-bound (7,8), the enzyme localization in figure 2 is modelled within the cleft space and within the membranes; see, e.g., ref. (9).

The reactions of AcCh in this reaction space cause the well-known electrical epiphenomena: the spontaneous miniature end-plate potentials, end-plate potentials and action potentials (or nerve impulses); see e.g. (10). The molecular mechanisms of the AcCh reactions with AcChR and AcChE are therefore an essential part of the complicated mechanism of the electric signal generation and transmission in neuronal, muscular, and secretory cell systems. In the following assay it will be shown how in particular the results of relaxation kinetic experiments with isolated AcCh-proteins (of electric fish) permit a deeper insight in the special type of the observed electrical epiphenomena. On the basis of molecular and electrophysiological data, possible interaction mechanisms are suggested for the sequence of AcCh reactions leading to bio-electric signals.

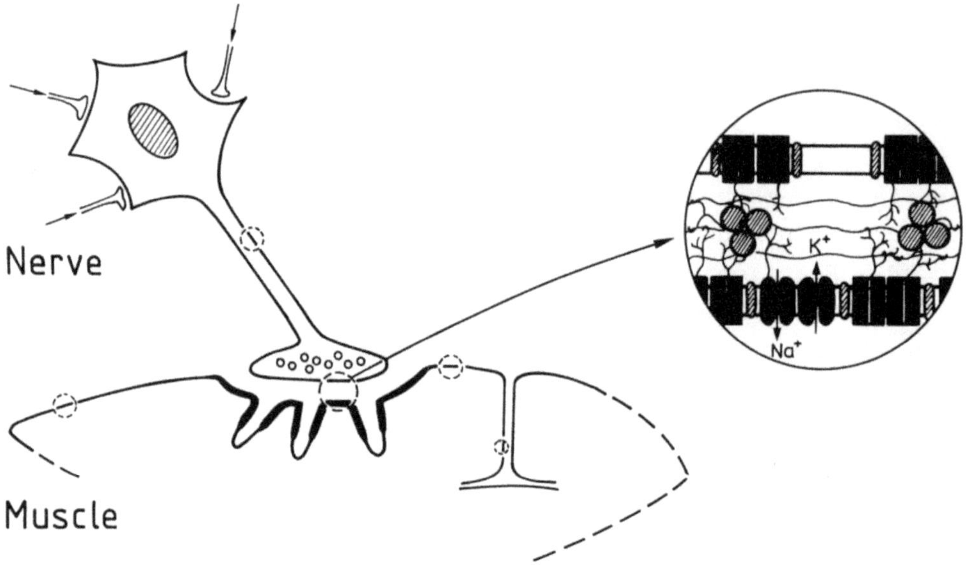

Figure 2: Scheme of a neuromuscular synapse, connecting a nerve and a muscle cell. The reaction products of acetylcholinesterase (AcChE) activity are found along all the plasma membranes, of the nerve, of the muscle, in the synaptic cleft, and in the muscular tubular system. Acetylcholine receptor as judged from reaction sites with α-bungarotoxin appear particularly accumulated in postsynaptic parts of the muscular membranes, but is also found presynaptically. The nerve terminal contains vesicles, the (possibly long-term) storage sites for AcCh synthetized in the cytoplasma.
The enlarged insert is an attempt to model possible locations of AcChE partially as intrinsic membrane protein (⊘), partially as extramembraneous 18S assemblies (⊘⊘⊘) bound to the basal structures via the collagen-like tails. The AcChR is modelled as a double-channel system (H-form; 500,000d), the glyco-parts of the proteins extending into the basal structures of the cleft.

A. AcCh induced elementary electric signals.

The probably most elementary epiphenomena resulting from the AcCh action are the ionic current blips due to single-channel fluctuations. When the concentration of AcCh increases, both the number of channels and the frequency of fluctuations increase. The spontaneous miniature end plate currents (m.e.p.c.) and the other more macroscopic electric signals represent a larger collection of single channels. The time course of a m.e.p.c. is suited for a comparison with the kinetic results of isolated AcCh proteins because the kinetic data of isolated molecules always reflect assembly averages. In figure 3 such a m.e.p.c. is redrawn from a review by Gage (11): a rapid growth phase (reflecting the rapid increase in the number of AcChR-channels) is followed by a slower decay phase reflecting the decrease in the number of open receptor-channels. A particular important observation is that 'the decay is exponential from the peak' (12), no rounding is observed. The growth phase probably reflects

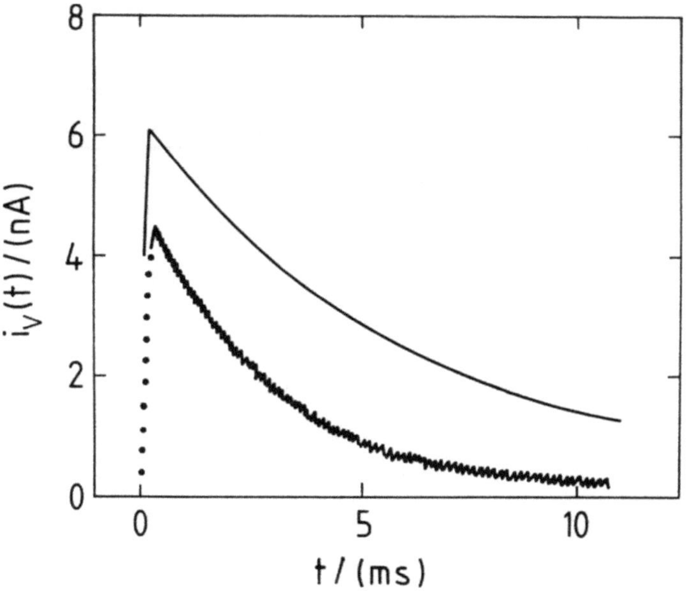

Figure 3: Miniature end plate current, mepc, in toad neuromuscular junction (redrawn from Figure 8 of ref.(12); and Fig. 2 of ref. (11); clamp potential - 70 mV, 293K in standard Ringer solution. Upper trace recorded after 30 min exposure to 1mg/ℓ neostigmine in

Ringer solution, a condition assumed to completely inhibit esterase activity: the slow decay reflects slow diffusion of acetylcholine in the junction (and probably also further receptor desensitization)

the rate of AcCh-induced conformational change in the AcChR. The decay phase is determined by esterase activity, but not in a direct rate-limiting manner.

It was found that the average life time, $\bar{t}_o$, of the open AcChR-channel does not depend on the concentration of the neuroactivator; see, e.g., ref. (13). At given temperature and membrane voltage, $\bar{t}_o$ is equal to the decay time constant τ_d of the m.e.p.c.; in addition, $\bar{t}_o$ and τ_d both have the same voltage and temperature dependence (12). It therefore appears that the closure phase of a m.e.p.c. is independent of AcCh (11,14). Furtheron, since practically complete inhibition of AcChE with neostigmine causes an increase of the peak amplitude of mepc by a factor of 1.4 and a prolongation of the decay phase by a factor of about 2 (see Figure 3 and ref. (12), the receptors in a 'normal mepc' appear not to be saturated. The independence of AcCh of the m.e.p.c. decay phase requires that during the decay phase the neuroactivator is much faster removed than it can return to AcChR (R). The effective binding of AcCh to AcChE (and hydrolysis) should therefore be faster than to AcChR, or in terms of the effective association rate constants:

$$k_{ass}(R) < k_{ass}(E) \qquad (1)$$

where $k_{ass}(R)$ reflects the overall reaction leading to the conducting conformation with a life-time of about 5 to 10 ms (15).

According to current knowledge the simplest reaction scheme describing main features of in vivo AcChR gating is given by

$$2A + R \rightleftharpoons \ldots\ldots \overset{K_1}{} \rightleftharpoons A_2R$$

$$k_c \upharpoonleft\!\downharpoonright k_o \qquad (2)$$

$$A_2R'$$

see also ref. (16).

Assuming rapid binding of AcCh (A) to form the complex A_2R, coupled to a slower conformational transition of the occupied receptor A_2R to the open channel configuration A_2R', normal mode analysis of the reaction equations (2) yields the relaxation time τ_{II} of the slow mode:

$$\frac{1}{\tau_{II}} = k_c + k_o \cdot \frac{[A]^2 + [R]}{[A]^2 + [R] + K_1} \qquad (3)$$

where k_o and k_c are the rate constants for the opening and closing steps, respectively, and K_1 is the overall dissociation constant in terms of assumed Hill-type cooperativity for the AcCh binding.

In equation (3) it is readily seen that τ_{II} can be independent of the activator concentration $[A]$ if $[A] \longrightarrow 0$. According to our gating concept the decay phase of a m.e.p.c. is determined by the slow receptor mode or

$$\tau_d = \tau_{II} = f(T,V) \qquad (4)$$

Because for $[A] \to 0$, τ_{II} is determined only by rate and equilibrium constants, the dependence of τ_d solely on temperature (T) and voltage (V) is obvious.

The essential condition $[A] \to 0$ during the decay phase of a m.e.p.c. may be fulfilled when the inequality (1) holds. In this context it is instructive to recall that under in vivo conditions not a trace of free AcCh is detectable, either at synaptic or at axonal parts of excitable membranes (3). These observations suggest that a very efficient, not purely diffusive but enzymatic, removal mechanism exists for AcCh. Indeed, it has been shown that the AcChE macromolecule has particular electrostatic properties such that already the diffusive association of cationic ligands like the AcCh to the enzyme surface is drastically accelerated (17,18).

We shall return to further details after the discussion of some kinetic properties of isolated AcChR and AcChE, because the rate constants of the effective binding of AcCh to the two proteins are of fundamental importance; see the inequality (1).

B. Acetylcholinesterase

A minimum estimate for $k_{ass}(E)$ may be derived from catalytic parameters of the enzyme. In the minimum reaction scheme for the enzyme (E) acylation by AcCh (A) according to

$$A + E \underset{k_{21}}{\overset{k_{12}}{\rightleftharpoons}} E \cdot A \xrightarrow{k_2} E \cdot acyl + Ch \rightarrow \ldots\ldots \qquad (5)$$

$k_{12} \geqslant k_{cat}/K_{app}$ is the bimolecular association rate constant for which a minimum value of $\approx 2 \cdot 10^8\ M^{-1}s^{-1}$ (at 0.1M ionic strength at 298K and pH 8) can be estimated from the catalytic turnover rate constant k_{cat} and the apparent Michaelis constant K_{app} (17).

Since $k_2 \approx 10^5\ s^{-1}$ and $k_{21} \approx 10^4 s^{-1}$, thus $k_2 > k_{21}$, we may safely set

$$k_{12} \approx k_{ass}(E) \geqslant 2 \times 10^8\ M^{-1}s^{-1} \qquad (6)$$

and obtain an estimate which is adequate for comparison with $k_{ass}(R)$ of the receptor.

Recent relaxation kinetic investigations demonstrated that cationic ligands bind extremely rapid to the enzyme active site (17,18). The observed bimolecular rate constants k_{12}

between 10^{10} and 10^9 $M^{-1}s^{-1}$ are unusually high for enzyme ligand interactions. In addition, the association rate constants k_{12} are very strongly dependent on the ionic strength, I_c, of the solution. Virtually the same strong I_c-dependence has been observed for a catalytic parameter proportional to k_{12} of acetylthiocholine, k_{cat}/K_{app}, a substrate whose structure and kinetic properties are very similar to those of acetylcholine (18).

The analysis of the I_c-dependencies shows that at least six to seven monovalent anionic groups contribute to the comparatively large values k_{12} for both the non-substrates and acetylthiocholine ($k°_{12}$ = 0.42 · 10^{10} $M^{-1}s^{-1}$), suggesting that an enzyme surface area larger than the ligand binding site itself is effective in trapping a ligand in encounter complexes. This larger surface area might include peripheral anionic sites from which ligand would move to the active site by surface diffusion. Thus due to a dominantly multi-anionic surface structure, this polyionic enzyme appears to be a powerful electrostatic sink for trapping and decomposing the acetylcholine cation.

C. Acetylcholine Receptor

The smallest, functionally intact acetylcholine binding protein which can be isolated under gentle experimental conditions from Torpedo fish, minimizing chemical modifications, is the socalled heavy (H) form of receptor rich membrane fragments; see, e.g. (19). This H-form of a molecular weight of roughly 500,000 d (Torp. cal.) is a dimer of two probably not identical monomers: the L- and the L'-form which are linked by intersubunit disulfide bonds. Provided that endogenous lipids remain attached to the isolated receptor-lipid complex, the H-form exhibits essentially the same positive-cooperative acetylcholine binding isotherms as biomembrane fragments (19,20).

Ca^{2+} and $AcCh^{+}$ binding. The isolated AcChR in detergent solution (probably largely in the L-forms) was found to bind large amounts of Ca^{2+} ions associated with high (μM) and low (mM) affinity sites. There is competition of Ca^{2+} binding with other cations; (see also ref.(29)). This competition has been used to estimate some thermodynamic and kinetic constants of acetylcholine binding to AcChR. As summerized in figure 4, upon binding of one AcCh-ion about 2 to 3 Ca^{2+} ions are released (21). The increase in the concentration of free Ca, $\Delta[Ca] \approx 10^{-5}$M occurs in a solution of $\approx 10^{-3}$M; the change of ≈ 1 percent is rather small and may be indicated with the help of metallochrome indicators and special spectrophotometers.

Relaxation kinetic studies have provided estimates for the overall rate constants of acetylcholine and of Ca^{2+} ion binding (5,22). As found by the Ca-relaxation, $k_1(R)=2.4(\pm 0.5)\times 10^{7}\,M^{-1}s^{-1}$ for AcCh suggests that the measured association rate constant is probably an overall, complex rate parameter involving several, more rapid elementary steps. In the simple case of very rapid pre-equilibria, the effective association rate constant $k_1(R)$ for the reaction model:

$$A + R \underset{k_{-1}}{\overset{k_1}{\rightleftharpoons}} A \cdot R \underset{k_{-2}}{\overset{k_2}{\rightleftharpoons}} AR \underset{k_{-3}}{\overset{k_3}{\rightleftharpoons}} AR' \qquad (7)$$

is given by $k_1(R)=k_3(k_1/k_{-1})\cdot(k_2/k_{-2})$ where the rate constants of diffusion controlled ion pairing may be estimated to be $k_1 \approx 10^8 M^{-1}s^{-1}$ and $k_{-1} \approx 10^7 s^{-1}$. The life time $t_0(R)$ associated with the overall process characterized by $k_1(R)$, is given by $t_0(R)=(k_{-1}(R))^{-1}=7$ms (5,22). The kinetic constants for acetylcholine so far characterize a receptor preparation (partially) delipidated) with overall dissociation equilibrium constant $\bar{K}_A \approx 10^{-6}$M (at 296 K, pH 8.5 and 0.1 M NaCl). This value is close to the acetylcholine concentration which causes the 'electrical half-response'. On the other hand, K_A for crude extracts, membrane fragments and recent receptor preparations where chemical modification could be largely reduced (20) is between 10^{-8} and 10^{-9}M, most likely representing the acetylcholine affinity to the inactivated receptor. Moreover, the rate constants for the bimolecular overall reaction, $k_1(R)$ and $k_{-1}(R)$, compare well with data from electric current relaxations (31): $k_{on} \approx 10^7\ M^{-1}s^{-1}$ and $k_{off} \approx 10^2$ to $10^3\ s^{-1}$ depending on membrane potential. The electrophysiological data further indicate that at least two acetylcholine ions must bind in order to open a single permeation site. This may be related to the fact that the H-form of the (freshly) isolated receptor protein has (at least) two binding sites for AcCh.

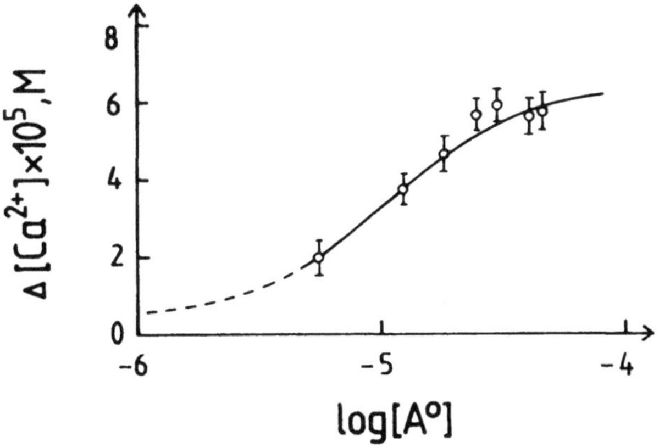

$$nA + RCa_x \rightleftharpoons A_nR + xCa$$

$$\alpha \equiv A_b/A_b^o = \Delta Ca/\Delta Ca^o \quad ; K_A = 10^{-6}M$$

$$\alpha[R_A^o] + \frac{\alpha}{1-\alpha}K_A = [A^o] \quad ; n = 2$$

$$x = 5(\pm 1)$$

Figure 4: The change in concentration of free Ca^{2+} ions reflecting release of bound Ca^{2+}, Ca_b^{2+}, ($\Delta[Ca^{2+}] = -\Delta[Ca_b^{2+}]$), from isolated acetylcholine receptor of Torpedo cal. (in 0.1M NaCl, 0.05 M Tris·HCl, 0.1% Brij, 0.0012 M Ca, pH 8.5, at 20°C) as a function of the total acetylcholine concentration [A°]. The receptor concentration is 2.6 mg/ml.

Among the various points of comparison , in particular the similarity between $k_{on} \approx 10^7\ M^{-1}s^{-1}$ and $k_{off} \approx 10^2-10^3\ s^{-1}$ from current relaxations on the one hand, and $k_1(R)=2.4(\pm 0.5)\times 10^7\ M^{-1}s^{-1}$ and $k_{-1}(R)=1.4\times 10^2 s^{-1}$ from studies on isolated receptors on the other hand suggests that the rate of coupled Ca^{2+} release (upon binding of AcCh not only reflects the overall rate of effective acetylcholine binding associated with a life time of 7ms, to isolated (partially delipidated) receptor, but may also be characteristic for the rate-limiting step in the conductivity increase of the membrane. Thus, stoichiometry of acetylcholine binding, equilibrium and rate constants suggest the low affinity receptor (with $K_A \approx 10^{-6}M$) as a candidate for the in vivo metastable, conducting receptor conformation, which by chemical modification (sulfhydryl-disulfide redox reactions) during isolation may be stabilized in detergent solution.

In contrast to the relatively low value for acetylcholine, the measured association rate constant for the binding of the dicationic inhibitor bis(3-aminopyridinium)-1, 10-decane (DAP) to isolated Torp. marm. AcChR is $k_{12}=1.2\times 10^8\ M^{-1}s^{-1}$ in 0.1 M ionic strength, pH 7.0 and 293 K. The ionic strength dependence of the association rate of k_{12} (DAP) suggests an effective charge of $-3(\pm 1)$ on the binding site of the protein (5, unpublished results). This value is somewhat less negative than that indicated for the esterase. But it seems that in both proteins of the permeability control system there are larger electrostatic contributions to the rate with which cationic ligands like acetylcholine are bound.

The estimates for the effective bimolecular rate constants k_{12} of AcChR-ligand binding appear to depend strongly on the type of ligand used; for decamethonium $k_{12}=2\times 10^8\ M^{-1}s^{-1}$ and for carbamylcholine and acetylcholine $k_{12} \approx 10^7\ M^{-1}s^{-1}$ (23), for suberyldicholine $k_{12}=0.98\times 10^7\ M^{-1}s^{-1}$ (24), for NBD-5-acylcholine $k_{12} \simeq 10^8\ M^{-1}s^{-1}$ (25), for Dns-C_6-Cho $k_{12}=9.5\times 10^7\ M^{-1}s^{-1}$ (26).

AcChR-lipid complexes. Recent studies with the isolated AcChR-lipid complexes from Torp. cal. confirm that the Ca^{2+}-binding isotherm is essentially two-physic with equilibrium constants in the µM and mM range (27), suggestive for intracellular and extracellular Ca^{2+} sites in AcChR. Ca^{2+} ions may be involved to preserve stability of the protein-lipid complex and may also bind to the anionic groups of the channel subunits. A larger number (10 to 20) of anionic, probably carboxylate, groups are suggested by the large Ca^{2+} ion binding capacity of AcChR. Provided that the density of the anionic charges locally exceeds a certain value, divalent ions like Ca^{2+} are preferentially bound. If AcCh induces a structural change which increases the average distance between the charged groups, this oligoelectrolyte preference for Ca^{2+} ions would be lost and ion exchange with, say, Na^{+} ions could occur (28). The 'indicator' of 'effective binding' of AcCh to the AcChR-gating macromolecule would therefore be the (allosteric) release of bound Ca^{2+}. However, prolonged exposure to receptor activators leads to definitely allosteric uptake of Ca^{2+}-ions; see also (29).

Transient release of Ca^{2+} ions followed by uptake of Ca^{2+} upon addition of activators to AcChR (unpublished results) suggest at least one metastable state in vitro, parallel to the electrophysiologically indicated in vivo, metastability for the conducting channel configuration, and parallel to the metastability suggested for the permeable state in sealed biomembrane vesicles (30).

The data suggestive for intrinsic asymmetry of AcChR structure and function (see, e.g. ref. (31)) invite speculation on a possible functional role. If the 'monomers' of the dimeric H-form have different cyclic sequences for the subunit positions, i.e. an L-form with $\alpha_2\beta\gamma\delta$, and an L'-form with $\alpha_2\gamma\beta\delta$ stoichiometry, a molecular weight of about 250,000 d for each monomer and of about 500,000 d for the asymmetric H-form would result, a value not inconsistent with recent estimates (32,33). Functionally, the L and L'-forms are candidates for two separate channels for Na^+-inflow and K^+-outflow, both, however, cooperatively controlled by the binding of at least two AcCh ions. Recent reconstitution experiments into planar lipid bilayers indeed indicate that the H-form leads to a 'double channel', whereas the conductivity contributions of the monomers are only half of those from the H-form (Schindler, Spillecke and Neumann, 1981, unpublished results). These characteristic features of the dimeric AcChR gating protein are only covered by more complicated reaction schemes (15).

D. Flow Concept for AcCh-Mediated Gating of Ion Flows

To the extent to which data on isolated proteins can be used to extrapolate to the cellular level, it is very tempting to compare the rate constant $k_1(R)=2.4(\pm 0.5)\times 10^7\ M^{-1}s^{-1}$ associated with a life time of $(k_{-1}(R))^{-1}=7ms$, with that of the enzyme $k_1(E)\geq 2\times 10^8\ M^{-1}s^{-1}$, probably $10^9\ M^{-1}s^{-1}$.

If, as suggested by the data, indeed $k_1(R)=k_{ass}(R)$ and $k_1(E)=k_{ass}(E)$, then the result $k_1(R)<k_1(E)$ parallels and quantifies the inequality (1) which was derived from electrophysiological data.

In order to model AcChE inhibitor effects on mepc consistent with the inequality (1), the elementary conductance increase must involve <u>at least two AcCh</u> molecules (5,34). Using several assumptions on receptor density in the synaptic cleft and applying the AcCh reactions in a competitive model, Rosenberry (1979) simulated main features of the time course of mepc; however, the sharp peak of mepc was not reproduced, and it cannot be modelled by any simple competitive model. Thus the particular shape of mepc indicates an essentially sequential processing of AcCh: the main part of neurally evoked AcCh binds first with AcChR in a microreaction phase 1. Because of the inequality (1) it appears that initially in the growth phase of a mepc the AcCh concentration $[A]_1$, close to activatable receptors is larger than the AcCh concentration $[A]_2$ in a second microreaction phase where AcChE fully competes with AcChR for activator. To fulfill the initial mepc condition

$$[A]_1 \gg [A]_2 \tag{8}$$

a partial separation of receptor and esterase sites (in the reaction phases 1 and 2) appears to be necessary; permitting,

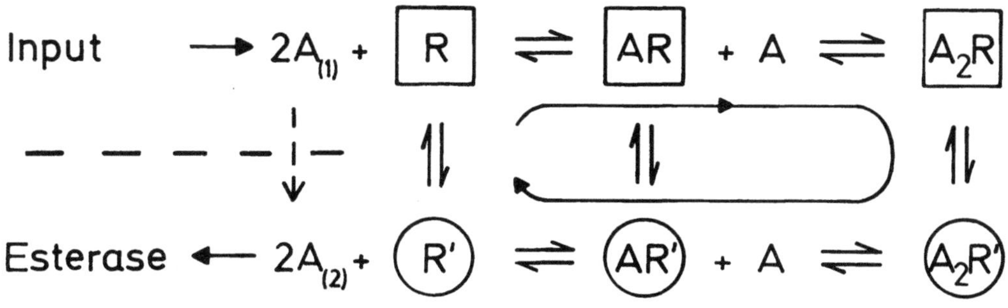

Figure 5: Flow scheme of the AcCh gating. Neurally triggered AcCh (input) flows toward the closed receptor (R) conformation, binds and induces the structural change to the ion transporting state A_2R' (reaction phase 1). In the second phase, AcCh which dissociates from A_2R' is rapidly hydrolyzed by the esterase (E). The receptors return to their activatable structure R. In phase 1, the concentration of free AcCh is initially much larger than in phase 2, where $[A] \rightarrow 0$; see text.

say, 90% of the available AcCh to reach the receptors and to bind; the rest of AcCh and all AcCh that dissociate from AcChR is rapidly removed by AcChE. These conclusions from purely electrophysiological data have been summarized in a flow scheme (35,5). The AcChR-gating cycle for neurally triggered AcCh is shown in figure 5; the desensitization processes are not included. It is readily realized that, once AcCh is more rapidly removed, i.e. $[A] \rightarrow 0$, closure of a channel can occur solely along intramolecular pathways, probably mainly <u>via</u> the $R' \rightleftharpoons R$ step and less <u>via</u> the $A_2R \rightleftharpoons A_2R'$ step; both pathways are consistent with first order decay of a mepc.

When AcCh is of non-neural origin, for instance applied artificially using a micropipette and in the presence of esterase

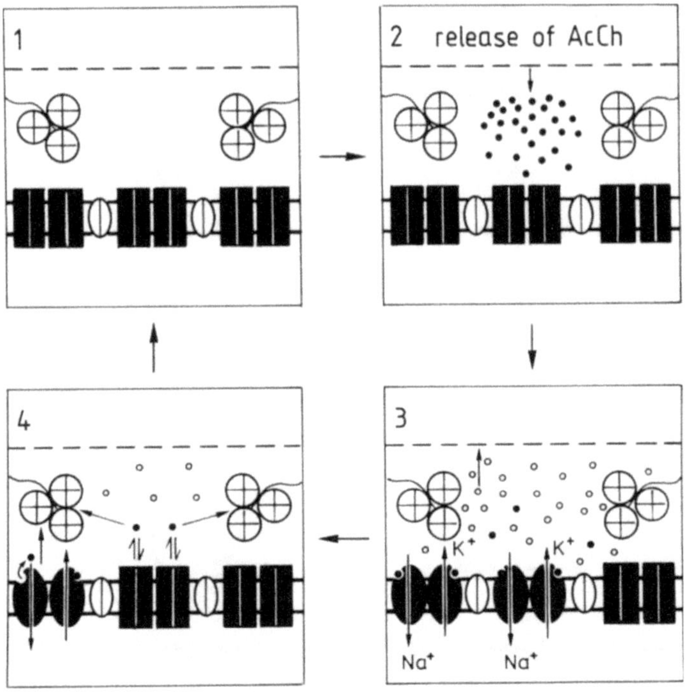

Figure 6: Model for the sequence of events causing the generation of a spontaneous postsynaptic miniature end-plate current (see figure 3) by acetylcholine (AcCh):

(6.1) resting state, [AcCh]→0, the receptor double channel (▮▮ ; H-form, binding ≥ 2 AcCh) is in the closed state;

(6.2) appearance of a pulse of AcCh (•);

(6.3) binding of AcCh to the receptors and channel opening, causing K^+-outflux and Na^+-influx; the remaining AcCh is rapidly hydrolized by esterase activity (⊕,⦶); predominantly presynaptic uptake of choline (o);

(6.4) dissociation of AcCh from the receptors and rapid hydrolysis by esterase activity; return of the receptors to the closed (resting state; 6.1).

inhibitors, AcChRs are multiply activated (10) and the decay phase of a mepc is prolonged. The inequality (4) may no longer hold for bath application of AcCh. The opening-closure kinetics is mainly determined by the kinetics of the $A_2R \rightleftharpoons A_2R'$ step which, due to the continuous presence of activator, becomes dependent on activator concentration, as suggested by experiments; (see, e.g., ref. (13).

The sequence of events underlying the time course of a m.e.p.c. (figure 3) may be viewed as schematically shown in figure 6. Neuronal activity releases a pulse of AcCh (part 6.2) which diffuses to the receptors causing a conformational change (part 6.3) with an average life time of a few ms (phase 1). Esterase activity rapidly hydrolyzes the remaining AcCh, $[A] \to 0$, causing the sharp peak in the m.e.p.c. When the AcCh ions which dissociate from AR'-sites of AcChR appear again in the reaction space (part 6.4), they are more rapidly attracted by the esterase than they can return to the receptors: the receptor channels close (phase 2).

In conclusion, we may describe the particularly characteristic time course of an AcCh induced elementary electric signal (the m.e.p.c.) in terms of appropriate kinetic constants which are observed for the isolated proteins AcChR and AcChE and assuming a microspatial separation of esterase activity and receptor reactions. Full esterase activity is necessary for both reaction phases discussed above, the growth and the decay phase of the spontaneous miniature end plate currents. The molecular properties of the two AcCh processing proteins appear to be the essential reason for the particular form of the electric signal.

Acknowledgement

The technical help of U. Santarius and financial support by the Deutsche Forschungsgemeinschaft, grant Ne 227, are gratefully acknowledged.

References

1. Dorogi, P. L., Neumann, E.: Proc. Natl. Acad. Sci. USA. 77, 6582-86 (1980).
2. Nachmansohn, D.: Harvey Lect. 1953, 49, 57-99 (1955).
3. Nachmansohn, D.: Chemical and Molecular Basis of Nerve Activity, Academic P., New York (1959); revised (1975).
4. Del Castillo, J., Katz, B.: Proc. Roy. Soc. London, Ser. B, 146, 369-81 (1957).
5. Neumann, E., Rosenberry, T. L., Chang, H. W.: in: Neuronal Information Transfer, eds. Karlin, A., Tennyson, V. M., V gel, H.J., Academic P., New York, p. 183-210 (1980).
6. Lentz, T.L., Mazurkiewicz, J. E., Rosenthal, J.: Brain Research 132, 423-442 (1977).
7. Massoulié, J., Bon, S., Vigny, M.: Neurochemistry Intern. 2, 161-84 (1980).
8. Viratelle, O. M., Bernhard, S. A.: Biochemistry 19, 4999-5007 (1980).
9. Brzin, M., Sketelj, J., Grubić, Z., Kianta, T.: Neurochemistry Intern. 2, 149-159 (1980).
10. Katz, B.: The Release of Neural Transmitter Substances. Liverpool University Press, pp. 55 (1969).
11. Gage, P.W.: Physiol. Rev. 56, 177-247 (1976).
12. Gage, P.W., and McBurney, R. N.: J. Physiol., Lond., 244, 385-407, (1975).
13. Neher, E., Stevens, C. F.: Ann. Rev. Biophys. Bioeng. 6, 345-81, (1977).
14. Stevens, Ch., F.: Cold Spring Harbor Symp. Quant. Biol. 40, 169-173 (1976).
15. Neumann, E.: Neurochemistry Intern. 2, 27-43, (1980).
16. Sakmann, B., Adams, P.R.: Adv. Pharmacol. Therapeut. 1, 81-90 (1979).
17. Rosenberry, T. L. and Neumann, E.: Biochemistry, 16, 3870-78 (1977).
18. Nolte, H.-J., Rosenberry, T. L., Neumann, E.: Biochemistry, 19, 3705-11 (1980).
19. Chang, H. W., Bock, E.: Biochemistry 16, 4513-20 (1977).
20. Chang, H. W., Bock, E.: Biochemistry 18, 172-79 (1979).
21. Chang, H. W., Neumann, E.: Proc. Natl. Acad. Sci. USA, 73, 3364-68 (1976).

22. Neumann, E., Chang, H. W.: Proc. Natl. Acad. Sci. USA 73, 3994-98 (1976).

23. Sheridan, R. Z., Lester, H. A.: J. Gen. Physiol. 70, 187-219 (1977).

24. Barrantes, F. J.: J. Mol. Biol. 124, 1-26 (1978).

25. Jürss, R., Prinz, H., Maelicke, A.: Proc. Natl. Acad. Sci. USA, 76, 1064-68 (1979).

26. Heidmann, T., Changeux, J. P.: Eur. J. Biochem. 94, 255-79 (1979).

27. Dorogi, P. L., Chang, H. W., Moss, K., Neumann, E.: Biophys. Chem. (1981), in press.

28. Neumann, E., Nachmansohn, D., Katchalsky, A.: Proc. Natl. Acad. Sci. USA, 70, 727-31 (1973).

29. Sugiyama, H., Changeux, J.-P.: Eur. J. Biochem. 55, 505-15 (1975).

30. Bernhardt, J., Neumann, E.: Proc. Natl. Acad. Sci. USA, 75, 3756-60 (1978).

31. Changeux, J. P.: Harvey Lecture (1980), in press.

32. Raftery, M. A., Vandlen, R. L., Reed, K. L., Lee, T.: Cold Spring Harbor Symp. Quant. Biol. 40, 193-202 (1976).

33. Reynolds, J. A., Karlin, A.: Biochemistry 17, 2035-38 (1978).

34. Rosenberry, T. L.: Biophys. J., 26, 263-289 (1979).

35. Neumann, E., Bernhardt, J.: Ann. Rev. Biochem. 46, 117-41 (1977).

36. Katz, B., Miledi, R.: J. Physiol., Lond., 231, 549-74 (1973).

Index

(authors in italics)

Bei Fragen zur Produktsicherheit wenden Sie sich bitte an:
If you have any questions regarding product safety,
please contact:

Walter de Gruyter GmbH
Genthiner Straße 13
10785 Berlin
productsafety@degruyterbrill.com